APHASIA AND KINDRED DISORDERS OF SPEECH

IN TWO VOLUMES

VOLUME II

APHASIA

AND

KINDRED DISORDERS OF SPEECH

BY

HENRY HEAD, M.D., LL.D. Edin., F.R.S.
CONSULTING PHYSICIAN TO THE LONDON HOSPITAL
HONORARY FELLOW OF TRINITY COLLEGE, CAMBRIDGE

VOLUME II

CAMBRIDGE
AT THE UNIVERSITY PRESS
MCMXXVI

CAMBRIDGE
UNIVERSITY PRESS

University Printing House, Cambridge CB2 8BS, United Kingdom

Published in the United States of America by Cambridge University Press, New York

Cambridge University Press is part of the University of Cambridge.

It furthers the University's mission by disseminating knowledge in the pursuit of education, learning and research at the highest international levels of excellence.

www.cambridge.org
Information on this title: www.cambridge.org/9781107419063

First published 1926
First paperback edition 2014

A catalogue record for this publication is available from the British Library

ISBN 978-1-107-41906-3 Paperback

CONTENTS

PART V

LIST OF ILLUSTRATIONS

INTRODUCTION

THROUGHOUT the previous volume examples of disorders of speech have been cited, presenting various forms and due to diverse causes. This volume is devoted to a series of clinical reports of illustrative cases arranged in numerical order. Each number corresponds to that employed to designate the patient throughout all my papers on this subject[1]. But, in order not to multiply these reports unnecessarily, I have omitted the records of certain cases in the series, which either failed to illustrate any new point, or were in some way incomplete. Thus, although the numbers run from 1 to 26, no account is given of No. 3, No. 12 and No. 16.

In most instances these reports represent drastically reduced versions of voluminous clinical records extending over considerable periods of time. Several of these patients have been under my care for some years and I have been compelled by exigencies of space to omit many observations of much interest, especially when they simply confirmed those made on some previous occasion.

Each case illustrates some one or more aspects of the problems dealt with in the previous volume and, in order that the reader may have some guide to their contents, I have summarised them shortly under the following descriptive headings.

§ 1. GRAVE DISORDERS OF SPEECH

When the disturbance of symbolic formulation and expression is acute in onset or unusually profound, the loss of capacity to employ language may be extremely gross. Speech is reduced to "yes" and "no" together with a few emotional expressions. The patient fails to understand exactly what is said to him and cannot execute any but the simplest oral commands. He is unable to read to himself with pleasure and fails to carry out orders given in print. Writing, whether spontaneous or to dictation, is affected, and printed matter cannot be copied in cursive script. The tests with the alphabet usually suffer severely and the patient finds it impossible even to arrange the block letters in due order. The free use of numbers may be gravely restricted and, in some instances, he cannot solve arithmetical problems, or indicate the relative value of two coins with uniform accuracy.

Such cases conform more or less to the type usually spoken of as "Broca's Aphasia." But the loss of function varies profoundly in degree. Should it be still more gravely diminished, the patient may be reduced to a condition of organic dementia in which it is impossible to carry out any systematic examination; for he is then deprived of almost every means of reproducing his mental processes in propositional terms both for internal or external use.

[1] [63], [64], [65].

On the other hand, a severe case of acute aphasia, such as No. 20, may pass in the course of recovery through a stage in which the defects are confined to acts of verbalisation. On the other hand, exactly opposite changes may occur in patients who are suffering from progressive organic lesions of the brain.

No. 26 (see p. 394) was a case of extremely severe aphasia of vascular origin in an unusually intelligent man of sixty. Speech was reduced to meaningless sounds with "Si, si" used correctly for affirmation. He could repeat nothing. He understood what was said to him and chose familiar objects correctly, although he could not execute more complex oral commands. He read to himself with pleasure and selected common objects slowly but accurately when shown their names in print; but he failed to execute more difficult printed orders. He could write nothing spontaneously, except his name and the first nine numerals; yet he could copy correctly, provided he was not compelled to transcribe print into cursive script. The use of the alphabet was defective; even when given twenty-six block letters he failed to arrange them in order. Arithmetical exercises were impossible and he could neither name coins nor express the simplest relation between any two of them. Orientation was not affected. Games, except draughts, were difficult or impossible. He enjoyed music and could sing without words. Vision was unaffected and there were no abnormal physical signs in the nervous system.

No. 21 (see p. 320) was a case of severe aphasia due to a vascular lesion in an elderly man. When first examined by me four days after the onset of the stroke, he was speechless except for "yes" and "no" together with a few emotional expressions. He could not say or repeat his name. He understood much of what was said to him, provided it did not convey an order, and seemed to comprehend the meaning of simple words in print. Writing was profoundly affected. There was no disorder of motion or sensation and the reflexes were normal. Vision was unaffected. The arterial tension was grossly raised and the vessel wall thickened.

He remained in fundamentally the same condition, and, eight and a half years after the seizure, I was able to make a complete examination with the following results.

He was still speechless, except for "yes" and "no" and a few automatic expressions. He could not repeat anything said to him, even "yes" and "no." He understood most of what he heard, choosing common objects and colours correctly to oral commands; yet he failed to execute more complex tasks, such as setting the clock and the hand, eye and ear tests. He could read nothing aloud and had difficulty in understanding what he read to himself; but he chose familiar objects to printed commands and on several occasions succeeded in selecting a printed card which bore words corresponding to the colour or to the simple pictures he had just seen. Thus, it is obvious that printed words conveyed some meaning to him, provided they did not imply a command. He could write nothing but his surname spontaneously, failed altogether to write to dictation and could not copy print in cursive script. He was unable to say, to repeat, to read or to write the alphabet. He succeeded in writing some of the letters to dictation and copied them with four errors only. He counted with extreme difficulty and failed to reach twenty. Simple problems in arithmetic puzzled him greatly, but he was able to indicate on his fingers with remarkable accuracy the relative value of two coins.

No. 1 (see p. 1) was a case of extremely severe aphasia, due to an extensive gun-shot injury of the left half of the head. The missile entered in the fronto-temporal and made its exit in the temporo-parietal region; at this point there was a small hernia cerebri (Fig. 15).

There was profound right hemiplegia, in which face and tongue participated; the upper extremity was flaccid, the lower hypertonic.

At first he was completely speechless except for "yes" and "no" and he could not repeat even these monosyllables. He understood much of what was said to him, but was unable to execute simple oral commands with certainty. He could not read and failed to carry out orders given in print; yet he was able to point to the word on a list which expressed the object he desired. At first he wrote nothing but his surname and a scrawl, which somewhat resembled one of his Christian names. Copying from print was impossible.

He recovered power rapidly and it then became obvious that his defects of speech were mainly of the Verbal type. He talked slowly and with obvious difficulty. When repeating anything said to him, his articulation, though defective, was better than with spontaneous speech. He understood all that was said and executed even complex oral commands correctly. Although he succeeded in carrying out printed orders, he still failed to comprehend exactly what he read to himself owing to defects of internal verbalisation. He wrote badly, employing the left hand because the right was powerless; not only was the act of writing difficult, but the words were badly spelt. To dictation the faults were of the same character though less gross. He could, however, copy print perfectly in cursive script, evidence that the defect was intellectual rather than mechanical. He was unable to say the alphabet spontaneously and had great difficulty in writing the letters in due sequence. In spite of his University education, he was puzzled by simple arithmetical problems. Orientation was in no way affected and he drew from memory a perfect ground-plan of his ward at the hospital. He could play simple card games, but not bridge; puzzles he enjoyed and solved with ease.

No. 20 (see p. 295) was a case of acute and severe aphasia in an elderly woman due to the removal of an extra-cerebral tumour, growing from the dura mater, which indented the brain around the meeting point of the inferior frontal and inferior precentral fissures.

The operation was followed by flaccid right hemiplegia, loss of movement in the same half of the face and tongue, together with the usual changes in the reflexes on the paralysed side. At the expiration of sixteen days all abnormal signs had passed away and there was no difference between the two halves of the body.

The loss of speech was at first profound and she could say "yes" and "no" only. The acts of speaking, reading and writing were all affected at first; even the power of understanding what was said to her was somewhat disturbed.

As she regained her capacity to use language, those aptitudes returned first which were least dependent on accurate word-formation. Clinically, within four months of the operation, she had been transformed from a severe example of loss of speech into one of Verbal Aphasia, so slight that it might have been mistaken for an articulatory disturbance only.

§2. SPECIFIC FORMS OF APHASIA

No two examples of aphasia exactly resemble one another; each represents the response of a particular individual to the abnormal conditions. But, in many cases, the morbid manifestations can be roughly classed under such descriptive categories as Verbal, Syntactical, Nominal or Semantic defects of symbolic formulation and expression.

(a) *Verbal Aphasia.*

The characteristic manifestations, which I have called Verbal defects, consist mainly of inability to discover the exact form of words and phrases necessary for perfect external or internal speech, together with want of power to transform them into written characters. Although verbalisation is profoundly affected, it is obvious that the patient can recognise names. For he chooses an object or colour in response to a printed order and, when shown some particular object, can select its name in print. Capacity to execute oral and printed commands is on the whole preserved unless the disturbance is severe. The patient can usually understand what is said to him in conversation or what he reads to himself, provided the sentences are not unduly long and complicated. But he cannot write spontaneously with ease and his spelling shows the same errors of verbal formation that are so evident in articulated speech. There is often extreme difficulty in transcribing print into cursive script. Numbers are grossly defective; yet he can recognise and express in some roundabout way the relation between coins of different value and has no difficulty with money. Orientation is not affected; he can usually construct a ground-plan of some familiar room. The power of playing games is not disturbed, although the defects of articulated speech may make it difficult to express the score.

The slighter the loss of function, the more closely does the disorder appear to be one of articulation. But spontaneous writing always shows defects of the same order as those of external speech. Moreover, the power of employing block letters in various ways to compose an alphabet or to form words is usually affected, showing that the fault lies in verbalisation and is not in origin simply "motor," "mechanical" or even purely "anarthric."

No. 6 (see p. 76) was a case of Verbal Aphasia, due to a gun-shot injury over the anterior portion of the left precentral gyrus, extending downwards on to the inferior frontal convolution (Fig. 7, Vol. I, p. 445).

There were no abnormal signs in the nervous system, except a transitory weakness of the right half of the lower portion of the face and some deviation of the tongue to the same side.

Four days after he was wounded he was speechless, but he soon began to utter a few badly articulated words. His power of speaking rapidly improved and throughout it was verbal structure and not nomenclature that formed his main difficulty. He could understand what was said to him and commands exacting a single choice were carried out accurately; but, as soon as two of these orders were combined, his response became slow and hesitating. Comprehension of printed phrases was obviously defective. Although he rapidly recovered the power of writing his name and address correctly, he could not write that of his mother with whom he lived. He was unable to count, but wrote the numbers up to twenty-one. Orientation was not affected. He drew well spontaneously and to command.

Seven years and eight months later, he had regained his power of carrying out all the serial tests, but still remained a typical example of Verbal Aphasia. He hesitated in finding words to express his thoughts, the pauses were unduly frequent and prolonged, and enunciation was defective. He could read aloud intelligibly, but stumbled at the longer words and complained that, when reading to himself, he was obliged to go over the same passage twice before he could grasp its meaning. As he said the words to himself silently, he was liable to mispronounce them and this confused him. In the same way, although he could write an excellent letter unaided, he did so slowly. He still failed to say or write the alphabet perfectly and even hesitated in putting together the twenty-six block letters; but he could repeat the alphabet after me, read it aloud and write it correctly to dictation. He counted slowly without mistakes, though articulation was somewhat slurred. He solved all the problems in arithmetic, except the most difficult of the subtraction sums, and he had no trouble with money. He drew excellently and produced a perfect ground-plan of the room in which we worked. He could play all games correctly.

Thus, the difficulty throughout lay with verbal construction, whether for external or internal speech, rather than with verbal meaning.

No. 9 (see p. 124) was a case of grave Verbal Aphasia due to an extensive gun-shot injury in the left parieto-occipital region. This produced profound right hemiplegia, both motor and sensory, with gross hemianopsia.

His speech was reduced to little more than the use of "yes" and "no" and he could not even pronounce his own name correctly. He had extreme difficulty in finding the names of common objects and colours, but the sounds he uttered bore a distinct relation to the words he was seeking. When he attempted to repeat what was said to him, articulation was extremely defective. His comprehension of single spoken words was good and he executed oral commands, provided they did not necessitate elaborate choice. He could select a familiar object in response to its name in print, but was slower and less certain with colours and failed grossly with the more complex tests. He wrote his own name, but could not add his rank, regiment or address, and was unable to write down the names of common objects. He could copy printed matter in capitals only. These defects of writing were not due to mechanical inability to form the letters, but rather to a difficulty in using them as appropriate symbols; for, if he were shown an object and asked to compose its name from a set of block letters, he was unable to do so. He counted up to ten, but could go no further and failed to solve simple problems in arithmetic. He succeeded in naming coins, although the words were badly pronounced, and in every case recognised their relative value. He showed a vivid appreciation of pictures and could draw on the whole correctly, even to command. He produced a ground-plan of his corner of the ward, but tended to draw some of the objects in elevation. Orientation was in no way affected. He played an excellent game of draughts.

Three years and nine months later, the defects of speech, though less severe, retained the same character, consisting mainly of loss of power to evoke words in a correct form and still greater difficulty in translating them into written symbols.

No. 19 (see p. 278) was a severe example of Verbal Aphasia due to an injury situated deep in the substance of the brain, unaccompanied by any external wound. The patient was unconscious for three weeks and recovered his senses to find that he was hemiplegic and was unable to say any word but "yes."

When he first came under my observation three years and nine months after the accident, the hemiplegia had passed away, except for some weakness and clumsiness of the right hand and to a less degree of the toes of the right foot. He was almost completely speechless and could not find words to designate familiar objects and colours. But he recognised their names; for he selected without fail a card bearing the appropriate designation of the object or colour shown to him. By this means he could name them correctly, although external verbalisation was almost impossible. He seemed to understand everything said to him and executed oral commands correctly. He showed remarkable power of comprehending printed words, provided he did not attempt to read them aloud or to spell out the letters of which they were composed, and he executed printed commands correctly. Writing was grossly affected and he could not write down unaided the names of objects or colours, the time shown on the clock, or movements made by me. But he succeeded better to dictation and copied correctly printed words in cursive script. He could not write the alphabet spontaneously and was unable to arrange the block letters in due order. Counting was defective and he failed to solve several simple problems in arithmetic; yet he could give the relative value of coins correctly. He drew to command and constructed from memory an excellent ground-plan of the room in which we worked. He played games well, provided he was not compelled to call the suit or number of the cards.

This case is an example of almost pure loss of verbalisation with no disturbance of the appreciation of verbal meaning. It shows that the power of forming words may be destroyed without loss of recognition of names. Were it not for the gross loss of capacity to write spontaneously and to carry out tests with the alphabet the case would correspond closely to one of "anarthria" as described by Marie.

No. 17 (see p. 248) was a case of Verbal Aphasia due to a severe gun-shot injury of the left hemisphere, followed by the formation of a cerebral abscess (Fig. 7, Vol. I, p. 445)

He showed gross spastic hemiplegia of the right arm and leg with some weakness of the same half of the face and tongue. This was associated with profound changes in sensibility. All the deep reflexes on the right half of the body were exaggerated, the abdominals were absent and the plantar gave an upward response. Vision was in no way affected.

He showed characteristic difficulty in finding words to express his thoughts and said that at first he had no more than a "twenty word vocabulary." Words were uttered singly or in short groups, isolated by pauses of varying length, and a single word of many syllables was liable to be slurred. Even a year after the injury, he could not say the alphabet perfectly and had much difficulty in counting. He named objects shown to him after considerable effort; this was due to defective power of verbal formation rather than to ignorance of nomenclature. He was able to repeat the content of what was said to him, but had the same difficulty in word-formation as during spontaneous speech. He seemed to understand what he heard and oral commands were executed with accuracy; he confessed, however, that, for a fortnight after he was wounded, he had difficulty in understanding things said to him unless they were "very simple and said very slow." He carried out printed commands correctly, but could not read to himself with complete understanding. When he read aloud, his articulation showed the faults evident during voluntary speech, though to a less degree. He wrote slowly and with great effort, using the left hand. His spelling was preposterous considering his education and the form of the written words showed the same defects that were manifested by spontaneous speech. Similar errors were present when he wrote to dictation, but he copied the same passage from print without mistakes in cursive script. He counted slowly and with effort, yet he showed remarkable powers of arithmetic. He drew excellently with his left hand. Orientation was not affected and he constructed a perfect ground-plan of his room at the hospital. He played card games well and, even if he uttered a wrong number, was not misled, but brought out the total score correctly.

No. 4 (see p. 55) was a case of slight Verbal Aphasia due to a severe gun-shot injury of the skull with thrombosis of the superior longitudinal sinus and hernia cerebri.

There was profound right hemiplegia with grave loss of power in the left lower extremity. Sensibility, especially to passive movement, was grossly affected on the right side and to a slighter degree in the left leg. Both plantar reflexes gave an upward response. The left upper extremity was in every way normal.

He talked fluently, but had difficulty in forming the longer words, and could repeat anything said to him, provided the sentence was not long and complicated. He understood almost all that he heard and executed oral commands correctly. He could carry out printed orders without mistakes; but he complained that, when reading to himself, he had a tendency to miss some of the words and this want of verbal exactitude was liable to confuse him. He wrote with the left hand comparatively fluently, but his spelling was faulty and he tended to omit some of the words. To dictation his writing showed the same kind of faults. Printed matter was copied with complete accuracy in cursive handwriting. He solved simple problems in arithmetic correctly after some hesitation and, although he had been a bank clerk, found difficulty in adding up long columns of figures; yet he could give the exact relation of two coins to one another. He drew excellently. Orientation and plan drawing were perfect. He played all games with ease.

It is important to notice that No. 20 (see p. 295), who suffered from a severe and widespread disorder of symbolic formulation and expression consequent on the removal of an extra-cerebral tumour from the frontal and precentral region, passed through a stage of pure Verbal Aphasia on her road to recovery. Finally, the only abnormal signs were a slight difficulty in articulated speech and some want of facility in writing spontaneously (p. 318).

In the same way, No. 1, an extremely severe case due to an extensive gun-shot injury of the head, became on recovery a straightforward though grave example of Verbal Aphasia (p. 10). He then talked slowly and with obvious difficulty in finding the words he required, although he named objects correctly. He understood all that was said to him and executed even complex oral commands. He still failed to comprehend exactly what he read to himself, owing to defects of internal verbalisation. He wrote with difficulty both spontaneously and to dictation, but copied print perfectly in cursive script. He was unable to carry out tests with the alphabet and was puzzled by simple arithmetical problems. Orientation was in no way affected and he drew from memory an excellent ground-plan of his ward at the hospital.

(b) *Syntactical Aphasia.*

This variety of aphasia is characterised by a more or less gross disorder of rhythm and syntax. The patient talks rapidly, his speech is jargon, and prepositions, conjunctions and articles tend to be omitted; polysyllabic words are slurred or badly pronounced. These defects are apparent whenever the patient attempts to talk spontaneously, to repeat what is said to him, or to read aloud. Internal speech is also disturbed in a similar manner, though to a less degree. He can write the names of common objects and, in the less severe cases, can compose a short letter; but he is liable to fail in writing down the gist of something he has been told or has read to himself. He writes badly to dictation, but can copy printed matter perfectly in cursive script. Orientation is not affected. The extent to which the power of solving problems in arithmetic is disturbed depends on the standard of education reached by the patient, but he has no practical difficulty in dealing with money.

No. 15 (see p. 227) was a case of Syntactical Aphasia due to injury by a rifle bullet, which traversed the left temporal lobe from before backwards to make its exit behind the ear (Figs. 8 and 9, Vol. 1, p. 449 and p. 451).

The left eye was destroyed, but the right showed loss of vision over the upper and outer quadrant of the field. There was no loss of motion or sensation. At first the movements of the right half of the face and tongue were a little weak, the right plantar reflex gave an upward response and the abdominals on this side were diminished; but these signs passed away within five months. He gradually developed attacks preceded by a "nasty smell" which nauseated him. Six years after he was wounded, this aura culminated for the first time in a seizure accompanied by loss of consciousness and characteristic chewing movements.

His speech was a perfect example of jargon due to disturbance of rhythm and defective syntax. He did not use wrong words, but he tended to talk with great rapidity and it was difficult to hear the prepositions, conjunctions or articles; these parts of speech were frequently omitted. The same errors marred his attempts to repeat what was said to him, or to read aloud; even when reading to himself he became confused by internal jargon and lost the significance of all but the simplest phrases. His power of naming was preserved, and he could state the time correctly. On the whole he understood what was said to him, unless he was compelled to repeat it to himself; simple oral commands were well executed, but he hesitated and made several errors over more complex tests. Spontaneous writing was poor, he wrote equally badly to dictation, but could copy perfectly. In the earlier stages, before the full development of the fits, he experienced little or no difficulty in counting and solved simple problems in arithmetic. He could name coins, knew their relative value and made no mistakes in the use of money. He evidently appreciated the full meaning of pictures, but found extreme difficulty in describing them in spoken or written words. He drew a spirit lamp both from the model and from memory, but failed to represent an elephant correctly. Orientation was unaffected and he drew a perfect ground-plan of a familiar room.

No. 13 (see p. 198) was a case of Syntactical Aphasia due to gun-shot injury of the left temporal lobe (Fig. 8, Vol. 1, p. 449).

There was slight want of power and incoordination of the right hand associated with distinct loss of sensibility; this subsequently passed away entirely. The lower extremity was unaffected and the reflexes were normal.

He talked rapidly; the rhythm of speech was disturbed and syntax was defective, whether the words were spoken or read aloud. If hurried, he tended to lapse into jargon. He named objects correctly and could repeat all that was said to him. Comprehension of spoken words was unaffected and he could execute oral and printed commands; yet, if he said the phrases over to himself in order to remember them, he was liable to forget what he had been told or had read silently. He could write a good letter spontaneously, but made many mistakes when he attempted to put down what he had read or when he wrote to dictation. Numerals were badly pronounced and arithmetic was defective. He could express the simpler relations between two coins, but had difficulty if he was compelled to employ higher numbers. Orientation was not affected.

Four and a half years later his condition had improved, but the form assumed by the loss of speech was identical with that revealed by the earlier observations.

No. 14 (see p. 215) was a case of Syntactical Aphasia due to a gun-shot injury in the region of the first temporal gyrus and the Sylvian fissure (Fig. 8, Vol. 1, p. 449).

He developed seizures in which he ceased to talk and his right arm fell powerless on the bed; he was never convulsed, did not appear to lose consciousness, but could not speak and was powerless to think. These attacks were preceded by a "tingling feeling" down the right side, accompanied by an hallucination of taste and smell and a peculiar mental state.

At first there was gross loss of power and incoordination of the right arm and leg; movements of the right half of the face were defective and the tongue deviated to this side. The deep reflexes on the right half of the body were brisker than those on the left, the right plantar gave an upward response and the abdominals on this side were diminished. Subsequent examination showed that there were profound changes in sensibility in the right upper and lower extremities.

From the first his speech was jargon. He knew what he wanted to say, but his words poured out in phrases which had no grammatical structure and were in most cases incomprehensible. He could not repeat a sentence said to him and, when he attempted to read aloud, uttered pure jargon. He was unable to find names for common objects and yet his correct choice to printed commands showed that he was familiar with their usual nomenclature. Comprehension of spoken words was obviously defective and he was liable to be puzzled by any but the simplest oral commands. In general conversation he frequently failed to understand what was said and to carry on a subject started by himself. Spontaneous thought was rapid and his intelligence of a high order, but his power of symbolic formulation and expression was hampered by defects of internal speech. He undoubtedly comprehended what he read to himself, even in French, but any attempt to reproduce it aloud resulted in jargon. Single words were for the most part more easily written than spoken and, when at a loss, he could frequently write something which conveyed his meaning. But he was unable to read what he had written, and this, together with his difficulty in forming phrases, made it impossible to compose a letter or coherent account of something he wished to convey. He could copy perfectly, but wrote badly to dictation, because of the rapidity with which he forgot what had been said to him. He added and subtracted without difficulty and enjoyed solving financial problems. He could not name coins, although he recognised their relative value. He played the piano, read the notes correctly and evidently recognised the constitution of a chord and changes of key.

(c) *Nominal Aphasia.*

Nominal Aphasia is more particularly characterised by want of power to discover appropriate names, or to find categorical terms in which to express a situation. Except in the acutest stages, the patient possesses plenty of words, but he cannot apply them exactly and verbal form may suffer in his efforts to discover the correct name. Internal speech is gravely affected and there is usually difficulty in understanding and executing oral or printed commands. The patient cannot comprehend what he reads to himself. Spontaneous writing is grossly affected; to dictation he writes somewhat better, and he can usually copy printed matter in cursive script, interspersed with irrelevant capitals. The use of numbers is defective and arithmetical problems are solved with difficulty. He may be unable to state the relative value of two coins and cannot calculate the price of the article he has bought, although he remembers exactly what he paid. Orientation is not fundamentally disturbed, but he tends to be puzzled, when, after taking a wrong turning, he does not see the familiar landmarks he expected. He can recall the position of objects in some familiar room, yet he frequently fails to represent them accurately on a ground-plan and tends to draw them in elevation. Card games are impossible in the more severe stages, but the patient may be able to play draughts or even chess. He cannot read musical notation, although he can sing without words and recognise whether music is correctly played by others.

No. 7 (see p. 89) was a case of Nominal Aphasia, due to gun-shot injury within the limits of the left angular gyrus (Figs. 10 and 11, Vol. I, p. 456 and p. 457). There were no abnormal physical signs.

Six weeks after he was wounded he was so grossly aphasic that it was impossible to obtain from him any coherent information. He could not express himself either in speech or in writing and had obvious difficulty in discovering a method of formulating his meaning. He rapidly regained sufficient use of language to permit of more complete examination. He then failed to say his name and address, or the days of the week and the months correctly. He could not name familiar objects and colours and was unable to tell the time. Repetition was gravely affected, though the sounds he uttered usually bore some remote resemblance to the words said by me. He showed obvious defects in comprehending the significance of spoken words and phrases. Oral commands were badly executed; he chose common objects or colours after great hesitation, and frequently gave up the attempt altogether. He had considerable difficulty in understanding the meaning of single words put before him in print and selected familiar objects and colours slowly with obvious effort. He failed grossly to execute more complex printed commands. With great effort he succeeded in writing his name imperfectly, but could not add his address and failed entirely to compose a letter. He was unable to write down the name of any of the colours shown to him and transcribed the time badly, although he employed numbers only. Writing to dictation was almost impossible, but he was able to copy correctly, using cursive script, interrupted by irrelevant capitals. He found it almost impossible to state the relative value of any two coins placed before him. Yet, in spite of his confused replies, he undoubtedly recognised their monetary value, for he was able to put together the equivalent of any one of them from amongst a heap of money on the table. Drawing to order was grossly affected and he failed to produce a ground-plan of the ward in which he lay, although he could indicate the position of the various objects visible from his bed. He played dominoes and draughts slowly but correctly. He sang in perfect time and tune, provided he did not attempt to pronounce the words.

Four years and nine months after he was wounded, his power to use all forms of language had greatly improved; yet although he could speak, read and write, he remained as definite an example of Nominal Aphasia as before. He managed to execute correctly all the serial tasks in which he had previously failed. But his powers of speech were obviously defective and he confessed that he had difficulty in finding names and that this confused him. Although he could carry out oral and printed commands, closer examination showed that any test, which demanded prompt recognition or formulation of differences in meaning between two or more words or phrases, was performed slowly and with effort. Above all he found difficulty in writing spontaneously, but he wrote well to dictation and copied excellently. He counted slowly but correctly and solved all but one of the simple arithmetical problems. He could name coins and state their relative value after some hesitation. He had recovered his power of drawing to command, but could not construct a ground-plan of the room in which we worked. Orientation was not affected. He could play draughts and billiards, but not card games.

No. 2 (see p. 14) was a case of Nominal Aphasia due to a fracture of the left half of the skull produced by the kick of a horse. The injury to the brain occupied mainly the region of the angular, superior parietal and parieto-occipital gyri (Figs. 10 and 11, Vol. 1, p. 456 and p. 457).

Right hemianopsia of a gross character was present from the first; but there were no other abnormal physical signs.

The patient was a highly intelligent, young Staff Officer. Throughout the many years he has been under my observation, his speech has steadily improved; but the defects, though less in degree, remained identical in character. He had no lack of words, but suffered from want of capacity to find the one which exactly corresponded to the meaning he wished to express, or was an appropriate name for some definite object. At the same time he failed to understand the significance of words presented to him orally or in print. He read aloud badly, especially if he attempted to spell out the words letter by letter. Writing was gravely affected; at first he wrote with extreme difficulty spontaneously or to dictation and could not copy print correctly in cursive script. Though he drew well spontaneously or from a model, he was unable to produce the figure of an elephant to command and he could not construct a ground-plan of some familiar room. Orientation was not fundamentally disturbed, although he had difficulty in formulating even to himself the way from one place to another. He failed to solve simple arithmetical problems and had much difficulty in calculating change. He could play chess even in the earlier stages. Throughout he showed a remarkable power of reacquiring knowledge. For example, he again mastered Hindustani, so far as to speak the language, and he recovered his power to play bridge. Superficially he would now pass for a normal, active man.

No. 11 (see p. 181) was a case of Nominal Aphasia due to a bullet wound in the left occipital region, running upwards and inwards, with a smaller opening in the skull situated in and just to the right of the middle line of the scalp (Fig. 24, p. 183).

Central vision alone was preserved in the right eye, whereas the left showed right hemianopsia with maintenance of central vision for 10° to the right of the fixation point.

There were no other abnormal physical signs. But the patient occasionally suffered from attacks in which, though consciousness was fully preserved, he either "felt numb" down the right side or seemed to go suddenly blind.

He talked slowly, but articulation and syntax were not essentially affected and he could repeat all that was said to him, if the sentences were not long and complex. He showed considerable hesitation in naming common objects and, at the first examination, failed several times with colours. He read to himself with difficulty and made many mistakes when reading aloud; in neither case could he obtain a clear notion of the meaning of the passage he had read. He wrote with great effort, employing capitals and small letters indiscriminately. Writing to dictation and even copying print into cursive script were very defective. He could count slowly up to a hundred, but hesitated over the higher decades. Numbers stated categorically seemed to convey little to him and he failed to place a certain coin into a definite bowl to orders given orally or in print. Moreover, his answers were equally defective, whether the command was printed in figures or in words, showing that it was the idea of number that was at fault. He failed to solve simple problems in arithmetic and had difficulty in stating the relative value of two coins, although he could build up the equivalent of any one of them from money placed before him. He was able to draw spontaneously, or from a model and from memory. But, asked to draw an elephant, he produced a figure without its most characteristic features; these he named and added one by one in response to my question as to what he had omitted. He could not construct a ground-plan, tending to represent all the salient objects in my room in elevation. In spite of the gross lesion of the visual centres, he still possessed visual imagery. There was no loss of orientation; he was liable to make mistakes, because he could not formulate to himself or to others the exact details of the route he should take. But he did not lose himself, for he recognised familiar landmarks, when they came into sight, and so guided himself to his ultimate destination correctly. He played draughts, but not card games, and was easily confused by puzzles.

No. 22 (see p. 329) was a case of Nominal Aphasia following a cerebral seizure in an elderly man with raised arterial tension and degenerated arteries. These defects of speech were associated with right hemianopsia, unaccompanied by any other signs of disease in the central nervous system.

Observations made eleven weeks and again three years after the attack, brought out results which were fundamentally identical in character. Words were not lacking, but he was perpetually held up for want of the one which exactly expressed his meaning. Articulation and syntax were not otherwise affected and he could repeat what was said to him, if it was not a long or complicated sentence. He had profound difficulty in naming an object shown to him. With colours he was particularly at fault; but, although he could not name them, he could describe how they would be composed from pigments. He understood most of what was said to him and oral commands were performed slowly, though on the whole correctly. The execution of printed commands was grossly defective and he failed to appreciate the meaning of a printed passage read silently. This was even more evident when he uttered the words aloud. He had never been able to write easily and with freedom and, although he wrote his name and address accurately, he could not compose a short letter. He failed to write down the names of familiar objects and colours, but on several occasions wrote some word of associated meaning, or the names of the pigments he would employ to make the colour. It was not the act of writing which was at fault, but the power to discover words of the exact meaning to fit a certain situation and then to transform them into appropriate written symbols. He could copy print exactly, although he could not translate it into cursive script. He counted up to twenty, then became somewhat confused, but ultimately reached a hundred without a mistake. He failed to solve simple problems in arithmetic. Coins were named and their relative value stated correctly. He could draw from a model, but was profoundly puzzled when asked to draw an elephant, and failed to construct a ground-plan of the room in which we habitually worked. He could, however, indicate the position of each salient feature relative to himself. Orientation was not affected, but he was liable to become confused if he did not see before him the landmarks and guiding points he expected. He had lost the power of reading musical notation and could no longer play his double bass.

No. 23 (see p. 348) was a case of congenital disorder of speech in an otherwise intelligent young man. There were no abnormal physical signs.

He had never been able to learn to read or write with ease, and his defects of symbolic formulation and expression were akin to those in certain cases of Nominal Aphasia. He did not lack words, but insisted that he could not find those which aptly expressed his meaning. He named common objects correctly after some hesitation, but was slower and less accurate with colours. He understood what was said to him in ordinary conversation and could carry out oral commands. Printed orders were less readily executed and he failed to comprehend exactly what he read to himself silently. He was unable to write down the name of an object or colour shown him; nor could he reproduce in writing the contents of a printed paragraph he had read. His writing was equally defective, even when the words were dictated by me. He could, however, copy print in cursive script, showing that the fundamental fault lay in the power to translate speech into written symbols rather than in the mechanical act of writing. He failed to say or to write the alphabet spontaneously, to write it correctly to dictation, or even to put together the block letters in due sequence. He could count, but was unable to solve simple problems in arithmetic. Coins were named correctly and, with some effort, he was able to state their relative value. Orientation was unaffected, but he failed to draw an accurate ground-plan of the room in which we worked. He could sing, provided he did not attempt to find the words, and had a keen ear for faults in music played by others.

(d) *Semantic Aphasia.*

These defects are characterised by lack of recognition of the full significance of words and phrases apart from their immediate verbal meaning. The patient fails to comprehend the final aim or goal of an action initiated spontaneously or imposed upon him from without. He cannot formulate accurately, either to himself or to others, a general conception of what he has been told, has read to himself, or has seen in a picture, although he is able to enumerate most of the details. Such patients understand what is said, can read and can write, but the result tends to be inaccurate and confused. Counting is possible and the relative value of coins may be recognised; but arithmetical operations are affected and the patient is commonly confused by the monetary transactions of daily life. Drawing, even from a model, is usually defective and in most instances construction of a simple ground-plan is impossible. Orientation is definitely disturbed. The patient finds considerable difficulty in laying the table, putting together portions of some object he has constructed, or in planning an operation he desires to perform. This interferes seriously with his activities in daily life and renders him useless for any but the simplest employment; and yet his memory and intelligence may remain on a comparatively high general level.

No. 10 (see p. 151) was a case of Semantic Aphasia, due to a wound with a hand-grenade in the region of the left supra-marginal gyrus (Figs. 12 and 13, Vol. I, p. 460 and p. 461).

There were no abnormal physical signs of any kind. But on two occasions, during periods of worry and mental distress, he suffered from a true epileptic attack, the first of which occurred five months after he was wounded, the second six years later.

He could name objects and colours shown to him and had no difficulty in finding or articulating words to express his ordinary needs; all his phrases were perfectly formed and spaced. But, in general conversation, he paused like a man confused, who had lost the thread of what he wanted to say. Words and sentences were repeated correctly, provided they did not contain a number of possible alternatives. He chose an object or colour named by me, but had obvious difficulty in setting the clock or in carrying out complex oral commands. He was easily puzzled and became confused with regard to the aim of the task set him. He understood the significance of printed words and short sentences, provided they did not contain a command. But he gave a poor account of a paragraph read silently to himself; his narration tailed away aimlessly, as if he had forgotten the goal for which he was making. He read aloud simple sentences without mistakes, but tended to doubt the accuracy of the words he had uttered correctly. He wrote with extreme rapidity, as if afraid of forgetting what he wanted to transfer to paper; at first, he tended to employ the same symbol for several different letters. He showed similar defects to dictation and not infrequently forgot what he had been told to write. Apart from the defects in handwriting he could copy correctly. Although he counted excellently, he was unable to carry out the simplest arithmetical operation; this was the more remarkable as he had been an accountant, accustomed to handle complex masses of figures. He was confused by the relative value of coins and had much difficulty with change in ordinary life. Although he appreciated the various details of a picture, he was liable to miss its general meaning. He could not draw from a model or from memory, nor delineate an elephant to command. He failed entirely to draw a ground-plan of a familiar room and was unable to express the relative position of its salient features. Orientation was gravely affected; he was liable to lose his way in the street and had difficulty in finding his own room in the hospital. He could play no games and puzzles worried him greatly.

Observations extending over seven years showed considerable variation in the degree but not in the character of the disturbance of function. In this case the sole disturbance produced by the lesion was want of capacity to comprehend and to retain in consciousness the general significance of some symbolic representation, or the intention of an act he was about to perform, either to command or on his own initiative. He could deal with the details of a situation, but not with its general aspects.

No. 8 (see p. 108) was a case of Semantic Aphasia in a young officer, who was struck in the left parieto-occipital region by a fragment of shell casing. The wound of entry, which lay over the supra-marginal gyrus and part of the superior parietal lobule, was alone accompanied by abnormal signs and symptoms (Figs. 12 and 13, Vol. 1, p. 460 and p. 461).

Four months after he was wounded seizures appeared and recurred at varying intervals dependent on whether he was worried or not. They usually consisted of loss of consciousness with or without slight convulsions; each attack was preceded by a period of confusion and "loss of memory."

There was definite right hemianopsia which assumed a peculiar form occasionally found with lesions of the cortex. The loss of vision over the defective half of the field was not absolute and he could appreciate moving objects. Moreover, if with both eyes open two similar objects were exposed at exactly the same distance from the fixation point, that to the right was frequently not appreciated, although it might be recognised if shown alone.

Reflexes, motion and sensation were unaffected; but on admission the edges of the optic discs showed distinct traces of previous swelling.

The disorders of symbolic formulation and expression were of the Semantic type. He frequently failed to recognise the intention of what he was told to do and was unable to combine details, duly appreciated, into a coherent whole. This was associated with difficulty in grasping a general idea. Articulated speech was unaffected, and he named objects correctly. He chose them to oral and printed commands and had no difficulty in comprehending the meaning of single words or short phrases. Yet he could not set the hands of a clock and frequently failed to gather the full meaning of general conversation. Reading aloud was unaffected, but he gave an imperfect account of what he had read to himself. Writing as such was perfect, although he had difficulty in putting down on paper exactly what he had gathered from conversation or reading. He was unable to solve problems in arithmetic and became confused over money. Drawing was defective. He could not find his way alone or plan where he wanted to go. Games, such as billiards, were impossible.

He recovered to a great extent and, six years after he was wounded, could carry out all the serial tests without a mistake. But he still showed in a minor degree those disabilities which made him so characteristic an example of Semantic Aphasia.

No. 5 (see p. 64) was a case of Semantic Aphasia, due to a wound over the inferior and posterior portion of the right supra-marginal gyrus in a strongly left-handed man (Figs. 13 and 14, Vol. 1, p. 461 and p. 463).

There was no disturbance of motion, sensation or reflexes. The visual fields were normal.

Articulated speech was not directly affected and he named common objects and colours correctly. The most striking feature was his inability to formulate, to appreciate and to retain in his mind the general meaning or exact intention of some act requiring symbolic representation. He understood simple statements and chose common objects to oral commands; but he made gross mistakes, when attempting to set the hands of a clock, or to carry out the hand, eye and ear tests. He failed more particularly to reproduce the sense of a simple narrative communicated to him by word of mouth. When he read to himself silently, his difficulty lay not so much in understanding a word or phrase as in gathering the general meaning of a group of statements; but he ultimately succeeded in executing all the tests to printed commands. He wrote spontaneously with remarkable ease. Yet the names of common objects and the time shown on a clock were written down badly; his handwriting deteriorated and his spelling was defective. To dictation, he was inaccurate and even made mistakes in writing the phrases of the man, cat and dog tests. On the other hand, he could copy print excellently in cursive script. All these faults in reading and writing were particularly evident, when he was tested with a short account in printed characters of his life before the war. If he was asked to render the general meaning of a picture and its accompanying legend, he was liable to become confused and to invent some fantastic explanation. He failed to solve two out of the six problems in simple arithmetic and was frequently unable to express the relative value of two coins to one another. He failed completely to draw an elephant to order. Orientation was defective. He could not produce a ground-plan of a portion of the ward in the neighbourhood of his bed, although he could recall to mind the essential differences in the uniform of Sister and Nurse.

No. 18 (see p. 259) was a case of Semantic Aphasia, produced by a gun-shot injury in the region of the left superior parietal lobule, combined with sub-cortical destruction due to an abscess in the substance of the brain. A sinus led down to fragments of bone which were removed by operation (Figs. 12 and 13, Vol. 1, p. 460 and p. 461).

My observations, made when he first came under my care in 1915, did not differ materially from those six and a half years later and they can therefore be summarised together. He suffered from no fits or seizures of any kind after the wound had finally healed. There was complete right hemianopsia and the pupils did not react to light thrown on to the blind half of the retina. There was no hemiplegia; face and tongue moved well on the two sides. Individual movements of the digits could be carried out perfectly with the eyes open; but, when they were closed, the fingers of the right hand performed finer movements clumsily. These digits were slightly atonic. The power of recognising posture and passive movement was diminished. The compass test, localisation, tactile sensibility and discrimination of shape, weight and texture were unaffected. All the reflexes, including the plantars and abdominals, were normal and equal on the two sides.

The defects of symbolic formulation and expression consisted in want of ability to recognise fully, to retain firmly and to act logically in accordance with the general meaning of a situation. Details could be appreciated correctly, but were not uniformly coordinated with certainty to form a total impression. No abnormality could be noticed in the course of ordinary conversation, beyond a certain hesitancy and diffidence in expression; there was a tendency for his talk to die out before it reached its full logical conclusion. He named correctly and repeated everything he heard with ease. He understood what was said to him and could carry out simple orders, although more difficult oral commands confused and puzzled him. He could read silently or aloud and understood the meaning of what he read, if it was not complex. He wrote his name and address correctly; yet, when he attempted to write down the gist of what he had been told or read to himself, he was liable to make curious errors. The act of writing was extremely rapid, as if he was afraid of forgetting what he wanted to express, and, even to dictation, he was liable to omit important words. He found difficulty in writing the alphabet, although he could say it correctly. Simple arithmetical exercises were badly performed and he started in each instance from left to right; it was not the detailed significance of numbers that was at fault, but the general conception of the acts of addition and subtraction. Once this had been rectified in his mind, the same problems were easily solved. In spite of the fact that he named coins and stated their relative value correctly, he was greatly puzzled by monetary transactions in daily life. Orientation was not so grossly affected as in some other patients of this group, but he did not like to go out unattended. The plan he drew of the room in which we worked was defective, although he could indicate orally its salient features. He understood straightforward pictures; those which demanded composition of detail, or the simultaneous comprehension of a printed legend, usually failed to convey to him their full meaning. He had the greatest difficulty in formulating the general intention of some act he was about to perform spontaneously or to order; but he was able to copy simple actions with ease, provided they did not demand recognition of several alternatives. Oral, pictorial and printed commands suffered to an almost equal extent. He could not put together the parts of a piece of furniture he had made under guidance and was unable even to lay the table with certainty. He could play no games with pleasure, and disliked puzzles, which confused him.

No. 24 (see p. 370) was a case of Semantic Aphasia, due to a vascular lesion in an elderly man. There were no abnormal signs beyond the affection of speech.

His principal defects of symbolic formulation and expression consisted in want of capacity to appreciate the general significance of details, however presented, and inability to deduce from them their logical consequences. He also failed to recognise, or was unable to retain in his mind, the full intention of an act he was about to perform spontaneously or to order. Thus, he frequently misunderstood the ultimate significance of pictures, especially in conjunction with a printed legend. During any series of tests he repeatedly forgot what he was expected to do and reflection of my movements in a mirror confused, rather than aided, him in imitating them correctly.

He talked rapidly, in somewhat slow and jerky sentences, as if afraid of forgetting what he wanted to say. He named objects slowly but correctly and did not lack words, although in ordinary conversation he occasionally used a wrong expression. He could repeat anything said to him, provided it did not consist of a long and complicated sentence. Single words and short phrases were perfectly understood and he executed even complex oral commands. If, however, he developed a false general conception of what he had heard, he was unable to correct it and became confused. Although he could carry out printed commands, he had great difficulty in understanding what he read to himself or aloud. Given a series of sentences which led by consecutive steps to some general impression, he was unable to reproduce what he had read. He wrote his name and address perfectly, but could not place on paper without the grossest mistakes his own ideas or the gist of something he had heard or read. To dictation he wrote well, except that he was confused by his errors in spelling. He copied slowly but perfectly. He counted with accuracy and wrote the numbers without difficulty; arithmetical problems puzzled him and were solved with effort. Coins were named correctly, but he expressed their relation to one another clumsily and was confused by the monetary transactions of daily life.

Drawing was very defective, even with a model before him. Orientation was gravely disturbed and he failed entirely to construct a ground-plan of the room in which we habitually worked.

No. 25 (see p. 379) was a case where the Semantic defects were of congenital origin. They were associated with no abnormal physical signs of any kind. From childhood the patient had recognised that she was unlike other persons. She had extreme difficulty in learning to read, to write and to carry out even simple calculations. But in spite of her disabilities, she was unusually intelligent and originated the idea of open-air schools, which she actually carried into execution. Her introspective notes formed a valuable addition to the results of my examination.

She could find all the words and names she required, even for the serial tests, and the syntax and balance of her phrases was unaltered. Repetition of words and short sentences was not affected. At first sight she seemed to understand everything said to her and she chose common objects and colours correctly and even executed the hand, eye and ear tests slowly to oral commands. But she complained that she could not "hold in her mind" a task explained to her in the course of conversation. Printed commands were on the whole well executed, but she was liable to miss the general significance of a passage read silently. Uttering the words aloud seemed to aid her greatly. The character of her handwriting and her power of expressing herself in this medium depended on the ease or difficulty of the task. When she wrote spontaneously, or attempted to reproduce what she had heard or read to herself, she was liable to omit essential points and her spelling was grossly defective; yet she copied printed matter in excellent cursive script. She had difficulty in solving simple problems in arithmetic and was confused with regard to the relation of two coins to one another. Orientation was distinctly affected and she had difficulty in finding her way.

§ 3. CASES ILLUSTRATING CEREBRAL LOCALISATION

(a) *Gun-shot and local injuries of the skull.*

In No. 6 (see p. 76) the wound was an almost vertical cut in the left temporal region of the scalp, 5 cm. in length, penetrating all the tissues, including the bone. In its deepest part the dura mater was laid bare, but the brain substance was not exposed. There was no wide-spread fracture of the skull and healing was complete in thirty days. No operation was performed at any time.

The upper end of this linear incision was 5·5 cm. from the middle of the scalp and 14 cm. behind the root of the nose; it lay 0·5 cm. anterior to the interaural line, whilst its extreme lowest point was 3 cm. in front. The whole nasion-inion measurement was 34·5 cm. and this was intersected at 14·5 cm. by the interaural line.

When the wound was plotted on the brain of a skull with approximately the same measurements, it was found to lie on the anterior portion of the precentral gyrus, extending downwards on to the inferior frontal convolution (Fig. 7, Vol. I, p. 445).

There were no abnormal physical signs, except a transitory weakness of the right half of the lower portion of the face and some deviation of the tongue to the right. All the reflexes, including the abdominals and plantars, were normal.

This patient was an excellent example of Verbal Aphasia.

No. 17 (see p. 248) was much less satisfactory from the point of view of anatomical localisation; for the extraction of a bullet from the brain was followed by formation of an abscess, which undoubtedly caused a considerable amount of deep destruction.

About ten days after he was wounded he was trephined and a rifle bullet was removed from the "left Rolandic region." When he came under my care five months later, the wound was represented by a sinus from which issued a considerable quantity of pus. The opening was situated 16 cm. backwards along the nasion-inion line, in the centre of an irregular area, from which bone had been removed; this measured 4·5 cm. vertically and 6 cm. horizontally and extended between two points 13 cm. to 19 cm. posterior to the root of the nose. The upper border of the bony opening lay 6 cm. from the middle line of the scalp. After removal of some fragments of bone from the substance of the brain and efficient drainage of an abscess cavity, the wound finally healed within eight months from the injury.

When the extent of this bony opening, which corresponded to those parts denuded of dura mater, was plotted on the surface of the brain, it was found to occupy an area extending between the inferior precentral and the lower third of the postcentral fissures. The destruction of tissue was not only superficial, but extended deeply into sub-cortical portions of the brain (Fig. 7, Vol. 1, p. 445).

For a time he suffered with Jacksonian convulsions, which began in the right hand and were always accompanied by some loss of verbal capacity. He showed the characteristic signs of a spastic hemiplegia; isolated movements of the right hand were impossible and the whole limb was hypertonic. The right leg was in a state of extensor rigidity accompanied by loss of power of dorsiflexion at the ankle. The lower portion of the right half of the face was somewhat affected and the tongue was protruded to this side of the middle line. Gross sensory changes of the cerebral type were present in both arm and leg of the affected half of the body. All the deep reflexes were greatly exaggerated on the hemiplegic side, the plantar gave an upward response and the abdominals were absent. The visual fields were unaffected.

His defects of speech formed a characteristic example of Verbal Aphasia.

In No. 15 (see p. 227) a rifle bullet had entered just to the left of the inner canthus of the right eye and had made its exit directly above the insertion of the left ear. A month later the wound of entry was represented by a minute perfectly healed white scar. On the other hand, the exit consisted of an irregular opening in the bone and tissues of the scalp, through which protruded a small pulsating hernia cerebri. Bone had been removed over an irregularly quadrilateral area about 3 cm. in vertical and horizontal extent; below, the opening reached the level of the insertion of the ear, and above, it was about 13 cm. from the middle line of the scalp, corresponding anteriorly to a point on the nasion-inion line 13 cm. from the root of the nose. The total distance from the nasion to the external occipital protuberance was 35 cm. The wound healed completely in eighteen weeks.

Thus the track of the bullet passed back through the left temporal lobe, entering its substance close to the tip and passing out at the level of the insertion of the left ear (Fig. 9, Vol. 1, p. 451). When plotted on the surface of the brain, the exit wound lay over the middle of the second temporal convolution, but must have produced some destruction both above and below the superior temporal fissure (Fig. 8, Vol. 1, p. 449). In its course it injured the extreme lower fibres of the optic radiations, producing upper quadrantic hemianopsia in the sole remaining eye.

A fortnight after he was wounded, there was a little weakness of the lower portion of the right half of the face and the tongue deviated slightly to the right. There was no loss of motion or sensation. The right plantar reflex gave an upward response and that from the right half of the abdomen was diminished. All these abnormal signs passed away entirely within five months from the date of the wound, leaving only the upper quadrantic hemianopsia, as far as such a condition could be observed in the one remaining eye. Ultimately he developed epileptiform attacks, preceded by an aura of smell and taste characteristic of a lesion within the temporal lobe.

His speech was jargon and the defects in the use of language assumed the form of Syntactical Aphasia.

No. 13 (see p. 198) would have been equally valuable from the point of view of localisation, had it not been for the uncertainty introduced by the operation carried out at the Front. He was struck by a shell fragment in the left temporal region and, when he came under my care some three weeks later, there was a linear surgical scar extending from the fronto-temporal to the parietal aspect of the scalp. On this healed incision was a pouting sinus, which lay 8 to 9 cm. from the middle of the scalp and was level with a point 16 cm. along the nasion-inion line. Here bone had been removed over an irregular area; when plotted on the surface of the brain it was found to lie just behind the central fissure.

But exactly below this area, 11 cm. to the left of the middle line, lay another fungating sinus penetrating the bone. This orifice in the skull was at a distance from the surgical incision and had not been subjected to operative treatment of any kind. It undoubtedly represented one of the original wounds and, when plotted on the surface of the brain, lay over the upper portion of the first temporal gyrus and the Sylvian fissure, on a level vertically with the foot of the postcentral fissure (Fig. 8, Vol. I, p. 449). I should like to suggest that this was the lesion responsible for the specific form of the loss of speech. The patient on receipt of the wound was obviously aphasic and the missile had probably injured the skull in the neighbourhood of the Rolandic region. The surgeon therefore trephined over the central fissure, but paid no attention to the small wound at a lower level over the temporal lobe, which had also perforated the skull.

He had no fits and showed very few abnormal physical signs of injury to the brain. At first the movements of the right angle of the mouth were slightly less than those of the other side and the tongue was protruded a little to the right; but this passed away quickly. The right hand "felt different"; the grasp was comparatively feeble, the fingers were somewhat hypotonic, but individual movements were possible. There was distinct ataxy of the fingers with the eyes closed, and the power of recognising passive movement and posture was defective in the right hand. All other forms of sensibility were perfect. The lower extremity was unaffected. All the reflexes were normal, including plantars and abdominals. These abnormalities of the right hand during the earlier stages are accounted for by the wound over the postcentral convolution.

On the contrary, the typical Syntactical defects of speech were probably due to the coincident injury of the first temporal convolution.

No. 14 (see p. 215) suffered from a much more severe injury, lying, however, exactly in the same situation as that of the effective wound in No. 13.

He was hit by a fragment of shell casing or by shrapnel just above the insertion of the left ear. When I saw him six weeks later, the wound was represented by a granulating surface of 2 cm. by 1·5 cm. situated 11 cm. from the middle of the scalp and 16 cm. backwards along the nasion-inion line. This unhealed patch was surrounded on three sides by a horse-shoe shaped incision, which had united firmly. Within, lay an irregularly quadrilateral area, where the bone had been removed; this was covered by normal scalp except over the site of the original wound.

When this was plotted on the surface of the brain, it was found to lie over the first temporal gyrus and the Sylvian fissure (Fig. 8 Vol. I, p. 449). But the trephined area was more extensive, especially in front and above, and there can be no doubt that it extended forwards to the lower portion of the central fissure.

The characteristic defects of speech were associated with extensive signs of cerebral injury. He developed seizures in which he ceased to talk and the right arm fell powerless on to the bed. He was never convulsed and did not always appear to become unconscious in these attacks, but he was unable to speak and found he was powerless to think. These attacks were preceded by a "tingling" feeling down the right arm and leg, accompanied by an aura of taste and smell and a peculiar state of mind, which he could not describe in comprehensible terms.

He did not suffer from headache or vomiting. The optic discs were normal and there was no hemianopsia. Movements of the lower part of the right half of the face were defective and the tongue deviated to this side. The deep reflexes on the right half of the body were brisker than those on the left and the right plantar gave an upward response; the superficial reflexes from this half of the abdomen were greatly diminished compared with those from the left. Even in the early stages there was no absolute paralysis of the right upper or lower extremity; isolated movements of the fingers were possible, but there was extreme incoordination of both arm and leg. Subsequent examination showed that the loss of power was mainly afferent in origin.

He was a severe instance of Syntactical Aphasia. His speech, both external and internal, was jargon and he could not write coherently.

No. 7 (see p. 89) was wounded by a fragment of a high-explosive shell, which produced a compound depressed fracture of the skull in the left parietal region, with laceration of the dura mater and protrusion of brain substance. He came under my care, nearly six weeks later, with a granulating stellate wound; in front this lay 7 cm., behind 9 cm., from the middle of the scalp and it extended between two points 19·5 cm. and 27 cm. on the nasion-inion line. An X-ray photograph showed an area of removal of bone in the anterior parietal region measuring 4 cm. by 2 cm. at its broadest part, with a fissured fracture running directly forwards. This wound healed finally eight weeks after it was inflicted.

When the extent of this opening in the bone was plotted on the surface of the brain, it was found to occupy an area shaped like an arrow head, pointing upwards and forwards within the limits of the angular gyrus (Figs. 10 and 11, Vol. I, p. 456 and p. 457).

There were no abnormal physical signs pointing to gross injury of the brain. The visual fields were normal; motion, sensation and the reflexes were unaffected.

His defects of speech formed a superb example of Nominal Aphasia.

No. 2 (see p. 14) was of much less value for purposes of anatomical localisation. The lesion was extensive and deep, at any rate in the centre; but the clinical observations were of unusual completeness and interest.

This young Staff Officer received a compound fracture of the skull in the left parieto-occipital region from the kick of a horse. Fragments of depressed bone were removed by operation, carried out within a few hours of the accident, and the brain below the injury was found to be reduced to pulp for a depth of about 7 cm.

At a subsequent operation to repair the opening in the skull, we were able to determine its exact limits. Its largest diameter, pointing upwards and a little forwards, was 10 cm., whilst horizontally it measured 5·5 cm. at its broadest part. Looked at from behind, its superior border was opposite a point 23 cm. along the nasion-inion and 3·5 cm. to the left of the middle of the scalp; below, it reached a point 33 cm. on the nasion-inion line and 3·5 cm. to the left.

Plotted on the surface of the brain this area of loss of bone occupied the angular, superior parietal and parieto-occipital gyri; its anterior border extended as far forward as the middle of the supra-marginal (Figs. 10 and 11, Vol. 1, p. 456 and p. 457). But we must bear in mind that this gives the extreme limits of the injury within which the destruction of brain tissue occupied a smaller extent.

Right hemianopsia was present from the first, but motion, sensation and the reflexes were unaffected.

He was a superb example of Nominal Aphasia.

No. 10 (see p. 151) was wounded in the left parietal region by the premature explosion of a hand-grenade. At the operation next day the dura mater was found to have been perforated in two places and two small fragments of bone were removed from the brain.

When he came under my care, thirty-four days later, the wound had healed completely. Bone had been removed over an oval area 2·5 cm. by 1·25 cm., extending between two points 15·5 cm. and 18 cm. along the nasion-inion line at a distance of 8 cm. from the middle of the scalp.

On plotting the site of this lesion, it was found to occupy the anterior portion of the supra-marginal gyrus, bounded in front by the postcentral fissure (Figs. 12 and 13, Vol. 1, p. 460 and p. 461). It was of small size and did not extend deeply into the substance of the brain; this was confirmed at an exploratory operation carried out whilst he was under my care.

There were no abnormal physical signs of any kind. But on two occasions in seven years, during periods of worry and mental stress, he suffered from an epileptiform seizure.

His defective use of language formed an excellent example of Semantic Aphasia.

No. 5 (see p. 64) was the only left-handed man in my series, and the wound, due to a rifle bullet, was situated in the right parietal region. On admission to the Base Hospital, this was a minute punctured opening, from which exuded cerebro-spinal fluid mingled with small quantities of disintegrated brain matter. The bullet had bored a circular hole in the skull, perforated the dura mater and was extracted from a point in the brain about 4 to 5 cm. in depth.

A fortnight later, when he came under my care, the wound of entry was healed and covered by a minute scab; it was situated 20·5 cm. backwards along the nasion-inion line and 11 cm. from the middle of the scalp.

This opening in the skull was found to lie over the inferior and posterior portion of the supra-marginal gyrus (Figs. 14 and 13, Vol. 1, p. 463 and p. 461).

There were no abnormal physical signs and the field of vision was not affected.

This patient also was an excellent instance of Semantic Aphasia.

In No. 8 (see p. 108) the lesion was more severe and of considerably greater extent. He was struck in the left parietal region by a fragment of shell casing, which traversed the brain almost directly from side to side and was removed through a small trephine opening over the right supra-marginal region.

When he first came under my care a month later, there was a small pouting wound of entry on the left side, which lay in the centre of a trephined area measuring 4 cm. by 2·75 cm. It extended between two points 26 cm. to 29 cm. along the nasion-inion; above, it was 2·5 cm., and below, 8 cm. from the middle line of the scalp, seen from behind. This healed in a fortnight. The opening on the right side, from which the missile had been removed by operation, had healed completely on admission.

When the extent of the opening in the skull surrounding the wound of entry was plotted on the surface of the brain, it was found to occupy the supra-marginal gyrus and part of the superior parietal lobule (Figs. 12 and 13, Vol. 1, p. 460 and p. 461).

Four months after he was wounded, he developed epileptiform attacks in which he became unconscious and was slightly convulsed. Under the influence of worry, confusion and noise these became somewhat frequent; but, with treatment and a quiet life in the country, they have been greatly reduced in number.

The most striking physical abnormality consisted of a peculiar form of defective vision characteristic of certain cortical lesions. Over the right half of the field a moving object could be appreciated up to the periphery, but a stationary white square was frequently unrecognised. Moreover, if two discs were exposed simultaneously, one to the left and the other to the right of the visual field, he never failed to appreciate the former, though he was frequently uncertain to the right of the middle line. This condition has remained unchanged throughout.

On admission, the optic discs were blurred at the edges, showing traces of previous swelling which had subsided. The pupils reacted well, even when the light was thrown on to the affected half of the visual field. Motion, sensation and the reflexes were unaffected. There were no abnormal signs on the left half of the body referable to the trephine opening on the right side of the skull through which the missile had been extracted.

His defects of speech formed an excellent example of Semantic Aphasia.

In No. 18 (see p. 259) the lesion lay somewhat higher and there was definite evidence of considerable sub-cortical destruction. He was struck by shrapnel and, when admitted under my care a month later, the wound consisted of a long granulating area which, at the site of its maximum breadth, covered a small stellate fracture of the skull. In the centre of this portion a small sinus led into the substance of the brain. This closed prematurely and suppuration continued in deeper parts. Finally, we explored the track, and several fragments of bone, lying about 1·5 cm. from the surface, were removed. The wound then became reduced to a minute sinus extending for 8 cm. downwards, forwards and inwards; this healed completely seven weeks after the operation and exactly eight months from the date of injury.

The opening in the skull occupied a roughly quadrilateral area, measuring 2 cm. in either direction. The superior border lay 1·5 cm. from the middle of the scalp and corresponded to two points 22·5 cm. and 24·5 cm. on the nasion-inion line. Plotted on the surface of the brain this area was found to lie over the superior parietal lobule (Figs. 12 and 13, Vol. 1, p. 460 and p. 461). But, when interpreting the signs and symptoms, we must not forget the definite evidence of sub-cortical destruction of tissue.

He suffered from no fits after the wound had finally healed. There was complete right hemianopsia and the pupils did not react to light impinging on the blind half of the field. Face and tongue moved equally on the two sides. Individual movements of the digits could be carried out perfectly with the eyes open; but, when they were closed, the fingers of the right hand performed these finer movements less perfectly than the left. Moreover, the right hand was slightly atonic. These defects were obviously afferent in origin and the power of recognising posture and passive movement was found to be somewhat diminished. Other forms of sensibility were unaffected. The reflexes were normal and equal on the two sides.

The defects in the use of language conformed to the Semantic type, but were somewhat less profound than in the previous cases. On the other hand, there was gross hemianopsia and some loss of sensibility in the right upper extremity.

(b) *Removal of an extra-cerebral tumour.*

No. 20 (see p. 295) was a woman of 56 in whom profound and extensive aphasic manifestations followed removal of a tumour which pressed upon the brain. Before the operation she suffered from occasional seizures which began in the thumb and index finger and, on the last occasion, the attack was followed by loss of speech lasting for several hours.

When she first came under my care in May, 1922, there were no abnormal physical signs of any kind except that I could not obtain the reflexes from the right half of the abdomen. Both plantars gave a downward response.

On June 20th, 1922, Mr Wilfred Trotter removed a smooth, lobulated, fibrous growth, which measured 5 cm. antero-posteriorly, 4 cm. vertically and 3·5 cm. in depth. Microscopically its structure was that of a fibro-endothelioma. It sprang from the dura mater, which was in turn firmly attached to the bone above it; this was soft and vascular, cutting like cheese. The tumour was so carefully extracted that not even the smallest fragment of cortical tissue adhered to the mass removed. The depression it had produced in the substance of the brain seemed to be centred around the meeting point of the inferior frontal and inferior precentral fissures.

The wound healed by first intention and the patient showed no evidence of surgical shock. The operation was, however, followed by profound aphasia accompanied by complete flaccid hemiplegia on the right side of the body with paralysis of the same half of the tongue and lower half of the face. The right plantar reflex gave a definite upward response, and arm- and knee-jerks were brisker than those on the normal side.

She improved steadily day by day both physically and in her powers of speech. At the expiration of sixteen days all abnormal physical signs had disappeared. Within four months after the operation she had been transformed from a profound example of aphasia into one so slight that it might have been mistaken for an articulatory disturbance only.

A little more than ten months after the operation, as the result of worry and consequent insomnia, she regressed to a condition resembling that found four weeks after removal of the tumour. Speech, reading and writing had grossly deteriorated and many of the serial tests were badly executed. There were no abnormal physical signs. The causes of her worry were removed and five months later she had recovered to a degree never reached before. This improvement continued, and has been steadily maintained.

§4. VASCULAR LESIONS

No. 26 (see p. 394) was a case of extremely severe aphasia in an unusually intelligent man of 60. On May 2nd, 1920, at 8 o'clock in the morning, he was suddenly seized with complete inability to express himself in words. He did not lose consciousness and within ten minutes had regained his speech completely. An hour later he exclaimed, "It's going again"; but he walked downstairs unaided and in a few minutes seemed to speak as well as ever. After driving for four miles in a motor-car, he became somewhat confused and asked where he was. From that moment he was unable to speak or to write normally. On alighting from the car his right arm was found to be paralysed and the right half of the face and tongue were affected; at no time did the weakness extend to the leg.

When I first saw him in November, 1923, he was an active, healthy-looking man. The pulse was 80 to the minute and regular, the systolic tension 160 mm., the diastolic 95 mm. The arterial wall was somewhat hard, but the vessel was not tortuous. The heart was slightly enlarged; at the apex the first sound was loud and over the base the aortic sound was a little exaggerated. The urine, of a specific gravity of 1022, contained no albumen or sugar.

I could find no signs pointing to disease of the nervous system, apart from the defects of speech. He could utter nothing but meaningless sounds with "Si, si" used correctly for affirmation, and could repeat nothing. He understood what was said to him and read to himself with pleasure, but could not execute complex oral or printed commands. He wrote nothing spontaneously except his name and the first nine numerals. Even when given the twenty-six block letters, he failed to arrange them in alphabetical order. Arithmetical exercises were impossible and he could neither name coins nor express the simplest relation between any two of them. Orientation was unaffected. Games, except draughts, were difficult or impossible. He enjoyed music and could sing without words.

No. 21 (see p. 320) was a man of 56 who suffered from a severe form of aphasia, lasting almost unchanged until his death nine years after the onset.

On May 13th, 1911, he rose in the morning well; but when he returned at 8 p.m. from his son's house, where he had been gardening, he seemed strange and was unable to find his words. He went to bed, slept heavily and next morning seemed in his usual health; but, as the day advanced, he became drowsy and strange in his manner. On the 15th he had obvious difficulty with speech. On the 17th he came to my out-patient department and was admitted to the wards of the London Hospital.

He was a grey-haired well-built man. His pulse was regular, but the arterial wall was thickened and tortuous. The systolic pressure reached 190 mm. There were no morbid signs in the heart. The urine was normal.

He was somewhat confused by the difficulty with his speech, but was otherwise intelligent. He complained of no headache, his optic discs were unaffected and I could discover no abnormal signs in the nervous system.

He could say nothing but "yes" and "no," together with a few emotional expressions, and could not even repeat his name. He understood to a remarkable degree what was said to him, provided it did not convey an order. He could not read aloud, but seemed to comprehend simple words in print. Writing was grossly affected.

He remained in fundamentally the same condition and, eight and a half years after the original seizure, I was able to make a complete examination by my serial methods.

He still showed signs of high vascular tension and degenerative changes in the arteries. The urine contained no albumen or sugar. He had suffered from no fits, seizures or other attacks since the initial stroke. He was free from headache, the visual fields were unaffected and there were no abnormal signs in the nervous system.

He was speechless, except for "yes" and "no" and a few automatic expressions, and could not repeat anything said to him. He understood most of what he heard, choosing objects and colours correctly to oral commands; yet he failed to execute the more complex tests. He could read nothing aloud and had difficulty in understanding what he read to himself. But printed words obviously conveyed some meaning to him; for he chose familiar objects to printed commands and on several occasions succeeded in selecting a printed card, which bore the name of the colour he had just seen. He could write nothing but his surname spontaneously, failed altogether to write to dictation and could not copy print in cursive script. He was unable to say, to repeat, to read, or to write the alphabet; he succeeded in writing some of the letters to dictation and copied them in capitals with four errors only. He counted with extreme difficulty and failed to reach twenty. Simple problems in arithmetic puzzled him greatly, but he was able to indicate on his fingers the relative value of two coins. He drew poorly from a model and failed completely to draw an elephant to command.

No. 22 (see p. 329) was a case of Nominal Aphasia in a man of 65. He woke on March 7th, 1920, to find he could no longer speak easily; there was no paralysis of arm or leg and he was ignorant of the hemianopsia discovered on examination some weeks later. Observations, made eleven weeks and again three years after the attack, brought out results which were fundamentally identical in character.

He was a somewhat worn-looking man, a highly intelligent artisan. By trade he was a house painter; but, as he played both the cornet and double-bass, he was in the habit of playing in an orchestra at one of the holiday resorts.

His pulse was regular, 68 to the minute, and the systolic tension reached 185 mm., the diastolic 100 mm.; the vessel was hard and tortuous. The heart was slightly enlarged, but nothing abnormal could be heard beyond an accentuation of the aortic second sound.

The optic discs were normal, but the arteries of the fundus were pale and evidently degenerated. There was gross right hemianopsia; form and movement were appreciated slightly to the right of the middle line and the pupils seemed to react to light thrown over the blind field. Motion, sensation and all the reflexes were normal.

His defects of speech formed an excellent example of Nominal Aphasia. He had profound difficulty in naming an object shown to him. With colours he was particularly at fault and, although he could not name them, he could describe how they would be composed from pigments he used as a house painter. Oral commands were executed slowly but he failed grossly to comprehend printed words and phrases. He could not write down the names of objects or colours or compose a short letter; it was not the act of writing that was at fault, but the power to discover words of the exact meaning to fit a situation and then to transform them into appropriate written symbols. He could count up to a hundred slowly, but failed to solve problems in arithmetic. Orientation was not affected, except that he became puzzled if he did not see before him the familiar landmarks he expected. He could draw from a model, but not a more complex figure or ground-plan to order. He had lost the power of reading musical notation and could no longer play his instruments.

No. 24 (see p. 370) was a case of Semantic Aphasia in a Doctor of Medicine aged 65. There had been no stroke or seizure of any kind; but, two weeks before I first saw him, he had begun to notice some difficulty in reading, which increased considerably a couple of days before he consulted me.

He did not look unduly old for his age. His pulse was 72 to the minute and regular, but the arterial wall was somewhat hard; the systolic tension was 220 mm., the diastolic 120 mm. The heart was distinctly enlarged. No murmurs were audible, although the second sound at the aortic area was accentuated. The specific gravity of the urine was 1030; it contained no albumen or sugar.

There were no abnormal physical signs pointing to disease of the central nervous system, except the defective use of language. This assumed a characteristic Semantic form. Although he appreciated details, however presented, he could not comprehend their general significance or deduce from them their logical consequences. He also failed to recognise, or was unable to retain in his mind, the full intention of an act he was about to perform spontaneously or to order. Thus, he frequently misapprehended the meaning of pictures, especially in conjunction with a printed legend. He named objects correctly and did not lack words. Single words and short phrases were understood and he executed even complex oral commands. Although he could carry out printed orders, he had great difficulty in comprehending what he read to himself or aloud. He wrote his name and address, but could not place on paper without the grossest mistakes his own ideas or the gist of something he had heard or read. He counted accurately and wrote the numbers without difficulty; arithmetical problems, however, puzzled him or were solved with effort, and he was confused by monetary transactions. Drawing was very defective. Orientation was gravely affected and he failed entirely to construct a ground-plan of a familiar room.

§5. CONGENITAL DEFECTS OF SYMBOLIC FORMULATION AND EXPRESSION

No. 23 (see p. 348) was a case of congenital disorder of speech in a healthy young man. Although highly intelligent, he had never been able to find words in which to express his thoughts and could not learn like other boys at school.

The visual fields were perfect, motion, sensation and the reflexes were unaffected, and he showed no abnormal physical signs of any kind.

His defects of symbolic formulation and expression were akin to those in certain cases of Nominal Aphasia. He did not lack words, but insisted that he was unable to find those which aptly expressed his meaning. He could not read or write with ease and had difficulty in solving the simplest arithmetical problems.

No. 25 (see p. 379) was an extremely intelligent woman in whom the defects resembled in character those found in Semantic Aphasia. They were accompanied by no abnormal physical signs of any kind.

From childhood she had recognised that she was unlike other persons. She had extreme difficulty in learning to read, to write and to carry out even simple arithmetical calculations. Yet, in spite of these disabilities, she became a professional gardener and originated the idea of open-air schools. Her introspective notes formed a valuable addition to the results of my examination.

APHASIA
AND KINDRED DISORDERS OF SPEECH

PART V
REPORTS OF CLINICAL CASES

No. 1

A case of extremely severe Aphasia, due to an extensive gun-shot injury of the left half of the head. The missile entered in the fronto-temporal and made its exit in the temporo-parietal region; at this point there was a small hernia cerebri. These wounds healed completely in fifteen weeks.

There was profound right hemiplegia, in which face and tongue participated; the upper extremity was flaccid, the lower hypertonic. The visual fields were not affected.

At first he was completely speechless except for "yes" and "no," but he recovered power rapidly and it then became obvious that the defects of symbolic formulation and expression were mainly of the Verbal type. Articulation was extremely bad and he could not repeat even single words with certainty. He failed to understand what was said to him and executed oral commands with difficulty. He did not comprehend exactly what he read to himself and carried out printed commands slowly and incorrectly. At first he could write nothing but his surname and was unable to copy print in cursive handwriting; this power of copying returned, however, long before he was able to write spontaneously or to dictation.

Recovery progressed with great rapidity and thirty weeks after he was wounded considerable power had returned to the right leg, but the hand was entirely useless; the tongue still deviated on protrusion. He had now become a straightforward example of Verbal Aphasia. He talked slowly and with obvious difficulty and, when repeating anything said to him, his articulation was better than with spontaneous speech. He understood all that was said and executed even complex oral commands correctly. Although he succeeded in carrying out printed orders with the exception of the hand, eye and ear tests, he still failed to comprehend exactly what he read to himself owing to defects of internal verbalisation. The right hand was powerless and he employed the left for writing; not only was the act of writing difficult, but the words were badly spelt. To dictation the faults were of the same character though less gross. He could, however, copy print perfectly in cursive script, evidence that the defect was intellectual rather than mechanical. He was unable to say the alphabet spontaneously and had great difficulty in writing the letters in due sequence. In spite of his University education, he was puzzled by simple arithmetical problems. Orientation was in no way affected and he drew from memory a perfect ground-plan of his ward at the hospital, in spite of its unusual and irregular form. He could play simple card games, but not bridge; puzzles he enjoyed and solved with ease.

Lieutenant A. C. A., aged 22, was wounded on October 18th, 1915, by a fragment of shrapnel, whilst sitting in a trench. No notes came through to England, except a temperature chart; but from this it was evident that an operation had been performed on the 21st, whilst he was still unconscious and that he subsequently suffered with irregular fever ranging between 98° and 101°–103° F. (38·4°–39·4° C.).

On November 10th, 1915, he was evacuated to England, where he came under my care at the Empire Hospital.

His injuries were confined to the left half of the head; they consisted of two granulating areas and a semicircular surgical incision, which had healed (Fig. 15). The anterior wound, representing the entry of the missile in the fronto-temporal region, was roughly triangular in shape, obliquely vertical in position and 4 cm. from the middle line. It was about 4·5 cm. in length and laid bare the superficial coverings of the brain.

Further back was the more important wound of exit, also roughly triangular in form with a herniating surface, from which cultures of streptococci and staphylococci were obtained. This area was 8 cm. in length horizontally and lay 5 cm. from the middle line of the scalp. It extended from a point 14 cm. to one 22 cm. along the nasion-inion line. The healed surgical flap lay between this portion of the wound and the centre of the scalp, with a descending limb running downwards in the direction of the ear.

Both wounds healed with unusual rapidity; by January 2nd, 1916, the anterior had closed completely, whilst the posterior was reduced to a deep pit with shelving edges leading down to a clean granulating area 2 cm. in length and not more than 0·75 cm. in breadth. By the end of the month even this portion had firmly healed.

On admission (Nov. 14th, 1915) his mental state was excellent and his temperature fell to normal in the first week. He was completely speechless except for "yes" and "no," which he could use in their proper sense, provided he was allowed to correct himself if he made a mistake; but he could not repeat them, when asked to do so.

He was unable to read, although he could point to the word on the list beside him, which expressed the thing he desired. If he was shown an object, such as an acid drop, he could not find the name on the paper; but whenever he wanted an acid drop he would ring his bell for the nurse and point correctly to the name. I also tested his power of asking in this way for a pear or an orange and repeatedly watched him employ this method for obtaining the bottle into which he passed urine.

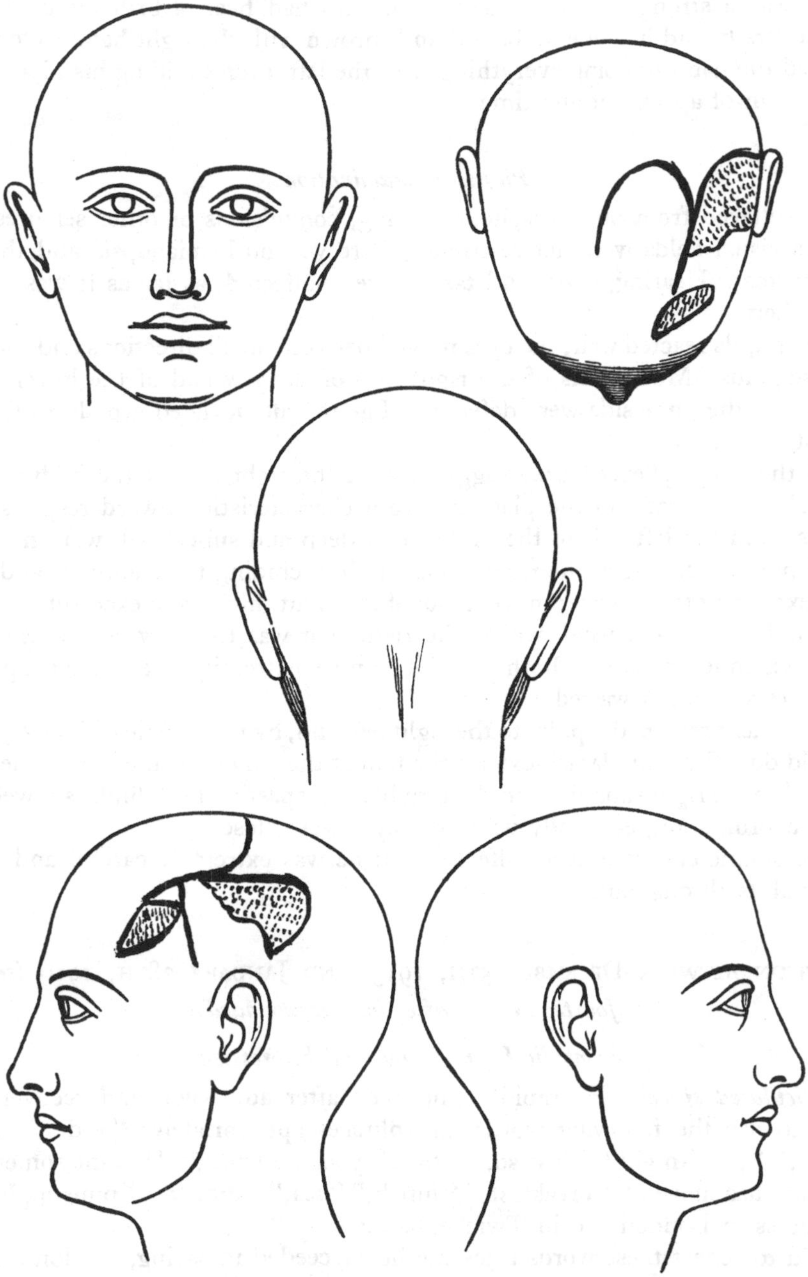

Fig. 15. To show the wounds of entry and of exit in No. 1.

He was a strongly right-handed man, who had been a brilliant cricketer at the University and had always batted and thrown with the right hand. He rapidly acquired the habit of doing everything with the left, even to filling his pipe. There was no sign of apraxia at any time.

Physical Examination.

He suffered from no headache, vomiting, convulsions or other seizures.

The visual fields were not restricted, there was no hemianopsia and the discs were normal. Hearing, smell and taste were unaffected, as far as it was possible to test them.

The pupils reacted well; the eyes moved perfectly in all directions and there was no nystagmus. Movements of the right half of the jaw and of the lower part of the face on the same side were defective. The tongue deviated grossly to the right on protrusion.

All the deep reflexes were exaggerated on the right half of the body; the abdominal was absent and the plantar gave a characteristic upward response. The reflexes from the left half of the body, both deep and superficial, were normal.

All power was lost in the right upper limb, including the shoulder, and in the lower extremity to the knee; movements of the right thigh were exceedingly feeble. The whole arm was flaccid, whilst the right foot was tonically contracted in the plantar-extended position. Both the right upper extremity and the leg up to the knee were somewhat wasted.

Movement returned rapidly to the right leg, and, by the middle of January, 1916, he could dorsiflex and plantar-extend the foot at the ankle. At the same time power returned to the right shoulder and the arm became spastic. Both limbs showed gross loss of coordination, especially when the eyes were closed.

The sphincters were never affected and he was extremely careful and cleanly in his habits throughout.

CONDITION BETWEEN DECEMBER 5TH, 1915, AND JANUARY 28TH, 1916 (*seven to fourteen weeks after he was wounded*).

Symbolic Formulation and Expression.

Articulated speech. He rapidly improved after admission and recovered the power to use the following words and phrases appropriately: "I don't know," "please," "good-night," "just so," "to tell you the truth," "I want something," "dressing has moved," "breakfast," "lunch," "tea," "dinner," "pine apple," and his address in London and in Twickenham.

Told to repeat these words after me he succeeded in saying, "I don't know," "dressing is moved" (instead of "has moved"), "tea," "breakfast" and "Cadogan

Gardens," a part of his London address. But he was unable to repeat any of the others including his own name.

Asked to give his name he laughed and made no sound; but when I said, "Is your name A. C. A.?" he at once replied, "yes." Then he added, "Twickenham," followed by the name of the road he had not been able to repeat.

When I suggested he should count he struggled vainly to do so, but emitted no sound. I then said, "One, two, three," and he still made no response. Ten minutes later, whilst I was preparing to test his power of naming common objects, he suddenly burst out, "One, two, three, four, five, six"; then he went back to "one, two," and after a pause counted rapidly, "One, two, three, four, five, six, seven, eight, nine, ten, eleven, twelve, thirteen, twenty-one, twenty-two..."

Reading. From the first it was obvious that he understood the significance of some printed words, although he could not read a book to himself with understanding. He chose the right object to printed commands in nine out of sixteen attempts and rapidly acquired the power to carry out more complicated actions.

With the hand, eye and ear tests he had some difficulty in reading the order aloud correctly, although the movements were executed faultlessly. From pictures, he read slowly but accurately.

Writing. In the earlier stages he was unable to write anything except his surname and a scrawl, which somewhat resembled one of his Christian names. At first he could not copy; but the power of transcribing print into cursive handwriting returned long before he was able to write spontaneously or to dictation. When he began to write again, he could do so better from pictures than if the words were dictated by me.

Serial Tests.

His condition changed so rapidly for the better during the period of nearly eight weeks, when he was subjected to more intensive examination, that the serial tests have been arranged according to their order in time, and the date has been added of the day on which they were carried out.

(1) *Naming and recognition of common objects*. (December 5th, 1915.)

He was extremely quick and certain in the choice of objects he had seen or held in his left hand out of sight. As the test proceeded he scarcely needed to see or touch for a moment the scissors, the match-box, the penny or the key, before he thrust out his left hand in the direction of the duplicate on the table in front of him. He remembered the order in which they lay and would point to their position even before the screen was removed.

He was extremely slow in selecting the right object from the set on the table in response to its name, whether said by me or printed on a card. He frequently seemed to forget the order in which they lay and moved his hand up and down the row as if testing whether they corresponded to the spoken or printed word. In both series, however, he succeeded in choosing more than one half correctly.

But he was completely unable to articulate, to write or to copy the name of any of these common objects. He remained silent and did not even attempt to utter any approximate sounds. The scrawled marks he made on the paper when writing, bore no obvious relation to the word he was trying to reproduce.

In order to discover how far his difficulties were due to lack of power to evoke and retain the symbols he required, I carried out the following experiments. Shown one of a set of common objects, he never failed to point out the duplicate amongst those on the table; this he did with remarkable quickness and certainty. But when two objects were exhibited at the same time, he was unable to choose both correctly except on one occasion only; he usually selected one of them and failed to make a second choice. For, when the test was carried out in this manner, it was no longer a simple act of matching; he was compelled to retain two symbols in his memory and to correlate them with two objects on the table.

Shown together.	*Objects indicated.*
Penny	Correct
Match-box	"No." No choice
Knife	No choice
Key	Correct
Pencil	Correct
Scissors	No choice
Match-box	Correct
Key	Correct
Scissors	Correct. Said "Yes and..?"
Penny	No choice
Knife	No choice
Pencil	No choice
Scissors	Correct
Match-box	Chose pencil
Pencil	Correct. Said "Yes and..?"
Key	No choice
Penny	No choice
Knife	No choice

Table 1.

	Pointing to object shown	Oral commands	Printed commands	Duplicate placed in L. hand out of sight	Naming an object indicated	Writing name of object indicated	Copying from print
Penny	Correct	Correct	Correct	Correct	Impossible	Impossible	Impossible
Match box	,,	,,	,,	,,	,,	,,	,,
Knife	,,	,,	,,	,,	,,	,,	,,
Key	,,	,,	,,	,,	,,	,,	,,
Pencil	,,	,,	Knife	,,	,,	,,	,,
Scissors	,,	"No"; then correct	Match box	,,	,,	,,	,,
Match box	,,	Correct	Correct	,,	,,	,,	,,
Key	,,	,,	,,	,,	,,	,,	,,
Scissors	,,	Correct; very slow	Match box	,,	,,	,,	,,
Penny	,,	Correct	Correct	,,	,,	,,	,,
Knife	,,	No response	Scissors	,,	,,	,,	,,
Pencil	,,	Key	Knife; then key	,,	,,	,,	,,
Scissors	,,	No response	Correct	,,	,,	,,	,,
Match box	,,	Correct	,,	,,	,,	,,	,,
Pencil	,,	Key	Penny	,,	,,	,,	,,
Key	,,	Correct	No response	,,	,,	,,	,,
Penny	,,	,,	Correct	,,	,,	,,	,,
Knife	,,	,,	No response	,,	,,	,,	,,

(2) *The hand, eye and ear tests.* (December 12th, 1915.)

Owing to the complete paralysis of the right arm this test was of necessity somewhat simplified; throughout he used his left hand only to touch the right or left eye or ear. But in spite of the fact that the task was easier, it was obvious from the way he failed to carry out movements reflected in the mirror that there was some defect of general understanding. This is not to be wondered at considering the severity of the lesion.

Table 2.

	Imitation of movements made by the observer	Imitation of movements reflected in a mirror	Pictorial commands	Pictorial commands reflected in a mirror	Printed commands read aloud and executed: He said	Printed commands read aloud and executed: Movements executed	Oral commands
L. hand to L. ear	No response. Then "Well yes"; correct	Reversed	Correct	Reversed	Correctly	None	No response
L. hand to R. eye	Correct	,,	,,	,,	,,	,,	,,
L. hand to R. ear	No response	Correct	,,	Correct	"L. hand to R. cheek"	,,	Reversed
L. hand to L. eye	L. hand to tip of nose	Reversed	Reversed	,,	"L. cheek to L. eye"	,,	R. *ear*
L. hand to R. ear	Correct	,,	Correct	,,	Correctly	,,	No response
L. hand to L. eye	,,	Correct	Correct; slow	,,	,,	,,	Reversed
L. hand to R. eye	,,	,,	Correct	,,	"L. hand to R. *ear*"	,,	,,
L. hand to L. ear	,,	Reversed	,,	,,	"R. hand to R. ear"	,,	No response
L. hand to R. ear	No response	,,	R. *eye*	R. *eye*	"L. hand to R. *eye*; no, ear"	,,	,,
L. hand to R. eye	Correct	Correct	Correct	Correct	Correctly	,,	R. *ear*
L. hand to L. eye	L. hand to R. eye; then to tip of nose	,,	,,	,,	"L. hand to R. eye"	,,	No response
L. hand to I.. ear	Correct	,,	,,	,,	Correctly	,,	L. cheek

(3) *The clock tests.* (January 13th, 1916.)

By the middle of January his condition had improved still further and his general intelligence was extraordinarily good. He set the clock perfectly not only in imitation, but also to both oral and printed commands. He was not satisfied to place the short hand exactly opposite the hour, but selected some point between the two figures on the clock face proportionate to the position of the minute hand.

He had recovered sufficient words to tell the time; but he was not only extremely slow in utterance, but confused "past" and "to" and stumbled over two of the numbers correcting himself each time.

Table 3.

	Direct imitation	Oral commands	Printed commands	Telling the time	Writing down the time shown on a clock face	Copying from print
Half-past 2	Correct	Correct	Correct	"Half..past..two"	Impossible	Correct
20 minutes past 9	,,	,,	,,	"Twenty..mints.. to..nine"	,,	,,
5 minutes to 2	,,	,,	,,	"Five..mints..to.. two"	,,	,,
5 minutes past 8	,,	,,	,,	"Five..mints..past ..eight"	,,	,,
Half-past 1	,,	,,	,,	"Half past..one"	,,	,,
20 minutes to 4	,,	,,	,,	"Twenty..to..four"	,,	,,
10 minutes past 7	,,	,,	,,	"Five..ten..mints.. to..five..seven"	,,	,,
20 minutes to 6	,,	,,	,,	"Twenty mints..to ..five..six"	,,	,,
10 minutes to 1	,,	,,	,,	"Ten..mints..to.. one"	,,	,,
A quarter to 9	,,	,,	,,	"Fifteen mints..to nine"	,,	,,

Although he was unable to write down the time shown on the clock, he could copy the printed cards in cursive handwriting.

He showed a strong sense of error and was not satisfied until the time was rightly given, especially when copying.

Asked to tell the time aloud and then to write it down, he failed not only in writing, but also in speech. Far from helping him, the fact that he knew he had to write confused him and rendered verbalisation impossible.

(4) *The man, cat and dog tests.* (January 26th, 1916.)

He read aloud from print and from pictures all the combinations of this test very slowly, but without a mistake.

Not only could he copy the printed words, but he was now able to write from pictures and to dictation; in both these acts the improvement due to practice was visible.

He repeated the words said by me accurately and his enunciation was much more rapid than when he uttered them spontaneously.

Throughout all the tests there was no tendency to reverse the order of the nouns or to substitute wrong names; his difficulty was in pronouncing the words or in writing them correctly.

Table 4.

	Reading aloud	Reading from pictures	Writing to dictation	Writing from pictures	Copying from print	Repetition
The cat and the man	Correct but very slow	Correct but very slow	A cat and the ma	the the	Correct	"Cat and the man"
The man and the dog	,,	,,	The ma and the dog	man dog	,,	"The dog and the cat"
The cat and the dog	,,	,,	Correct	Correct	,,	Correct
The dog and the cat	,,	,,	The dog and the	,,	,,	"Dog and cat"
The man and the cat	,,	,,	The mat	,,	,,	"The man..and the cat"
The dog and the man	,,	,,	The dog and the ma	,,	,,	"Dog and the..man"
The cat and the man	,,	,,	The cat and the	,,	,,	"The..cat and the man"
The man and the dog	,,	,,	The ma and the dog	,,	,,	"The..man and the dog"
The cat and the dog	,,	,,	Correct	,,	,,	Correct
The dog and the cat	,,	,,	,,	,,	,,	,,
The man and the cat	,,	,,	The m and the cat	,,	,,	"The man..and the..cat"
The dog and the man	,,	,,	The dog and the ma	,,	,,	Correct

(5) *Naming and recognition of colours.* (January 28th, 1916.)

Here again he was not only able to match a colour he had seen, but could carry out correctly oral and printed commands.

He found great difficulty in evoking words to designate the colours and, although he never used wrong names, failed six times in sixteen attempts. At the termination of this sitting I carried out another naming series and his power of finding the right word had obviously improved owing to the many occasions on which he had heard or read the colour-names in the course of these tests.

Table 5.

	Pointing to colour shown	Naming colour shown	Oral commands	Printed commands	Printed name read aloud and colour chosen		Writing name of colour shown	Naming colour shown [2nd series]
					He said	He chose		
Blue	Correct	No response	Correct	Correct	Correctly	Rapidly and correctly	Blue	Correct
Yellow	,,	,,	,,	,,	Very slow; correctly	,,	Ye	,,
Green	,,	Correct	,,	,,	Slow; correctly	,,	No response	No response
Orange	,,	"Red"	,,	,,	Correctly	,,	Orog	Correct
Red	,,	"Red, I suppose"	,,	,,	,,	,,	ret	,,
Black	,,	Correct	,,	,,	Slow; correctly	,,	Bla	,,
Violet	,,	"Heliotrope"	,,	,,	"Vi-let"	,,	vi	,,
White	,,	Correct	,,	,,	Correctly	,,	wo	,,
Red	,,	No response	,,	,,	,,	,,	rd	,,
Green	,,	Very slow; correct	,,	,,	,,	,,	y	No response
White	,,	Correct	,,	,,	,,	,,	whi	Very slow; correct
Orange	,,	No response	,,	,,	,,	,,	oro	Correct
Violet	,,	"Heliotrope; red"	,,	,,	Slow; "vi-let"	,,	vi	"Heliotrope"
Yellow	,,	No response	,,	,,	Slow; correctly	,,	Illegible scrawl	Correct
Black	,,	Very slow; correct	,,	,,	Slow; correctly	,,	ble	,,
Blue	,,	No response	,,	,,	Correctly	,,	blu	,,

When he was permitted to read the printed card aloud, he showed the same verbal inability; and yet the choice of the colour was rapid and correct. He thrust out his hand in the right direction long before he could find the name. The response to printed commands was immediate and did not come through the uttered word.

He wrote the names of the colours extremely badly; in fact he completed the word he was writing on one occasion only. But the fragmentary scrawls on the paper indicated that he knew the name, although he was unable to reproduce it at will. Thus "bla" was black, "oro" orange and "vi" violet.

CONDITION FROM MAY 21ST TO MAY 27TH, 1916 (*thirty to thirty-one weeks after he was wounded*).

Considerable power had returned to the right leg and he walked with a characteristically hemiplegic gait. He was able to dorsiflex and plantar-extend the right foot, though feebly compared with the normal limb. The hand was entirely useless, but some movement was possible at both shoulder and elbow. The whole of the right upper extremity was strongly hypertonic.

Some weakness of the lower part of the face was still present on the right side, and the tongue deviated somewhat on protrusion.

Otherwise his physical condition was not materially changed.

Before he joined the army he had been an undergraduate at one of the older Universities, reading for a classical degree, and he had now regained his old intellectual vigour. He was bright, cheerful and in no way cast down by his disabilities. He maintained an amused attitude towards the tests, as if he were playing a game; he knew when he was wrong and determined to find the right answer. Sometimes he was able to rectify his mistakes; but not infrequently he failed to do so in spite of repeated attempts, although he would never accept a false solution as correct. His memory was now excellent and his temper equable.

He had become extremely clever with his left hand; he wrote with rapidity and ease, buttoned his clothes, filled his pipe and carried out many other complex acts with one hand alone.

Articulated speech. He talked slowly and with obvious difficulty, but the pauses were less frequent, the words were emitted in larger groups and were more perfectly pronounced. Asked what he had been doing at our Convalescent Hospital he said, "Walking a little...talking difficult a bit...five or six times in the car...that's all I think." Q. "What games have you played?" A. "Picquet...and whist...but it was not much good...About two months ago..." Q. "Have you played bridge?" A. "Oh! no...not bridge...gave up...patience...two months ago." By this he intended to imply that he had begun to be able to play patience, a simple single-handed card game, two months before.

Understanding of spoken words. He had regained the capacity to comprehend what was said to him and could execute even the complex hand, eye and ear tests to oral commands without mistakes.

Reading. It was obvious from the manner in which he executed printed commands that he could read with understanding. But he still found little pleasure in reading to himself, owing to defective internal verbalisation.

When he was permitted to say the words aloud, orders were better carried out than if he remained silent; the spoken word was a definite help to his understanding.

Writing. He could copy printed matter perfectly in cursive handwriting. Words written spontaneously were very badly spelt and the faults, e.g. "machts," for matches, exceeded all normal limits. On writing to dictation these mistakes were less frequent but, when they occurred, belonged to the same class (cf. also the clock tests, p. 13).

The alphabet. He said the alphabet rapidly, but omitted U and V. Asked if he had left out any letters, he answered, "I don't think so." He had great difficulty in writing the letters in due sequence; on the first attempt he wrote, *a b c d e f g k l j* and the second time, *a b c d e f g* followed by several other letters which he erased. He knew he was wrong and perpetually tried to correct himself, until he became muddled and ceased altogether. On the other hand he wrote the alphabet to dictation with one mistake only; he made an *x* for *w*; but when the whole series was completed, seeing that there were two *x*'s, he went back and corrected this error.

Arithmetic. He was given the following simple sums in addition and subtraction. As they increased in difficulty, he grew slower and the last two contained actual errors.

Addition.

123	158	186
236	429	546
359	587	732

Subtraction.

543	641	512
321	228	267
222	427 (wrong)	355 (wrong)

Orientation. He had no difficulty in finding his way about and was able to describe the exact position of his bed and its relation to other objects in the ward. "This bed...in the corner...opposite the...the...the door...er..facing the... er..door..It's a big room..picture...over fireplace," etc. He described accurately the colours of the uniforms worn by the matron and by the nurses. He evidently possessed a strong visual memory.

He drew a perfect ground-plan of the large ward in spite of its somewhat irregular and unusual form.

Games, etc. He could play picquet and various simple forms of patience. Whist he had tried but found it difficult and Bridge he could not play at all. Jigsaw puzzles he enjoyed.

Serial Tests.

(1) *Naming and recognition of common objects.*

Table 6.

	Oral commands	Printed commands	Duplicate placed in L. hand out of sight	Naming an object indicated	Writing name of object indicated	Copying from print	Writing to dictation	Repetition
Penny	Correct	Correct	Correct	Correct	Correct	Perfect	Correct	Perfect
Match box	,,	,,	,,	,,	Maths	,,	,,	,,
Knife	,,	,,	,,	"Pen-knife"	Key	,,	,,	,,
Key	,,	,,	,,	Correct	Correct	,,	,,	,,
Pencil	,,	,,	,,	,,	Pensel	,,	,,	,,
Scissors	,,	,,	,,	,,	Scissers	,,	Scissirs	,,
Match box	,,	,,	,,	,,	Machts	,,	Correct	,,
Key	,,	,,	,,	,,	Correct	,,	,,	,,
Scissors	,,	,,	,,	,,	Scissers	,,	Scisse	,,
Penny	,,	,,	,,	,,	Correct	,,	Correct	,,
Knife	,,	,,	,,	,,	Knike	,,	,,	,,
Pencil	,,	,,	,,	,,	Correct	,,	,,	,,

He chose an object placed in his left hand out of sight and executed oral and printed commands without a moment's hesitation. The whole series was named slowly, but correctly, except that on one occasion he called the dinner knife a "pen-knife."

He wrote these names badly; they were wrongly spelt, although each one obviously corresponded to the true nomenclature. Writing to dictation was less faulty, whilst he copied the printed words perfectly in cursive script.

Repetition was correct and his articulation was better than when he named the objects voluntarily.

(2) *The man, cat and dog tests.* The various forms of these tests could be carried out with little or no difficulty. He read the simple words and phrases easily, both from print and pictures, copied them correctly and wrote them to dictation without a mistake. Told to write from pictures, he gave the two nouns accurately, but did not fill in the other words. He repeated all the sentences after me and his articulation was better than when he said them spontaneously.

(3) *The clock tests.* He was able to set the hands of one clock in direct imitation of another, and to execute oral and printed commands without hesitation. Asked to tell the time, he answered correctly, employing the usual nomenclature; but

there was much hesitation and difficulty in finding the words he required. When he attempted to write down the time without saying anything aloud, this was still more evident and he wrote as follows:

Time set.	*He wrote.*
2.30	"Two thich"
9.20	"Twenty — nine" (said "past" but wrote a line)
1.55	"Five minutes to two"
8.5	"Five parts eith"
1.30	"Ha one."
3.40	"Twer to four"
7.30	" se "
5.40	"Twe to six"
12.50	"Ten minutes to one"
8.45	"Eith fouthy fixe"

Here it was obvious that he recognised the time, but could not find words in which to express it.

(4) *The hand, eye and ear tests.*

Table 7.

	Imitation of movements made by the observer	Imitation of movements reflected in a mirror	Pictorial commands	Pictorial commands reflected in a mirror	Oral commands	Printed commands	Printed commands read aloud and executed	
							He said	Movement executed
L. hand to L. ear	Correct	Correct	Correct	Correct	Correct	R. ear	Correctly	Correct
L. hand to R. eye	,,	,,	,,	,,	,,	L. eye	,,	,,
L. hand to R. ear	,,	,,	,,	,,	,,	L. ear	,,	,,
L. hand to L. eye	,,	,,	,,	,,	,,	R. eye	,,	,,
L. hand to R. ear	,,	,,	R. *eye*; corrected	,,	,,	Correct	,,	,,
L. hand to L. eye	,,	,,	Correct	,,	,,	R. eye	"L. hand to R. eye, to L. eye"	,,
L. hand to R. eye	,,	,,	L. eye; corrected	,,	,,	L. eye	Correctly	,,
L. hand to L. ear	,,	,,	Correct	,,	,,	Correct	,,	,,
L. hand to R. ear	,,	,,	,,	,,	,,	,,	,,	,,
L. hand to R. eye	L. eye; corrected	,,	,,	,,	,,	,,	,,	,,
L. hand to L. eye	Correct	,,	,,	,,	,,	,,	,,	,,
L. hand to L. ear	,,	,,	,,	,,	,,	,,	,,	,,

This series showed a profound improvement compared with the observations made during the acute stage. He could imitate my movements, when we sat face to face, and carry out pictorial commands accurately, although in both cases his actions were somewhat uncertain and hesitating. With reflections in the glass, on the other hand, he was quick and definite in his movements.

Given a command orally, he repeated it in a whisper and then slowly carried it out correctly. To printed commands he made several mistakes; but, when permitted to read aloud, every movement was accurately performed.

No. 2

A case of Nominal Aphasia, due to severe and extensive fracture of the left half of the skull, produced by the kick of a horse. The injury occupied mainly the region of the angular, superior parietal and parieto-occipital gyri and at the operation the brain was found to have been reduced to pulp for about 7 cm. below the level of the wound. Right hemianopsia of a gross character was present from the first, but there were no other abnormal physical signs. Subsequent repair of the opening in the skull with bone from the tibia was followed by excellent results physical and mental.

The patient was a highly intelligent, young Staff Officer. Throughout the whole time he has been under my observation, his speech has steadily improved; but the defects, though less in degree, remained identical in character. He had no lack of words, but suffered from want of capacity to find the one which exactly corresponded to the meaning he wished to express, or was an appropriate name for some definite object. At the same time he failed to understand the significance of words presented to him orally or in print. Writing was gravely affected; at first he wrote with extreme difficulty spontaneously or to dictation and could not copy print correctly in cursive script. Though he drew well spontaneously or from a model, he was unable to produce the figure of an elephant to command and he could not construct a ground-plan of some familiar room. Orientation was not fundamentally disturbed, although he had difficulty in formulating even to himself the way from one place to another. He failed to solve simple arithmetical problems and had much difficulty in calculating change. When he first came under my care, he could play chess, but not card games; puzzles always pleased him and enabled him to exhibit his mental ingenuity.

Throughout, he showed a remarkable power of re-acquiring knowledge; for example he again mastered Hindustani, so far as to speak the language, and he learnt to play bridge. Superficially he would now pass for a normal, active man.

Captain E. N. C., aged 30, was on the Staff of the army in Mesopotamia. On February 19th, 1918, he was riding in the early morning, when the saddle slipped and, as he fell, the hoof of his horse struck him in the left parieto-occipital region.

There was an extensive compound fracture of the skull and at the operation, which appears to have been carried out the same night, fragments of depressed bone were removed over a large area. A fissured fracture was found to extend towards the base of the skull and another in the direction of the occipital region. The brain below the injury was reduced to pulp for a depth of about three inches (about 7 cm.). After the operation cerebro-spinal fluid poured out to a considerable amount and a hernia cerebri developed which, however, subsided after lumbar puncture had been carried out three times.

On June 13th, 1918, a Medical Board assembled in Bombay reported that the wound was completely healed. The patient was bright and cheerful and complained of no headache. Right hemianopsia was present, but otherwise there were no abnormal signs; motion and sensation were not affected. There was some degree of aphasia; the patient could not remember the name of objects, and agraphia and word-blindness were present, though he could copy letters unintelligently. Considerable improvement had already occurred, and the patient was keen to learn to read and write again. He was intelligent and could understand everything said to him.

With this somewhat scanty history he was admitted to the Empire Hospital for Officers under my care on September 6th, 1918.

Condition in September 1918 (*twenty-eight weeks after the accident*).

Physical Examination.

There was a perfectly healed wound in the left parieto-occipital region, roughly oval in shape and 10 cm. by 5·5 cm. in size. Looked at from behind, the opening in the bone extended forwards to a point on a horizontal level with the 23rd cm. along the nasion-inion line and about 3·5 cm. to the left; it reached as far back as the 33rd cm. and at its termination was also about 3·5 cm. from the middle line (Figs. 10 and 11, Vol. 1, pp. 456 and 457). The scar was firm and depressed; it did not pulsate unless he lowered his head, as in doing up his boots, when it became nearly level with the surface and a slight impulse could be felt.

He suffered occasionally from a dull headache over the wound, especially if he was tired or had slept badly. Exertion did not seem to bring it on, but he disliked stooping or any movement or posture which produced pulsation.

There was complete right hemianopsia to movement, form and colour (Fig. 16). Vision was otherwise excellent.

I could discover no other abnormal physical signs in the central nervous system and he was in splendid general health.

He had always been strongly right-handed and could not cut a piece of paper, when the loose-jointed scissors were placed in his left hand.

Symbolic Formulation and Expression.

He was an extremely intelligent man who at the time of his accident knew several oriental languages particularly Hindustani. He is still under my care and during the last five years has subjected himself on many occasions to complete examination, evincing throughout the greatest interest in elucidating his condition. He showed remarkable introspective powers and frequently gave me information which was of the greatest value in directing my observations.

It is impossible to give more than a tithe of the experiments carried out during the last five years; but I shall begin by describing in full his condition in September 1918, when he first came under my care.

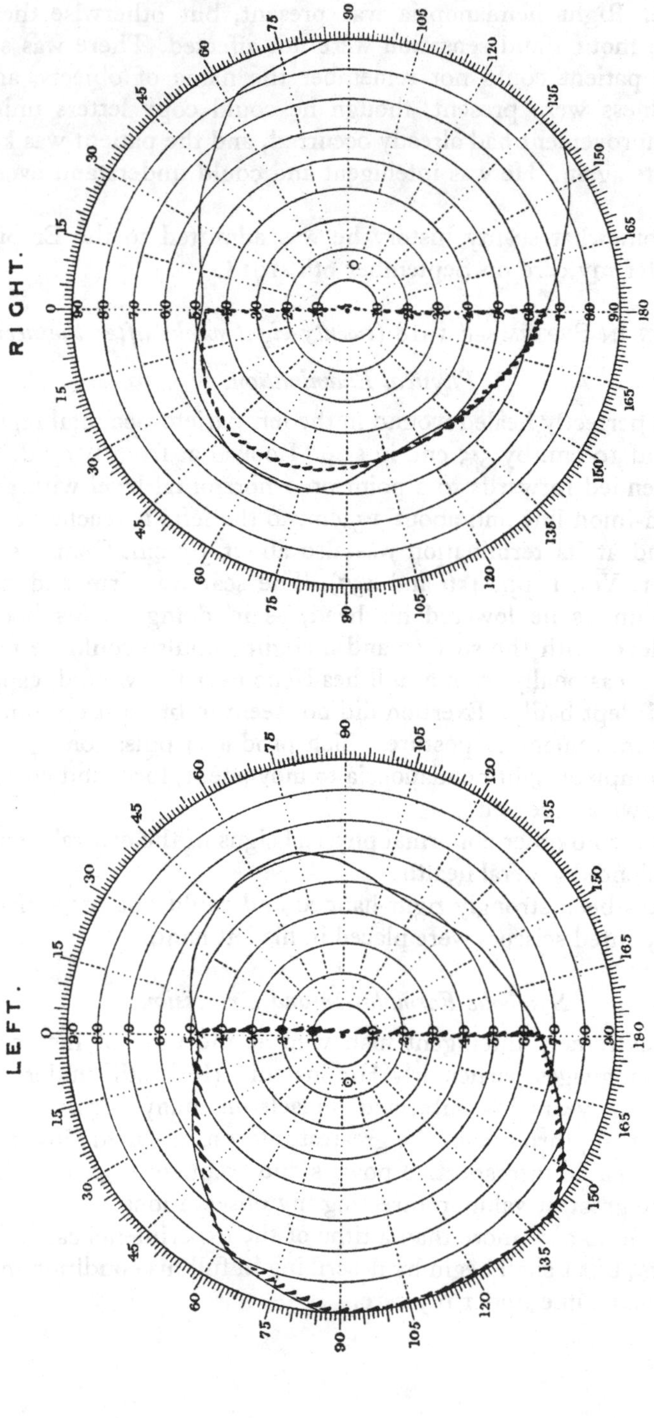

Fig. 16. To show the limitation of the fields of vision in No. 2.

Articulated speech. Most of the words in ordinary conversation were well pronounced and intonation was normal. But, when he had difficulty in finding a name or some nominal expression, he would try various combinations of sound more or less related to the word he was seeking. Thus, blue was called "ber-loo," orange "or-ridge"; but this seemed to be due to difficulty in finding the significant expression rather than to lack of verbal aptitude. For he was able to give long explanations of his inability to find the right names; e.g. in order to show that he recognised black, he said, "I remember that now, because people who are dead... the other people who are not dead, they usually have this colour." The syntax of his phrases was not affected except in so far as he was perpetually at a loss for names; this frequently necessitated the recasting of the structure of the sentence before it could be brought to a conclusion.

Asked to repeat a series of words or some simple phrase he had no difficulty in enunciation; but the content of the sentence was frequently incorrect (see the man, cat and dog tests, pp. 26–27). Although the same words might be badly pronounced in spontaneous speech, they could be repeated accurately (cf. Table 1).

Understanding of spoken words. He succeeded, after considerable hesitation, in choosing the common object named by me, but he frequently failed to select the correct colour to oral commands. As soon as the order demanded some more complex action, such as setting the hands of a clock, placing a certain coin into a definite bowl, or executing the hand, eye and ear tests, he made many gross errors.

Moreover, he was often unable to appreciate the exact significance of ordinary conversation. Although unusually intelligent, he was liable to become confused, because certain words were incomprehensible on a single hearing. If, however, care was taken to speak slowly and to repeat anything he did not at once understand, he was able to grasp the meaning of what he heard.

Reading. He could not read the newspaper to himself nor could he comprehend the contents of a letter. So long as he did not attempt to spell the printed words, he chose correctly from amongst a number of common objects the one indicated on the card; but, when it was a question of separate colours, he not infrequently fell into error.

When a command was given to him in print, he failed entirely to carry it out and tried in vain to spell the words of which it was composed.

Single words were read aloud badly and he failed to reproduce simple phrases. It was not, however, words that were lacking, for he would sometimes employ those required for a correct answer though in a wrong order. Thus he read The cat and the dog as "The dog and the cat, yes, the dog and the cat"; The man and the cat became "The dog and the cat. It might be anything. I have to think."

He was greatly hindered by attempts to spell out the printed words letter by letter; this confused him and he then made a guess at the significance of the word. This was particularly evident during the man, cat and dog tests (vide pp. 26–27).

Writing. He wrote his usual signature "E. N. C..., Capt. 112th Inf." with ease and rapidity, though quite unable to add his address. He was incapable of writing a letter or a sentence of any length, but amused himself by making lists of words, especially those which came into his head spontaneously that he wished to remember; of these the following may serve as examples: "Post offest" (Post Office), "The King One" (The King's Own Regiment), "Arbes" (Arabs), "Turskes" (Turks), "Masptmeren" (Mesopotamia).

He found it easier to write from pictures; every sentence was written throughout in ordinary handwriting, although the structure of some of the words was defective.

Writing to dictation was extremely faulty; even his name and address were reproduced as follows:

Capt. Eric Nelers C....
Hill Colmn,
Haill Sopst
Banternter
Sarris

instead of:

Capt. Eric Nelson C....
The Corner House
High Street
Brentwood
Essex.

Similarly, when dictated, the days of the week were written in an extremely faulty manner, although each one bore a recognisable relation to the word said by me. If, however, he was asked to write some extremely simple phrase conveying no command, as in the man, cat and dog tests, the fault lay in the substitution of one noun for another and not in the structure of the written word.

If I said the days of the week, he could repeat them perfectly, but wrote them almost as badly as when he attempted to produce them spontaneously. Self-dictation did not seem to make the task easier for him.

He could copy printed words in capitals, letter by letter, as if drawing from a model, but was unable to transcribe them into cursive handwriting correctly.

The alphabet. He had no difficulty in saying the alphabet, pronouncing each letter perfectly. He read it aloud rather slowly, but articulation and enunciation were accurate. Asked to write the alphabet he started to do so in capitals; when he reached H in this manner, he began again and wrote the whole in cursive handwriting somewhat slowly and carefully. Given the printed letters to copy he transcribed them rapidly and correctly.

The days of the week.

Table 1.

Said spontaneously		Copied from print		Read aloud	Written to dictation	Written spontaneously	Words said by the observer, repeated by the patient and then written	
1st series	2nd series	In cursive handwriting	In capitals				He said	He wrote
"Monday"	"Monday"	Mondey	Correct	Correctly	Munder	Mandern	Correctly	Mal Merinder
"Tuesday"	"Tuesday"	Tuersty	"	"	Tusdernd	Tuederny	"	Tuedery
"Wednesday"	"Wednesday"	Wednersty	"	"	Wesdend	Wersteney	"	Wednersty
"Thursday"	"Thursday"	Thersteay	"	"	Thirstin	Thirsteny	"	Thursdy
"Frys-day"	"Friday"	Freray	"	"Frys-day...Friday"	Fridery	Frerny	"	Frdernd
"Secon-day"	"Second-day"	Satereay	"	"Secon-day...Saturday"	Stersdery	S. Serkeng	"	Saternd
"Sutton-day"	"Sunday"	Sun Day	"	Correctly	Saterstn	Saterney	"	Sondery

When he tried to say the days of the week in order, he became somewhat confused and I therefore made a set of several observations, recorded on Table 1. On the first attempt he became muddled over the last three days, but on trying again he failed over Saturday only. He could read them aloud, stumbling somewhat over Friday and Saturday but repeated them with absolute correctness and perfect enunciation. Told to write the days of the week spontaneously, or to my dictation, or in response to the words he had repeated correctly, he made many mistakes. He could copy the names on a printed card in capitals, imitating letter by letter, but he was unable to transcribe them into cursive handwriting.

Numbers. He could count accurately with perfect enunciation and wrote with fair rapidity numbers up to twenty in their correct order. But, when he attempted to write them in words, he made the same sort of mistakes as those described for the days of the week. Thus, he wrote "one," "to," "twe," "forn," and "far," five was illegible, "six," "nenn," "nert," "nerv," "ten," "alon," "walm" and "walr," "netr," "forn," "farst," "six," "santen," "aten," "geten," "tenwa." With each numeral he whispered or said aloud the name with absolute correctness as he attempted to write it.

Arithmetic. Six exercises in simple arithmetic were given to him with the following results:

Addition.

231	648	856
356	326	275
567 For the second figure he said "eight" correctly but wrote first 7 and then 6.	974	1031 (wrong)

Subtraction.

865	782	523
432	258	284
433	536 (wrong)	399 (wrong)

He was aware of the processes involved in addition and subtraction, though his method of carrying them out was peculiar. When about to add 8 and 6, he did not take these numbers as entities, but counted up to eight and then on for another six, saying finally "fourteen." This was a difficult task and required several attempts before he reached the answer; with 3 and 6 on the other hand he simply counted up to nine.

By this cumbrous method he frequently forgot to carry over from the previous addition; when the answer was given correctly, as for example 7 + 5 and 1 to carry over, he called the 7 "eight," counted eight and then on for five more. But, when he came to add 8 + 2 and 1 to carry over, he counted eight and then two, thus bringing out the answer incorrectly.

Coins and their relative value. He had some difficulty in naming the various coins, especially those of higher value. A series of observations produced the following results:

Sixpence—Correct.
Shilling—Correct.
Penny—Correct.
Half-penny—"Half-pence," "Hăf-pence."
Two-shilling piece—"Two shillings. I call it a plozens; it's another name I can't remember." (Florin.)
Ten-shilling note—"It's half of a pole; half of a pound; ten shillings."
Half-a-crown—"Two and a half; the name I couldn't tell you."
One-pound note—"That's twenty-shillings or a pown, or a pown, a pound."
One shilling—"Twenty shillings. No, no, that's a..."
Sixpence—"That's half a shilling."
Half-penny—"Half a penny."
Half-a-crown—"Two and a half. One, two, two shillings."
Two-shilling piece—"That is two shillings."
Penny—Correct.
One-pound note—"That's a pown."
Ten-shilling note—"Half a pown or ten shillings."
Sixpence—(Very slow). Correct.
Two-shilling piece—Correct.
One-pound note—"Pown."
Half-penny—"Hăp-perny, hăp-perny."
Half-a-crown—"Two shillings, two and a half."
Penny—Correct.
Ten-shilling note—Correct.
Shilling—Correct.

I then laid a coin on the table and asked him, "How many of this, go into that?" placing beside it one of higher value. He was evidently conscious of their fundamental relation, but became confused in attempting to express it; sometimes he added the one to the other, at others he gave the right number but touched the wrong coin. For example:

One penny and sixpence—"Seven pennies. Oh! one penny and a half shilling—Oh! I see...No, I can only say that one...sixpence and a penny or seven pennies."
Sixpence and a shilling—"One and a half." I asked, "How many of that (sixpence) would you have to give me for that (shilling)?" He answered, "You would have to give...sixpence from there and twelve from there."
Ten-shilling note and one-pound note. "You'd have to give two of that (ten shillings). No, you'd have to give two of these (one pound). I think you'd have to have two for ..."; he then laughed and gave up.
Half-penny and penny—"You'd have to have one more. You'd have to get one more like this (half-penny) to get one of those (penny)."
Sixpence and shilling—"Two. One more of those (sixpence) to get one more of those (shilling)." Then he suddenly exclaimed, "One more sixpence to get a shilling."
Sixpence and two-shilling piece—"Three more shillings. No, one, two, three, you'd have to get three more sixpence to make two shillings."
One shilling and ten-shilling note—"Oh yes! ten shillings...No, one, two, three, four... nine shillings. For nine shillings you'd get one more shilling to get ten shillings; you'd have to take nine shillings and a shilling."
Two-shilling piece and one-pound note—"Eighteen shillings."
Sixpence and shilling—"Two of those (sixpence)."
Sixpence and half-a-crown—"Five of those (sixpence)."
Shilling and one-pound note—"Nineteen of those (shilling) to make a pown."
Two-shilling piece and ten-shilling note—"Eight of these (two shillings) to get one of these."
Two-shilling piece and one-pound note—"Eighteen of these to give one of these (one pound)."
Penny and shilling—"Eleven of these (penny)."
Penny and two-shilling piece—"Twenty-three to make one of these (two shillings)."
Half-crown and one-pound note—"One, two, three, four, five, six, seven, eight, nine, ten, eleven, twelve...It'll be about fifteen but I'm not sure—No it won't. I think it will be eight of these (half-crown) to get that (one pound)."

From these experiments it is obvious that at bottom he recognised the relative value of the various coins to one another. But in five only out of the sixteen tests did he give a direct answer, such as two sixpences in a shilling or five in half-a-crown. In eleven instances he stated correctly the additional number of the lower coin required to make up the value of the higher one; in one case, given a penny and a two-shilling piece, he went so far as to say "twenty-three." It was evidently easier for him to work with numbers as part of a series than as abstract symbols.

Pictures and drawing. His appreciation of pictures was remarkably good and he not only noticed the various details but recognised their significance for the general conception.

He made an excellent drawing of a spirit-lamp, placed on the table in front of him; the complex relations of the wick and other parts were admirably indicated. Later on he reproduced this drawing almost exactly from memory.

He had always been fond of drawing and amused himself by making pictures of the animals he had shot in Cashmir; on one occasion when trying to describe the difficulties of transport in the East he drew spontaneously a spirited rough picture of a camel (Fig. 17).

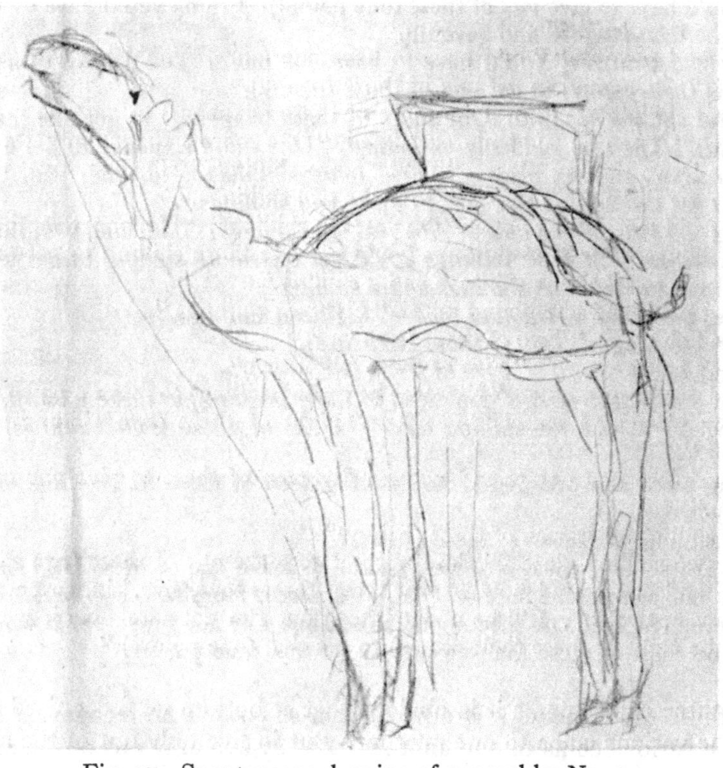

Fig. 17. Spontaneous drawing of a camel by No. 2.

When, however, he was told to draw an elephant he produced an absurd figure without trunk, tusks or ears (Fig. 18). Asked what he had left out he added a tail, two more legs and marks on the forehead evidently intended for horns. He was extremely troubled about the trunk and the tail, saying, "Oh! that certainly comes from there (pointing to the tail and then to the mouth); this I know he generally takes from there (rump) and brings round to there (mouth) to eat with; with that on there he can generally eat." He added two marks on the head, saying, "They are his eyes" but at the same time touched his own ear; "He's got two of them," pulling his own ears, "two big ones."

I then drew the rough outline of an elephant and asked him to point to the various parts as I named them; trunk, tusk, ear, fore-foot, eye, tail and hind-foot were all indicated without hesitation.

Orientation, etc. He had no difficulty in finding his way about the hospital and showed by his actions that he knew the position of his room on the second floor. When, however, we walked together from my house in Montagu Square to the Empire Hospital he made frequent mistakes, even after he had made the journey on foot several times. He would take the wrong turning and look round puzzled; what he saw did not correspond to what he expected and he retraced his steps

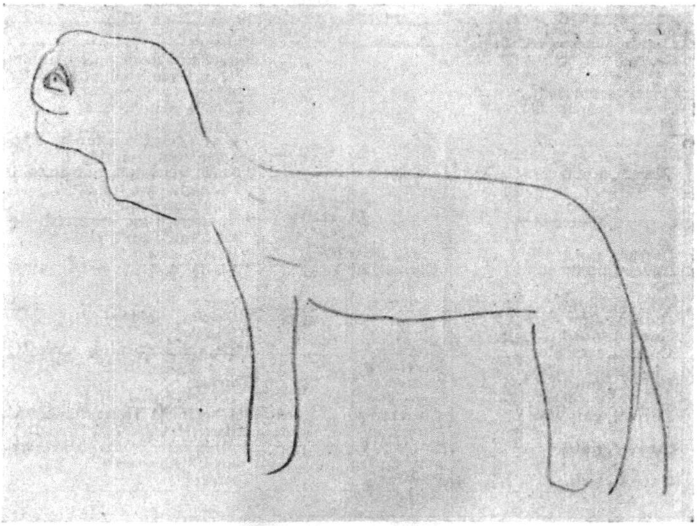

Fig. 18. Attempt by No. 2 to draw an elephant to command.

slowly. At certain salient points he said, "I passed by here with my sister this morning," and proceeded to describe some incident he had seen there correctly. After several mistakes he turned into the street which led to the hospital; he looked up and said, "That's it." I asked, "How do you know?" and he replied, "There you see that?...where the Padre is (pointing to the spire of a church); that's near the hospital." He then walked along rapidly, took the right turning to the hospital, which he recognised at once, and ran up to his room without hesitation.

The persistence of the conception of right and left, in spite of his inability to express the idea in abstract terms, is shown by the following conversation. As we were walking along the street he said, "I've been so long out of the Old Country that I don't know which way cars come. If I was riding in one up the street I should be riding there"; he swung round to face the direction in which a vehicle would move keeping to the left-hand side of the road and tapped the left curb with his stick. Then he added, "But that's not it there," waving his stick to signify a foreign country.

Serial Tests.

(1) *Naming and recognition of common objects.*

Table 2.

	Pointing to object shown	Oral commands	Printed commands	Duplicate placed in hand out of sight	Naming an object indicated	Writing name of object indicated
Knife	Perfect	Correct (whispered "knife")	Correct	Perfect	Correct	Jan
Key	,,	Correct	,,	,,	Pulled keys from pocket, saying, "No, I can't tell you that"	Gave up
Penny	,,	Correct (repeated "penny")	,,	,,	Correct	panin
Matches	,,	Correct (repeated "matches")	,,	,,	"That's match, mat, mats, match"	Machin
Scissors	,,	Correct, hesitated	,,	,,	"That's knap, ker, kur-te...No, I can't tell you that"	Nare
Pencil	,,	Correct, quick	,,	,,	"Pentl, permitch, not quite it. Pě-night; no, I can't"	Knelers
Key	,,	Correct, slow	,,	,,	"That's mer, may"	No, karest
Scissors	,,	Correct, hesitated	,,	,,	"No idea. I know exactly what it is, but I can't tell you"	Gave up
Matches	,,	Correct, quick	,,	,,	"That's match"	No Merest
Knife	,,	Correct, hesitated	Correct, slow	,,	"Nĕ-ife, ker-nife"	Knerreg
Penny	,,	Correct, slow	Correct	,,	Correct	pe, peuner
Matches	,,	Correct, slow	,,	,,	"That's...match"	mar, matare
Scissors	,,	Correct, quick	,,	,,	"That's...no"	Gave up
Pencil	,,	Correct, very slow	Correct, very slow	,,	"It's a p. something...No"	,,
Penny	,,	Correct, quick	Correct, very slow	,,	Correct	penne
Knife	,,	Correct, very slow	Correct, very slow	,,	"Kě-ṅife. I always remember that...It's Canif in French"	Kerrert
Key	,, ,,	Correct, quick	Correct, very slow	,,	Pulled keys from pocket and said, "Mat, latch"	wer, karet
Matches	,,	Correct, quick	Correct, quick	,,	Correct	Marest, maters

Asked to point to the object on the table that I had named, he showed a tendency to repeat the name, although he fully understood that he was to say nothing; in most cases, however, he made his choice silently. But, even if no word was uttered or whispered under his breath, his lips not uncommonly moved soundlessly.

During this test he remarked, "When you say one of them to me, I look along and see it there on the table. If it wasn't here on the table I couldn't tell you. I can't remember what they are unless I think." It was in fact the object in front of him that made him able to appreciate the significance of the name said by me.

In the same way, when the command was given in print, he held the card in his left hand, referring back to it from time to time as his right forefinger swept over the objects on the table; suddenly he pounced on the one which corresponded to the printed name. But if he was asked to point to that shown to him, or if a duplicate was placed in his hand, there was none of this hesitation; his finger indicated the correct object at once without passing backwards and forwards along the set in front of him. Evidently his choice was now made directly without the intervention of words.

During his attempts to write the names of the various test-objects his lips moved although he uttered no sound and he was obviously verbalising silently.

(2) *Naming and recognition of colours.*

Table 3.

	Pointing to colour shown	Oral commands	Printed commands	Naming	Writing name of colour indicated	Printed name read aloud	Printed names copied	
							In cursive handwriting	In printed capitals
Black	Perfect	Pointed to white, saying "black"	White	"Green...red; no, not red. I can only call it dead"	Red	"Red"	Correct	Correct
Red	,,	Correct; whispered "red"	Correct; very slow	"Ber-lu. I know what it is. It's what the Staff ... the same colour I had here. I think it's red"	Bell	"Green. No, its red, blue. No it isn't blue its red"	,,	,,
Blue	,,	Correct; whispered "ber-lu"	Violet	"Ber-lu"	No response	"Green"	,,	,,
Green	,,	Correct; whispered "green"	White	Whispered "Green." Compared it with the blue band on his arm and rejected it. "I don't know this one... Ber-lu"	Green	"Green"	Gerry	,,
Orange	,,	Chose yellow, saying "O-age"; then corrected	Correct	"It's like pil... I think that's red"	Read	"Red"	ORange	,,
White	,,	Chose yellow silently	Yellow	"That's green"	Gernd	"Red, that's red"	Whore	,,
Violet	,,	Correct	Correct	"Ber-lu, ber-loor... It's more like mauve"	Moved	"Blue, green; no mauve"	Vioney	,,
Yellow	,,	"I have no idea. Yellow, I don't know." Finally chose orange	White	"That's red"	Grena	"Red"	Correct	,,
Red	,,	Correct; said "pred"	Correct	"What the Staff is again. I can't remember what it is"	Blead	"Red"	,,	,,
White	,,	Correct; said "white"	Correct	"Green"	Red	"Green"	,,	,,
Yellow	,,	Correct	Violet	"That is... I know what I'm trying to remember... kark-too, tark-loon, kar-ki... that's right"	Run	"Red"	,,	,,
Blue	,,	Correct; said "ber-lu" and chose very slowly	Looked at blue band on his arm and very slowly chose correctly	"Ber-lu"	Movy	"Ber-lu"	Blur	,,
Green	,,	White; said "dreen, green"	Black	"Mauve. It's not quite mauve, but it's rather like, I think"	Gernat	"Red"	Correct	,,
Black	,,	Correct; said "black"	Blue	"That's red"	Mat	"I know it is an ordinary one. Green, no, red, no"	,,	,,
Orange	,,	Yellow; said "orridge"	Correct	"I think it's pink"	Grend	"Mauve"	,,	,,
Violet	,,	Correct; said "violet" and chose very slowly	,,	"Mauve"	Moved	"This one is mauve"	Vinolet	,,

Table 4.

	Reading aloud	Reading from pictures	Writing from pictures	Copying from print
The dog and the cat	"The only thing I can tell you is horse; no, dog was and the cat"	Correct	Correct	THE Dog AND THE Cat
The man and the dog	"It was a dog"	,,	The as the man an the dog	THE Mat AND THE Dog
The cat and the man	"The cat...I know that is the dog" (pointing to CAT)	,,	The cat an the man	The Cat ane THE MAN
The cat and the dog	"The dog and the cat. Yes, the dog and the cat"	,,	Correct	THE Cat and THE Dog
The dog and the man	"The dog...the dog was ...I've no idea"	,,	The dog an the man	The Dog and THE Mat
The man and the cat	"The dog and the cat. It might be anything. I have to think"	,,	The man and the do cat	Thy Mat and THE Cat

Table 5.

	Direct imitation	Oral commands	Printed commands		Telling the time
			Ordinary nomenclature	Railway time	
5 minutes to 2	Perfect	"Five, five, one, two. I think it's that; I'm not sure" Set 1.30	2.5	Correct	"Two; from half past two"
Half-past 1	,,	"Half past. That is half past two" Set 1.30	Correct	,,	"That's half past two"
5 minutes past 8	,,	"No idea"	Finally correct	,,	"Seven and just a little"
20 minutes to 4	,,	Short hand at 4; long hand at 5 min. to the hour	Short hand at 4; long hand at 20 min. past	,,	"Three and twenty; no, not quite four"
10 minutes past 7	,,	7.5	Short hand at 7; long hand at 10 min. to the hour	,,	"Six and seven"
20 minutes to 6	,,	4.55	8.20	,,	"Nearly six; that's the nearest I can get"
10 minutes to 1	,,	Short hand at 1; long hand at 5 min. to the hour	1.15	,,	"Nearly one; not quite. I know it but I can't tell you"
A quarter to 9	,,	"I've no idea"	Hour hand at 8; long hand at half past	,,	"Eight, nine, half for nine"
20 minutes past 11	,,	Short hand at 10; long hand at half past	10.20	,,	Pointed to the half hour saying, "In getting from here it will be half twelve"
25 minutes to 3	,,	"I'm not sure about this" Set 1.5	3.35	,,	"Two and a half and just a little more"

Table 4 (*continued*).

Reading what he had written	Repetition	Choosing the card corresponding to the words said by the observer	Writing to dictation
"The dog and the horse... the dog and the cat"	"Dog and the...the dog and the cat"	Chose: The cat and the man	The dog and it cat
"The dog...that's the dog" (pointing to dog)	Correct	Correct	The dog and the man
"Cat...the cat was...and the dog"	"Cat and the dog"	Chose: The cat and the dog	Correct
"Oh! the cat and the dog"	Correct	Chose: The man and the cat	The dog and the cat
"The dog was...I think this is was...was with the cat"	,,	Correct	Correct
"It was...and the cat"	"The man and the dog"	Chose: The man and the dog	The dog and the cat

Table 5 (*continued*).

Choosing a printed card corresponding to the time shown		Copying from print	Writing down the time	Telling the time aloud and writing it down afterwards	
Railway time	Ordinary nomenclature			He said	He wrote
Correct and quick	Correct	Correct	2.5	"Half past two"	[2 and then 51] 51.2
,,	,,	,,	[1 and then 6 to left] 6.1	"Half past two"	[1 and then 5] 1.5
,,	,,	,,	[6 and then 5 to left] 5.6	"Fourteen, only I don't know what it is"	[6 and then 5] 6.5
,,	Correct; but doubtful if he was right	,,	3. Said "I don't know whether to put it here (L.) or there (R.)" finally 3.40	"Three and a half, thirty, whatever it is"	[3 and then 8] 8.3
,,	,,	,,	7.2	"Half past six; but not quite right. It's as near as I can get"	[7 and then 2] 7.2
,,	Correct; very slow	,,	[6 and then 6 to left] 6.6	"Five and a half"	[5 and then 8] 8.5
,,	Correct; hesitated	,,	[1 and then 10 to left] 10.1	"One; not quite one"	[1 and then 10] 10.1
,,	Correct; very slow	,,	[9 and then 51 to left] 51.9	"Nine; half past nine"	[First R. then L.] 9.9
,,	,,	,,	"It's not so much," pointing to quarter 11.4	"That's eleven; past eleven"	[First L. then R.] 11.11
,,	Correct; slow, uncertain	,,	[3 and then 7 to left] 7.3	"Two and a half past. Two and a half"	[3 and then 7] 7.3

At first sight it might seem from the observations that he was colour blind; but this is excluded by the rapidity and correctness with which he matched colours in the first series of tests. The defect was one of names and their significance and his gross errors were due to want of nominal recognition.

Both oral and printed commands were followed by the same kind of mistaken answers.

During his attempt to name the colours shown to him he began to use descriptive expressions, when at a loss for the word; for instance, he could not remember red and said, "It's what the Staff...the same colour I had here," pointing to the lapel of his tunic. I therefore laid before him the printed cards one by one, asking him to tell me, "What sort of thing is this?" His answers were as follows:

Black—"That is the dead."
Red—Holding the lapel of his tunic, "Where the Staff have it."
Blue—"This is this," pointing to the blue band on his arm.
Green—"That is up there," pointing to the trees.
White—Took hold of my white coat.
Yellow—"This one," holding his khaki tie. (Notice that this is the key to his use of the word "karktoo" when naming yellow.)
Black—"Oh! yes, that is the dead."
Red—"That's the Staff."
Blue—"That one is this," pointing to his left arm.
Green—"This is up there," pointing to the trees.
White—He caught hold of my coat.
Yellow—"Yes I know this is...," picked up his tie.

In many of these tests, as for instance when he seized hold of my white coat, he was in reality not naming but matching two coloured objects. I therefore carried out the experiment in another way in order to test the nominal value of these descriptive expressions. The colours were laid out on the table as usual, omitting orange for which he could find no comparison. He had agreed that the lamp-shade was violet and, in order to avoid as far as possible direct matching, I had removed it from the room and taken off my white coat and his khaki tie. I had also turned his back to the window so that he could not see the trees. I then said, "The dead," and he chose black; "What the Staff wear," red; "What is on your arm," blue; "What is out there," green; "What I wear," white; "Like the lampshade," he answered, "I know it was mauve," and chose violet; "Your tie," he hesitated and then chose yellow. This series of tests was repeated and his answers were uniformly correct. Thus, although he hesitated greatly when I said the name of the colour, he chose rapidly and with certainty when the command was given in a descriptive phrase or similitude.

(3) *The man, cat and dog tests.*

When he was shown the printed cards, he tried to spell out the words letter by letter and failed entirely. With "The dog and the cat" he began, "I know that's T the first one; H E. This is D O." Then tracing a G, with his finger on the table he said, "I know that's dog." He continued, "This one is A; this is N; this one is D; the next one is T H, the other E; next is C A T cat." These attempts seemed to convey little or nothing of the general contents of the sentence for he concluded, "The only thing I can tell you is horse; no dog was and the cat."

In many cases he succeeded in spelling out the whole correctly but could not say what was on the card. Thus with the third example he spelt "T H and E. The next is C A T; A N D. The next is T H E. M and A and N." He summed up, however, "The cat...I know that is the dog (pointing to cat). No, I cannot tell you any more." In the last of the series he was equally correct with the letters but said, "The dog and the cat. It might be anything. I have to think."

During his attempts at repetition he volunteered the following information. "If you say dog to me, I can see the dog; but if you say the dog and the cat I think of the dog and can't think of anything else." This inability to hold the two leading names in his memory for a sufficient time to reproduce them was evidently responsible for his errors in repetition, writing to dictation and choosing a card corresponding to the sentence said by me. On the other hand, the context was correct, when he read aloud, wrote from pictures or copied a printed card, because the objects were continuously in front of him; the writing was faulty but he never confused the man, the cat or the dog.

(4) *The clock tests.*

Whenever he was in doubt or difficulty with these tests, his errors tended to assume three forms. He mistook "to" the hour for "past" and vice versa, he confused the significance of the two hands or he set the short hand exactly opposite the hour mentioned in the command. But if the task was one which he could carry out with ease (column 1 and 4 Railway time of Table 5) none of these mistakes appeared, even in the preliminary movements; the hour hand was set at some point between two figures on the clock face corresponding roughly to the number of minutes past or to the hour.

If the test was an easy one, his answers were extraordinarily certain and definite. For instance, when he was choosing from among the cards printed in numbers the one which corresponded to the clock set by me, I inadvertently placed the hands at 6.20; he shook his head to signify that it was not on the table; but as soon as I made the correction to 5.40 he picked out the right card.

Whenever he attempted to write down the time, he first wrote the hour and then tended to place the number of minutes past the hour on the right and to the hour on the left. Thus ten minutes to one became "10.1," twenty minutes past eleven "11.4" (for the long hand placed at twenty minutes past pointed to 4). In the same way, twenty-five minutes to three was "7.3," for the hour mentioned in the command was "3" and 7 corresponded to twenty-five minutes to.

These tests show particularly well the want of recognition of the significance of such symbols as the numbers on the face of the clock and the long and short hands.

(5) *The coin-bowl tests.*

He failed completely to execute this test either to oral or printed commands and did not recognise that the number of the coin was not identical with that of the bowl into which it was to be placed. The words in quotation marks were said by him under his breath.

(6) *The hand, eye and ear tests.*

During the explanation which preceded these tests he said, "I can't remember which is my right hand; but I know if I were going to fight I'd go like this," throwing himself into a correct boxing attitude with the left hand leading. Then he exclaimed, "Now I know, this is the right, this is the one with which I used to do this," making the movements of writing.

Condition between October 1918 and October 1920.

From September, 1918, when he first came under my care, he steadily improved. He lived in the country, played golf, went for occasional walking tours and spent most of his life in the open air. At the same time his sister, who was a trained Froebel teacher, dedicated herself entirely to his welfare; she adapted her knowledge to the task of re-educating him and under her care he progressed greatly in speaking, reading and writing. But from beginning to end his difficulties and disabilities remained the same in kind as those already described.

I shall, therefore, summarise shortly the observations of the first two years and then pass on to detail more fully those made in October 1920, two years and six months after the injury.

He was throughout in perfect physical health and suffered from no headache or other abnormal symptom except the hemianopsia. But we came to the conclusion that so large an opening in the skull produced a deleterious mental effect, and on October 17th, 1919, Mr Wilfrid Trotter closed it with three bone grafts from the shin. This operation was a brilliant success; the wound healed by the first intention and no one could now tell that the skull had ever been opened. The moral result was equally satisfactory; he ceased to be conscious of changes in posture and no longer wondered whether this or that physical act would affect his head.

Articulated speech. His power of voluntary expression steadily improved and by September, 1919, he was able to name common objects and colours correctly, though with considerable hesitation. If in want of a name, he would make repeated attempts to capture the right sound, frequently with success; articulation was not otherwise affected.

He showed a tendency to employ ready-made phrases and slang which came more readily to him than orthodox expressions, although this was not his habit

Table 6.

	Oral commands	Printed commands [Not read aloud]
1st into 3rd	1st into 1st; 2nd into 2nd; 3rd into 3rd	3rd into 3rd
2nd into 1st	"Second penny"; 1st into 1st	1st into 1st
4th into 1st	4th into 4th	1st into 1st
3rd into 2nd	3rd into 3rd	3rd into 3rd
2nd into 3rd	"Second"; hesitated; then 1st into 1st	"Two, three" 3rd into 3rd
4th into 3rd	4th into 4th	"Three, three, four" 3rd into 3rd
1st into 2nd	3rd into 3rd	2nd into 2nd
2nd into 4th	"Second...one, two..." 2nd into 2nd	2nd into 2nd
3rd into 1st	3rd into 3rd	"Three, three" 1st into 1st
4th into 2nd	4th into 4th	"Two" 2nd into 2nd
1st into 4th	1st into 1st	4th into 4th
3rd into 4th	3rd into 3rd	3rd into 3rd

Table 7.

	Imitation of movements made by the the observer	Imitation of movements reflected in a mirror	Pictorial commands	Pictorial commands reflected in a mirror	Oral commands	Printed commands
L. hand to R. ear	R. hand to R. ear	L. hand to L. ear	L. hand to L. ear	Correct	"I can't remember; left something"	"No idea"
R. hand to L. eye	L. hand to L. eye	Correct	R. hand to R. eye	R. hand to R. eye	L. hand to L. eye	"That's your eye; can't"
R. hand to L. ear	R. hand to R. ear	Correct; slow	R. hand to R. ear	R. hand to R. ear	L. hand to L. ear	"I see eye again," pointing to ear
L. hand to L. eye	L. hand to R. eye	Correct; slow	R. hand; then correct	Correct	R. hand to R. *ear*	"No, I see eye again"
R. hand to R. ear	Correct	,,	Correct; slow	,,	R. hand to R. *eye*	"No, I can't do it"
L. hand to R. eye	L. hand to L. eye	Correct; slow	L. hand to L. eye	,,	L. hand to L. eye	"No"
L. hand to L. ear	Correct; slow	Correct	Correct	,,	L. hand to L. *eye*; corrected	"Ear, I think that's ear, but I can't be sure"
R. hand to R. eye	Correct	,,	,,	,,	Correct	"That will be eye"
L. hand to R. ear	L. hand to L. ear	,,	L. hand to L. ear	L. hand to L. ear	L. hand to L. ear	"Is that face?" pointing to ear
R. hand to L. eye	R. hand to R. eye	,,	R. hand to R. eye	R. hand to R. eye	R. hand to R. *ear*	"Eye, eye"
R. hand to L. ear	R. hand to R. ear	,,	R. hand to R. ear	L. hand to L. ear	L. hand to L. ear	"R...E A R... E A T...No"
L. hand to L. eye	Reversed	,,	Reversed	Correct	R. hand to R. *ear*	"E W E...Eye, yes"
R. hand to R. ear	Correct	,,	Correct	Reversed	L. hand; the R. to R. *eye*	"E A O..." pointing to his ear
L. hand to R. eye	L. hand to L. eye	,,	L. hand to L. eye	R. hand to R. eye	L. hand to L. *ear*	"Eye, eye"
L. hand to L. ear	Reversed	,,	R. hand; then correct	Reversed	L. hand to R. *eye*	"E A R... A E A R...eye"
R. hand to R. eye	Correct	,,	Correct	,,	R. hand to R. *ear*; then eye, then *ear*, uncertain	"Eye...that's eye and that is T O...to"

before he was injured. He would say, "I made a priceless blob" (a mistake in tact); "The question of going to St Ives is a good egg" (a good idea). He was particularly fond of "putting heavy guns on to it," whenever he intended to imply that much effort had been used.

The following conversation forms a good example of his difficulties in expression. He was trying to explain to me how he would walk from the Empire Hospital, Westminster, to the War Office in Whitehall and said, "I have no streets in London; no names at all. Suppose I was going from the Army and Navy, that's what it is called, just round here (the Army and Navy Stores), I should then say some place to a hospital about a quarter of a mile away. I remember the hospital is on the left on the way to the War Office, about half way. I believe it's the Abbey. No, it's near the Abbey on the way to the War Office." Later he added, "I saw the hospital." I put the question, "The Abbey?" and he replied as follows: "It's here, but then it's gone again and I have to feel for it again. The only thing I can remember of it is the opening, the big opening, where everybody goes in. I can get that" (moving his hand in the form of a large arch). Since it was obvious that he had described Westminster Hospital and Westminster Abbey, I asked, "Have the hospital and Abbey anything to do with one another?" He answered, "Nothing except my focus, the place of them; the distance, that is all. I should say how far the hospital is to the Abbey in re-, in re-, that's where I go wrong. I want to say in re- something (relation). There are just little bits in expressing what I want to say; little bits in which I have to turn my brain another way to get what I want to say, whereas a year or two ago I should have said it without thinking. You see, it's like this; with me it's all in bits. I have to jump like this," marking a thick line between two points with his pencil, "like a man who jumps from one thing to the next. I can see them but I can't express. Really it is that I haven't enough names. I've got practically no names. The easiest thing is what I do now. I say what I can, it's all wrong; but they get an idea of what I want to say." (Oct. 1919.)

It is evident from this conversation that he was able to recall visual images of objects on his way to the War Office in Whitehall. First of all, he saw the Army and Navy Stores and then Westminster Hospital on his left with the great door of Westminster Abbey on the right; but want of names prevented him from connecting the two, except in position and he was forced to jump from one image to another without the cohesive links of verbal formulation.

Understanding of spoken words. He still had difficulty in grasping the exact meaning of "to" and "past," "high" and "low," "up" and "down," "back" and "front," when contrasted with one another. Asked, "Would you like to stop in or go out?" he would reply, "Either," in order to hide his want of exact comprehension. But, if the question was put directly, "Do you want to stop in?" he would answer, "No"; "Do you want to go out?" "Yes," showing that he had definitely made up his mind to one course of action, but was puzzled by the two alternatives in the same sentence.

He liked to have everything that was said to him illustrated as much as possible in a drawing or diagram. Thus, when his sister was teaching him music, she told him that the scale consisted of three tones, a half tone, two tones and another half tone. This puzzled him completely; she played the scale and he still failed to grasp it. But as soon as she drew the following diagram, where each horizontal line

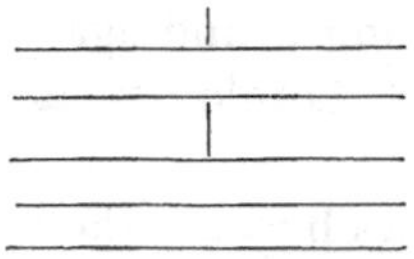

represented a tone and each short vertical one a half tone, he understood and from that time (Dec. 15, 1918) never forgot it.

He was accustomed to say, "I understand pretty well now what anybody says, unless it's anything that's rather...that's what I can't say...rather tricky, rather heavier...I can't quite get what I want to say. Everything I say is very little, like a child; I can't express what I want to say."

One day, after having tea with us, he made the following comment on a fellow guest, "I like that young man; he's clever. I notice that clever people say everything in a few words so that I can understand. Stupid people take a lot of words and I can't remember what they have said; it confuses me."

Writing. By repeated practice and with the help of his sister's instruction he recovered to a considerable extent his power of writing spontaneously. But he was extremely slow and inaccurate; he was accustomed when composing a letter to put it aside for correction and then to re-copy it. The following is part of a long letter he wrote to me in November, 1919. "About 8 days ago a young Navy officer here, one of your {patrons / pashents} came to see me and told me about his escape from death. It was soon after the 'abrooge' fight, he said I think that he was incharge of a small motor boat near the Dutch couest. Four Hun aeroplan's sighted the craft and quickly smached it into Tinder by mashen gun fire. All three were wounded. Life saving apparaters luckily being obtained on the nick of time. The motor boat was on fire too, to say nothing of themselves being on fire. All so they had a number of pounds of T. and T., in the boat which might go off at any minute. What accueley happened it blow up a hundred yards after they had swam away from it. The rest can be told in a minuete—how a small Duch smak found them. And that is how the officer in question became a spin case, three or four times badely wounded and paraliesed."[1]

[1] This was intended to convey the following story: "About eight days ago a young naval officer here, one of your patients, came to see me and told me about his escape from death. It was soon after the 'Abrooge' fight. He said I think that he was in charge of a small motor boat near the Dutch coast. Four Hun aeroplanes sighted the craft and quickly smashed it to tinder by machine-gun fire. All three were wounded, life-saving apparatus luckily being obtained in the nick of time. The motor boat was on fire too, to say nothing of themselves being on fire. Also they had a number of pounds of T.N.T. (trinitrotoluol) in the boat, which might go off any minute. What actually happened was that it blew up after they had swum a hundred yards away from it. The rest can be told in a minute—how a small Dutch smack found them. And that is how the officer in question became a spine case, badly wounded three or four times and paralysed."

A printed paragraph read silently or aloud, written spontaneously or to dictation, and copied. The nature of his disabilities came out particularly clearly when, after reading a series of printed sentences, he was asked to reproduce their meaning in different ways.

(1) For instance, in October 1919, he was given the following extract from an advertisement:

"Partridge Shooting. Birds are fairly plentiful this year thanks to a warm late May and June. It is a pleasure to see the 'old hands' gathering round again and, as before the war, the cars bringing the guns were fitted with Dunlop tyres, so the cars of to-day are similarly equipped."

After he had occupied ten minutes in poring over these sentences he was asked, "What have you read?" He answered, "It takes me an awful long time. In the early summer there are lots of young partridges...I think it is...That's as far as I've got."

He then read aloud slowly and syllabically, "Partridge Shooting. Birds are fairly plentiful this year thanks to a warm late May and June...June. It is a... pleasure to see the old hands gathering round again and as before the war the cars bringing the guns were fitted with Dunlop tyres, so the cars of to-day are simul... simerly...simuly...ecuped...whatever that means...yes, equipped."

I demanded, "What is it all about?" He replied, "It has been a good warm May and June, from which the young pheasants are...are...I should say in thousands. The rest is about Dunlop tyres. I don't quite see the joke...quite what it is about. I suppose because people...No, I don't see why they should have Dunlops at all."

I then dictated the passage to him and he wrote: "Partritgh Shouting. Beards are vearly plentiful this year thanks to the worm late May and June. It is a pleshore to see the old gathering round again, and as before the War the cars bringing the cars were fittedy by Dunlop tyres so the cars of the day are similley exclipted."

I then asked him to write a short account of what he had just written to dictation and he produced the following: "As the May and...There are a lot of young Phesionts this year at June and May and as there are many Dunlop cars running out for shooting." He then ceased to write and exclaimed, "As a matter of fact this is quite wrong because it is not the time you shoot partridges."

He copied the printed matter slowly but accurately in cursive handwriting, correcting any errors he may have made.

I then said, "Can you tell me what you have just copied?" and he replied, "That's the...because there's been a good warm summer, for instance, there will be a lot of partridge shooting and there will be a lot of...a lot of...I suppose wanted for Dunlop tyres for the shooting, to take the shooters...to...get their shooting."

(2) Another excellent example appeared when he was asked to read to himself the following account of a famous prize fight a few days after its occurrence (Dec. 8, 1919):

"Carpentier, the French champion met Beckett, heavy weight champion of England, on Thursday, Dec. 4th, at the Holborn Stadium. Becket was knocked out in 74 seconds by a right-hand hook to the jaw."

At the end of six minutes he returned the paper and started to tell me what he had read in the following words. "Carpentier met Beckett in the Holborn...say ...so...Sadium, I used to know it, and Carpentier being the Champion now... who is...oh no...who met Beckett...now the champion of England...knocked ...er...knocked...er...Beckett out in 74 seconds...with a right...with a right hook to the jaw." He then added, "I wasn't thinking so much of the fight...but what I had been reading...I saw the picture of 74...seconds...saw what I had read."

I then said, "Can you see the fight?" and an extraordinary change came over his narration. "Now I think about the fight I see the picture of Carpentier. I see Beckett falling...I see the ref...ref...what you call it...referee...The last thing I can picture is Carpentier standing like this with both hands like this." He sprang from his bed and assumed an attitude, with both hands on his hips looking down towards the ground, in the position assumed by Carpentier in the photographs of the termination of the fight. The change in manner from the puzzled aspect of a man slowly recalling what he had read to the brisk, vivid, smiling person describing what he saw was remarkable.

I then gave him the paper and asked him to read it through again and to write me an account of what he understood. He wrote as follows: "Carpanter the Hevey Chanpion of (Phrance) France met Beckett the English Hevey waite at the Holbon (Sadeon) Stadion on Thursesday the 4th Dec. after 74 minutes fight, (with) Carpomter (nockered) knocked out Beckett with a right hand nunch in the (gor) jaw." The words in brackets are those he wrote and then erased.

To dictation he wrote: "Carpanter the French champshain met Beckett hevey champion of England on Theresday 4th Dec. at the Holborn Stadion. Beckett was knocked out in 74 seconds (wil) by a right Hand Hook to the (Jo) Jaw."

He could, however, copy the printed matter in cursive handwriting accurately but slowly.

Numbers. From the first he could say the numbers in order and write them in figures although he had difficulty in using them as direct symbols. Told to pick out five objects he did so by counting them in the usual way; but asked to add five to any written numeral, he made five dots on the paper and then counted them up starting from the given number. This he did with all numbers up to ten; above this a number such as eighteen had no meaning for him unless he had reached it by counting.

This corresponds with another experience which throws light on the nature of his disability. Suppose he were told that something had happened on Thursday, March the 12th, it conveyed nothing to him until he had repeated to himself Monday, Tuesday, Wednesday, Thursday, and then January, February, March, finally counting up to twelve. Telling him the day or the month did not convey to him at once the part of the week or of the year in which it fell.

A set of observations made with the *coin-bowl tests* on September 25th, 1919, is worthy of reproduction because of the light it throws on his method of executing commands given either orally or in print. The results are given in Table 8.

Table 8.

	Oral commands	Printed commands: In figures only (e.g. 1st into 3rd)	In a complete phrase (e.g. First penny into third bowl)	In verbal numbers (e.g. First into third)
1st into 3rd	Very slow. Repeated command aloud. Then correct	Correct and extremely rapid	Finally correct (45 sec.)	Correct (6 sec.)
2nd into 1st	Very slow, correct	,,	,, (60 sec.)	,, (5 sec.)
4th into 1st	1st; then 4th into 1st bowl; correct	,,	,, (50 sec.)	,, (10 sec.)
3rd into 2nd	Hesitated. Then correct	,,	1st into 2nd (80 sec.)	1st into 2nd; corrected (25 sec.)
2nd into 3rd	Correct	,,	Finally correct (55 sec.)	Correct (5 sec.)
4th into 3rd	Correct; slowly	,,	3rd into 3rd; corrected (70 sec.)	,, (8 sec.)
1st into 2nd	Correct	,,	Correct (5 sec.)	,, (3 sec.)
2nd into 4th	,,	,,	,, (5 sec.)	,, (15 sec.)
3rd into 1st	,,	,,	,, (12 sec.)	,, (7 sec.)
4th into 2nd	4th into 3rd	,,	,, (7 sec.)	,, (5 sec.)
1st into 4th	Correct, quick	,,	,, (25 sec.)	,, (4 sec.)
3rd into 4th	Correct, very slowly	,,	,, (30 sec.)	,, (3 sec.)

Throughout his attempts to carry out oral commands he made movements of his lips without uttering a sound; he was evidently repeating the order to himself silently. He explained, "It is an extraordinary thing. With some of them I do it without thinking; then if I think too much and say to myself 'third into fourth' I don't know what it means. Now if I say 'the first into the fourth,' I pick up this (the first coin) and then I have to think what is 'fourth.' If I do it myself I can do it as quickly as you like; but you tell me to do it and I have to think what it means even if I say it to myself. I think the whole thing is it gives me one more...what do you call it?...if you do two or three things together...what do you call that?... factus, factor...do you call it factor when I can get two or three things together? It's a word I often use."

"I know exactly what it is. It's this; the name...what do you call this?...a tumbler, a glass (in reality a brass bowl)...I don't want to call it anything. I want to say 'the first to the fourth.' I don't want to say what that is (pointing to bowl) or what that is (pointing to coin). I want to do the first to the fourth, or whatever it is, without saying it."

When it came to carrying out printed commands, I gave him first of all cards on which the form of the order was "1st into 3rd," etc. This he carried out with great rapidity and certainty; the action of placing the coin in the bowl was completed in every case within five seconds. Next he was given cards on which the command was printed in full, e.g. "First penny into third bowl," etc. His actions became slower and less certain and he complained, "I see where the trouble is. I can't get its name. You see the first is like writing in numbers; with the other I have to read it. For the moment I didn't know that was a penny. Then I got that, but I don't know what that means" (pointing to FIRST BOWL on the card) "F I R S T, that's first. I don't know what the other means, B O W L, oh! yes, bowl." I then printed a series of orders omitting the words penny and bowl; for example, "First into third," etc. His responses again became much quicker. Omission of the two names, which had little effect in determining the actual nature of the choice, reduced the average time of the act from 40 secs. to 8 secs.

Thus the form assumed by the verbal task has a greater effect on the ease and correctness of the response than the character of the action performed by the patient.

This was particularly evident from the records of certain *Clock tests* carried out in October, 1919. (Table 9.)

Table 9.

	(A) In full (e.g. five minutes to two)	(B) Railway time in letters (e.g. one fifty-five)	(C) Railway time in figures (e.g. 1.55)
5 minutes to 2	Correct (10 sec.)	Correct (35 sec.)	Correct (5 sec.)
Half-past 1	,, (6 sec.)	,, (28 sec.)	,, (2 sec.)
5 minutes past 8	,, (18 sec.)	,, (30 sec.)	,, (2 sec.)
20 minutes to 4	,, (5 sec.)	,, (30 sec.)	,, (4 sec.)
10 minutes past 7	Set 7.5 (12 sec.)	,, (12 sec.)	,, (3 sec.)
20 minutes to 6	Correct (25 sec.)	,, (12 sec.)	,, (4 sec.)
10 minutes to 1	,, (15 sec.)	,, (50 sec.)	,, (2 sec.)
A quarter to 9	Set 9.15 (12 sec.)	Set 8.35 (32 sec.)	,, (12 sec.)
20 minutes past 11	Set 11.40 (20 sec.)	Set 10.40 (16 sec.)	,, (6 sec.)
25 minutes to 3	Correct (33 sec.)	Correct (50 sec.)	,, (5 sec.)

First I gave him a series of commands set out fully in words and he executed them somewhat slowly with three mistakes; throughout his lips moved but he uttered no sound. I knew from previous experience that he could set the clock quickly and accurately if the order was given in figures or what might be called "railway time," e.g. 1.55. I therefore varied the procedure as follows: using the same nomenclature the words were printed in letters instead of figures, e.g. "One forty-five." This puzzled him profoundly; his lips moved and he wrote in the air with his finger, as if he were trying to trace the equivalent numbers. Then I handed him a series of cards on which the time was expressed in figures and his answers were rapid and correct; moreover he did not move his lips or make any movements with his hand. The average times required for each act according to the mode of command were as follows: railway time in figures, 4·5 sec.; ordinary nomenclature in words, 15·6 sec.; railway time expressed verbally, 29·5 sec.

CONDITION IN OCTOBER 1920 (*two years and eight months after the injury*).

He was in superb physical health, bright, gay and happy. His powers of speaking, reading and writing had greatly improved. He was more conscious of his errors and tried hard to correct them, frequently with success; at the same time this led to greater fatigue. If he had been acquiring a foreign language, I should have said that he knew more and was therefore more concerned to rectify his mistakes. This was exactly what happened when playing golf; he used to play three rounds poorly without fatigue. Now, he would be tired at the end of one round because as he said, "I do too much thinking," but at the same time his game had greatly improved.

Articulated speech. Asked to name common objects or colours placed before him, he stumbled and hesitated, but was ultimately successful and could tell the time without mistakes.

His greatest difficulty was in finding the exact word to express the meaning he was anxious to convey. He complained, "It's the names that trouble me. When I'm writing a letter, I worry a long time to remember what the expression is... 'euphonic'...properly spelt. I can often get it so close that a lot of people can understand what it is...I mean spelt properly...I should have called it 'topography,' if you had asked me." Here "euphonic" and "topography" were wrongly employed, evidently in place of phonetic and calligraphy. This was characteristic of his defects of speech; it was not words that were lacking, but words appropriate to the particular situation. As he said, "There is a little kink in the brain so that I can't focus it; the fact of thinking too much, I can't say what I want to say."

He could repeat anything said to him faithfully, provided he was not required to remember more than three or four words at a time, and his enunciation was perfect.

Reading. He still had extreme difficulty in appreciating the complete meaning of what he read to himself (vide infra, p. 39) and he read aloud inaccurately and with considerable effort. An attempt to "spell out" the words not infrequently confused him more than if he tried to decipher each one as a whole.

Writing. He wrote with much effort and many corrections. The letters were well formed, but the spelling was deplorable. Having slowly written down what he wanted to say, he read it through, made certain corrections and then copied the whole again; but even this final version was full of mistakes.

His writing was almost equally defective to dictation and he complained that he was puzzled by the names and spelling of the words.

He could, however, copy accurately from print and his handwriting under these conditions improved greatly in character.

A printed paragraph. He was handed the following account of a prize fight in print: "Carpentier, the French champion, met Beckett, heavy weight champion of England, on Thursday, December 4th, 1919, at the Holborn Stadium. Beckett was knocked out in 74 seconds by a right-hand hook to the jaw."

This he read to himself making movements of the lips and tongue, but uttering no sound. At the end of ten minutes he said, "Yes, I think I've got it. Carpentier... the French champion...met...the English champion, Carpentier, Beckett...at the Holborn...Stadium...After...oh! it was...on the twenty...no, fourth of December 1919. Er...Carpentier knocked er...Beckett...out in seven, in seventy-four seconds by a right hand hood...I think it was a hook...to the jaw."

He added, "I can see thousands of people all round. Then I see Beckett... knocked clean out and Carpentier standing at ease. He was just standing like this (placing his hands on his hips and looking down). Beckett is 'pura,' that's a Hindustani name for knocked out...'be-hosh' without any sense, no life or sense in him. I can see that."[1]

After reading the printed sentences again silently he wrote, "Carpation the french Champain met Bekett the English Champion heavy weight on Desember 4th. 1919. Carpantier nocked out Becket in 74 secionds with a right hand hook to the jaw."

To my dictation he wrote the same passage as follows: "Carpantia the frinch champian met Beckett heavey weight champian of England on Threrstay Desember 4th. 1919 at the Hoberian Staidian. Becket was nocked out in 74 secends by a right hand hook to the jaw."

He copied the whole accurately though somewhat slowly from print; there were no errors in spelling and his handwriting improved greatly.

When he repeated the words after me, intonation was perfect; but he could not hold more than three or four words in his head at the same time and frequently asked me to say the phrases over again.

Numbers and arithmetic. His power of using numbers had greatly improved, but he still tended to count up on his fingers or by means of dots rather than to use the figures as a direct symbol.

Asked to write the various numbers in sequence he formed all those above ten by writing 2, 3, 4, etc., and placing a 1 in front of them.

He still added and subtracted slowly and incorrectly, saying, "I really don't know whether any of them are right"; but he never mistook one arithmetical process for the other.

When he had finished he said, "I don't understand the words, the names yet. Addition, that is taking away—no, that is making it more. These (pointing to the

[1] Both the Hindustani words were used correctly.

subtraction sums) are making it smaller. It's just those names which worry me a lot. I understand if someone gives me some money, or if I have to spend some more; it's just the names of them that worry me."

He was able to fill up a cheque spontaneously, but could not be certain that the written words and the figures corresponded with one another. On the occasion (Dec. 17th, 1919) when he drew a cheque in my presence for "Eighty-five pounds, ten shillings and sixpence" he filled in the figures "£80. 10*s.* 6*d.*"; he noticed this discrepancy and succeeded finally in making the correction.

Drawing. Asked to draw an elephant, he produced a poor outline of its body to which he slowly added the salient features of the animal after much hesitation. The ear was called "the eye," he was uncertain about the position of what he called the "tufks" (tusks) and for the trunk he employed the Hindustani name "sung,"[1] adding "that's not exactly, but a fellow who knew would understand." He could not find a name for the tail, which he placed correctly, saying, "I don't know; I've no idea in any language."

Orientation and plan drawing. From the time when he first came under my care there was no doubt that he recognised the spacial relation to one another of the various pieces of furniture in some familiar room. If I drew a four-sided figure on paper to represent its ground-plan, he could point to the position of the tables, chairs, cupboards, windows, etc., correctly. But as soon as he was asked to draw a ground-plan of the room he failed entirely; he drew a number of objects in elevation, the table, the desk, the mirror on the wall and the electric light pendant from the ceiling. He was, however, unable to transpose these visual images onto a plan.

On one occasion (Oct. 11, 1919) he said, "I can see the outside of your house. I could make a picture of that." He drew four vertical lines, saying, "First, second, third," evidently intended to represent the first three houses of our Square. He then started to block out my house, saying, "No. 4," added the roof and chimneys and drew the number of floors correctly. Pointing to the first storey he said, "I know that floor, it's a very big room (drawing-room). This one (dining-room on the ground floor) is different." Here he became confused and could not draw correctly the relation of the front door to the ground-floor window.

He had exactly the same difficulty in showing me how he came from the Marble Arch Station to my house, a distance of five minutes' walk, although he could find his way without fail.

When he was asked to point to an object corresponding to one he had just seen or held in his hand out of sight, he did so with great rapidity and certainty; during these tests, I noticed that he did not pass his hand along the series on the table in front of him, but pointed straight to the object he wanted. So certain was he of its position, that I repeated the experiment without removing the screen. He still indicated the place of the thing he was seeking, in spite of the fact that

[1] Sund.

it was covered from his sight; and yet he was unable to express correctly in words the serial order in which the objects lay, though he could name them correctly. He said, "If you hold it up I see it at once. The fact of thinking too much...I can't say what I want to say."

Evidently, when the act was one of those he could perform easily, he not only selected the true duplicate of what he had seen or felt, but knew its position in space. If, however, he was compelled to formulate its relation to the other objects of the series, he was unable to do so.

Music, etc. When he first entered the hospital he could not whistle a note; "I did not seem to know where to get the tune from." One day in October, 1918, he started on his own initiative to whistle, "The little grey Home in the West," but invariably became lost after a bar or two. In December, 1918, when on a walking tour, he passed a mill and asked his sister what it was. On her replying that it was a mill he began to whistle, "She was a miller's daughter," and continued in perfect tune to the end.

During the winter of 1918–19, he would stand beside his sister when she was playing the piano and could sing several songs through without words.

Games, etc. From the first he was able to play chess well, and in 1919 taught his sister the game. He was extremely clever at draughts, "fox and geese" and all games that did not necessitate the comprehension or expression of names. Once he had found the solution to a puzzle he never forgot it and could solve the problem time after time.

He was quite unable to play any card game until Feb. 1920; he then re-learnt Bridge and could play well without saying the names of the cards, although he could not score.

Golf he found very helpful; for, from the first, he had no difficulty in hitting the ball and he found keeping his own score "very educative." Except that he was blind over the right half of the visual field, he shot as well as ever; a partridge got up to the right out of sight, he heard someone call, swung round and brought it down easily.

Serial Tests.

(1) *Naming and recognition of common objects.*

He was able to indicate quickly and with certainty from amongst the objects on the table the one which corresponded to that shown him or placed in his hand out of sight.

Asked to name them one after the other, he stumbled and hesitated but was ultimately successful in every instance. In the same way the words he wrote obviously corresponded to the objects he was trying to name, although they were badly spelt.

When the command was given orally, his hand hovered in the air whilst he thought and then pounced on the object named by me; he did not go straight for it as when he had to find the duplicate to one seen or felt. He said, "I can do it but it takes some seconds to get my brain straight."

This delay for consideration was an equally striking feature with printed commands and he volunteered the following explanation. "It's the interpreting words into pictures; when you give me KNIFE (printed card) I can't see the picture in my brain. All these things (passing his hand over the objects on the table) have no names at all until I really read K N I F E and say 'knife' to myself; then I can say what it is." I showed him the card bearing the word KEY and he replied, "I'm

Table 10.

	Pointing to object shown	Oral commands	Printed commands	Naming an object indicated	Writing the name of an object indicated	Duplicate placed in hand out of sight
Knife	Perfect	Correct, slow	Correct, slow	Correct	Correct	Perfect
Key	"	"	"	"	"	"
Penny	"	"	"	"	Penney	"
Matches	"	"	"	"	Correct	"
Scissors	"	"	"	"Kīnshi, Scissors"	Sissers	"
Pencil	"	"	"	Correct	Pensil	"
Key	"	"	"	"	Correct	"
Scissors	"	"	"	"Kīnshi again"	Sissers	"
Matches	"	"	"	"Box-er-matches"	Correct	"
Knife	"	"	"	Correct	"	"
Penny	"	"	"	"	Penney	"
Matches	"	"	"	"	Correct	"
Scissors	"	"	"	"	Sissers	"
Pencil	"	"	"	"	pencel	"
Penny	"	"	"	"	Penney	"
Knife	"	"	"	"	Correct	"
Key	"	"	"	"	"	"
Pencil	"	"	"	"This, er, pencil"	Pencel	"

not quite sure of that; I was not certain if it was a key or a knife. I have to spell it K E Y and I say 'key' and look down on the table and then I know that's the key" (pointing to it). "I still puzzle what K E Y means; if I see that (pointing to the key on the table) then I don't have to worry, I know K E Y is that...is a key."

I then handed him two cards, one bearing the word MATCHES, the other WATCH; he pointed to the match-box and holding up the latter card said, "nothing here," which was correct. Asked, what is the difference, he replied, "They are both written (printed); this one is here (pointing to the matches), the other there is nothing. I focus this one (matches) because it is here (pointing to the box). I can't focus this (the watch card) so well because it is not so clear." He then moved his eyes round my room as if seeking something and added, "When I look at that big one (my consulting room clock), that helps me. I want to interpret the reading 'Watch' into a picture or into that (pointing to the clock) watch. If I think of a watch and don't have to read it, I see a picture of my own watch. If you say it to me I see it at once, the picture is alright; if you show it me like that (printed) I have to think, I don't get the picture easily." Later he added, "Suppose you had shown me 'looking glass,' written like this (printed), I should have had to think a long time. But if I looked up and saw that looking glass (pointing to the one on the wall) I should have known it at once."

(2) *Naming and recognition of colours.*

Table 11.

	Pointing to colour shown	Oral commands	Printed commands	Naming colour	Writing name of colour indicated	Name read aloud and colour chosen	
						He read	He chose
Black	Perfect	Correct	Correct	Correct	Correct	Correctly; certain	Correctly; quick
Red	,,	,,	,,	"White, red"	,,	,,	,,
Blue	,,	,,	,,	Correct	,,	,,	,,
Green	,,	Correct; slow	,,	,,	,,	,,	,,
Orange	,,	Violet. "I should call that orange"	Correct; very slow	"Cerise or orange"	Bereis	,,	,,
White	,,	Correct	Correct	Correct	Correct	,,	,,
Violet	,,	,,	Orange. "No, no, that's it"; correct	"Mauve or purple"	Purple	,,	,,
Yellow	,,	,,	Correct	Correct	Correct	,,	,,
Red	,,	,,	,,	,,	Ded. Then replaced D by R	,,	,,
White	,,	,,	,,	,,	Correct	,,	,,
Yellow	,,	,,	,,	,,	,,	,,	,,
Blue	,,	,,	,,	,,	,,	,,	,,
Green	,,	,,	,,	,,	,,	,,	,,
Black	,,	,,	Blue	"Black or the dead I would call it"	,,	,,	,,
Orange	,,	No choice	Violet	"Cerise; yellow; no I mean orange"	Saruse	,,	,,
Violet	,,	Correct	Correct. "That was wrong," pointing to orange	"Purple"	Purple	,,	,,

Here again his powers had obviously improved, although the nature of his disability was fundamentally the same.

Asked to point to a colour shown him he went directly for the duplicate on the table; but in answer to oral or printed commands, he started at one end and moved backwards and forwards over the colours until his hand finally came to rest over the one corresponding to the order. The difference in his actions was extremely definite; in the first case he pounced on the colour at once, in the second he ranged over the series with movements of greater or less extent until he could make up his mind to a choice. At the same time he moved his lips and occasionally the name was just audible. When, however, he chose the duplicate of a colour he had seen, there was no sign of verbalisation.

If he was made to read the printed cards aloud he did so correctly; articulation was perfect even of words such as violet and orange, but he spoke deliberately like one careful of his enunciation. It was remarkable how rapid and certain was his choice as soon as he had said the word aloud; he pointed to the colour without any of that hesitation, so pronounced a feature of silent reading. He said, "It was much easier. I think I know the name of the colour; having said it to myself, I focus the attention on to the colour."

(3) *The man, cat and dog tests.* Throughout the two years his power of carrying out these tests had steadily increased. He was now able to read aloud these simple phrases and could both read and write correctly from pictures; but in attempting to repeat the words said by me he twice failed to give an accurate reply in twelve observations. This he explained as follows: "I say them one after the other and I don't think. I don't have a picture; I say them like, what is that animal, the parrot, yes the parrot." Dictation and copying were now perfectly executed and his handwriting was distinctly better than when he wrote from pictures.

(4) *The clock tests.*

Table 12.

	Direct imitation	Oral commands	Printed commands: Railway time	Printed commands: Ordinary nomenclature	Telling the time	Writing down the time
5 minutes to 2	Perfect	Correct	Perfect	Correct	Correct	Correct
Half-past 1	,,	,,	,,	,,	,,	,,
5 minutes past 8	,,	5 minutes *to* 8	,,	,,	,,	,,
20 minutes to 4	,,	Correct	,,	10 minutes to 4	,,	,,
10 minutes past 7	,,	,,	,,	Short hand at 7; long hand at 10 minutes *to* the hour	,,	,,
20 minutes to 6	,,	6.0. On repetition correct	,,	Short hand at 6; long hand at 10 minutes to the hour	,,	,,
A quarter past 12	,,	12.30	,,	Hesitated between a quarter to and a quarter past; finally correct	"Fifteen minutes past 12"	,,
10 minutes to 1	,,	Correct	,,	Correct	Correct	,,
A quarter to 9	,,	,,	,,	,,	,,	,,
Half-past 2	,,	,,	,,	,,	,,	,,
20 minutes past 11	,,	,,	,,	,,	,,	,,
25 minutes to 8	,,	,,	,,	Short hand at 8; long hand at 25 minutes *past* the hour	,,	,,
A quarter past 6	,,	6.30 "No"; 6.15. Then again 6.30; corrected to 6.15	,,	Correct	"Fifteen minutes past 6"	,,
25 minutes to 3	,,	Short hand at 3; long hand at 25 minutes to the hour	,,	Short hand at 3; long hand at 25 minutes to the hour	"25 minutes to 2"; corrected	,,
10 minutes past 4	,,	10 minutes *to* 4	,,	Correct; much hesitation	Correct	,,

Here again the improvement was obvious. He still hesitated over setting the clock to oral commands or to one printed in letters; but if it was given in the form of figures it was carried out exactly. His power of telling the time had increased and he was now able to write the time correctly.

There was, however, still a tendency to confuse "to" and "past" and to set the hour hand opposite a number on the clock face and not in proportion to the position of the minute hand.

(5) *The coin-bowl tests.* The improvement in his power of carrying out these tests has been so fully dealt with on p. 36 that it is only necessary to say that to oral commands he corrected himself three times in twelve observations, whilst to printed commands, whether in figures or in words, his answers were correct.

(6) *The hand, eye and ear tests.*

This is in some ways an even more instructive series of observations than those made when he first came under my care (see Table 13). For he still showed difficulty in imitating my movements, sitting opposite to him, and in carrying out pictorial commands; but as soon as either set of actions was reflected in the glass he executed them without fail, saying, "That's easier, doing exactly the same as you; before I didn't know which was the right and the left, now I'm copying. Looking at the glass I don't think if it's right or left; it's just copying."

To oral and printed commands his answers were slow, hesitating and he made many mistakes; but, when he read the printed cards aloud, he carried out the orders perfectly. "What worries me," he said, "is the name of ear and eye; they are very similar. It is names that bother me."

Although he could imitate perfectly movements made by me reflected in the glass, he was unable to write them down. This gave him more trouble than any other form of the hand, eye and ear tests. He tried to imitate the movement with his hand and then to write it down; but, although the action might have been correctly performed, it was wrongly described in writing or he was so puzzled that he gave up the attempt.

Condition in March 1921 (*three years and one month after the injury*).

He was leading an open-air life in the country and his executive capacity had steadily improved.

The opening in the skull had been so perfectly filled in with bone, that it was impossible to discover by ordinary methods of examination that it had ever been injured.

Beyond the gross hemianopsia over the right half of the field of vision to movement, form and colour, I could discover no abnormal physical signs.

Symbolic Formulation and Expression.

The main interest in the series of observations made at this time consisted in the comments by the patient, when attempting to explain his disabilities. These are given under the heading of the various tests which evoked them; but the actual records obtained did not differ materially from those set out above.

Table 13.

	Imitation of movements made by the observer	Imitation of movements reflected in a mirror	Pictorial commands	Pictorial commands reflected in a mirror
L. hand to L. eye	Correct	Correct	L. hand to R. eye	Correct
R. hand to R. ear	,,	,,	Correct	,,
R. hand to L. eye	R. hand to R. eye	,,	R. hand to R. eye	,,
L. hand to R. eye	L. hand to L. eye	,,	L. hand to L. eye	,,
L. hand to L. ear	Correct	,,	Correct	,,
R. hand to R. eye	,,	,,	Correct; very slow	,,
L. hand to R. ear	Correct; slow	,,	L. hand to L. ear	,,
R. hand to L. ear	Reversed	,,	R. hand to R. ear	,,
L. hand to L. eye	L. hand to R. eye	,,	Correct	,,
R. hand to R. ear	R. hand to L. ear	,,	,,	,,
R. hand to L. eye	R. hand to R. eye	,,	R. hand to R. eye	,,
L. hand to R. eye	L. hand to L. eye	,,	R. hand to R. eye	,,
L. hand to L. ear	Correct	,,	Correct	,,
R. hand to R. eye	,,	,,	,,	,,
L. hand to R. ear	,,	,,	R. hand to R. ear	,,
R. hand to L. ear	,,	,,	L. hand to L. ear	,,

Speech, reading and writing. He talked with greater ease, although he frequently had difficulty in discovering the exact word to fit a situation. He named common objects and colours slowly and deliberately, insisting that he was more successful if he did not concentrate on the act he was performing. After reading the story of the prize fight to himself (p. 35), he made the following attempt to convey to me what he had gathered; this was characteristic of the worst aspect of his disorders of speech at this period: "Carpentier...the French...heavy champion... champion heavy weight...met...er...the English champion heavy weight boxer ...Carpentier...Beckett...at the Holborn...Studi...Stadium...Carpentier knocked...Beckett...out...on...after seventy-two seconds fight...with a right hand hook to the jaw...I forgot to say it was Saturday...it was Thursday the...I can't remember what day it was."

He understood almost all that was said to him and carried out oral commands slowly but in the end correctly, except in the case of the complex hand, eye and ear tests. When making his choice, he insisted that he must first obtain an image suggested by the word I had said and that this must then be fitted to the appropriate object on the table before him.

He read to himself slowly and with difficulty. The simpler printed commands were executed with many corrections, but he failed with the hand, eye and ear tests. He set the hands of a clock, if the order was given in railway time, but failed when it was printed in the ordinary nomenclature. If he was asked to select a card bearing the name of an object shown to him, he explained that choice was

Table 13 (*continued*).

Oral commands	Printed commands	Reading aloud printed commands and executing them: He read	Reading aloud printed commands and executing them: Movement made	Writing down movements made by the observer reflected in a mirror
L. hand to R. eye	L. hand to L. *ear*; corrected	Correctly	Correct	Left eye
Correct	Correct	,,	,,	right
,,	,,	,,	,,	right eye to
L. hand to L. eye	L. hand to L. *ear*	,,	,,	left hand to left eye
L. hand to R. ear	Correct	,,	,,	left hand to
Correct	Correct; slow	,,	,,	right ear to left eye
L. hand to L. ear	L. hand to L. ear	,,	,,	left eye to ear
R. hand to R. ear	Correct	,,	,,	right hand to lef ear
Correct; slow	,,	,,	,,	left ear to eye
Correct	R. hand to R. *eye*	,,	,,	right hand to ear
,,	Correct	,,	,,	right hand to left eye
L. hand to L. eye	,,	,,	,,	left hand to right eye
Correct	L. hand to R. ear	,,	,,	left hand to left ear
,,	R. hand to L. eye	,,	,,	right hand to right eye
,,	Correct	,,	,,	left hand to right ear
,,	R. hand to L. *eye*	,,	,,	right hand to left ear

impossible unless he could get the "picture" (image) and the "name" to "synchronise."

He used to be a fluent Hindustani scholar, but after the accident lost all knowledge of the language. Some power of speaking had returned, although he could neither read nor write it.

His handwriting showed the same kind of faults noticed on previous occasions though to a less degree. For instance, after reading to himself the account of the prize fight he wrote, "Carponta, the French Heavy weight champion met Beckat in the Holbon Stadum Dec. 4th. 1919. Carpanta knocked out Becket after 74 minutes fight with a right hand hook to the jaw." He then remarked, "I think I could remember more by going over it again quietly." In fact he now writes excellent letters by drawing up a rough draft, correcting it repeatedly and finally making a fair copy.

He wrote equally badly to dictation, but copied print in cursive script accurately and without corrections.

Numbers and arithmetic. He counted with ease and rapidity and wrote the figures correctly; but between 10 and 20 he first put down the number, say 3, and then placed 1 before it to represent 13. He had re-learnt in a fortnight his power of counting in Hindustani in order to teach his sister, who was going to India.

He still had much difficulty with arithmetic and failed to solve the last two problems in subtraction. Moreover, he was not always certain if the answer was right or wrong.

Drawing and plan. He now drew an excellent picture of an elephant to command and named the various parts on the whole correctly (Fig. 19).

Asked to construct a ground-plan of the room in which we habitually worked, he represented the various objects in elevation; he could not reduce his visual images, which were unusually accurate, to a diagrammatic form. But, when I traced a quadrilateral figure on the paper and asked him to show me the position of the salient features, he did so without mistakes, at the same time describing them one by one.

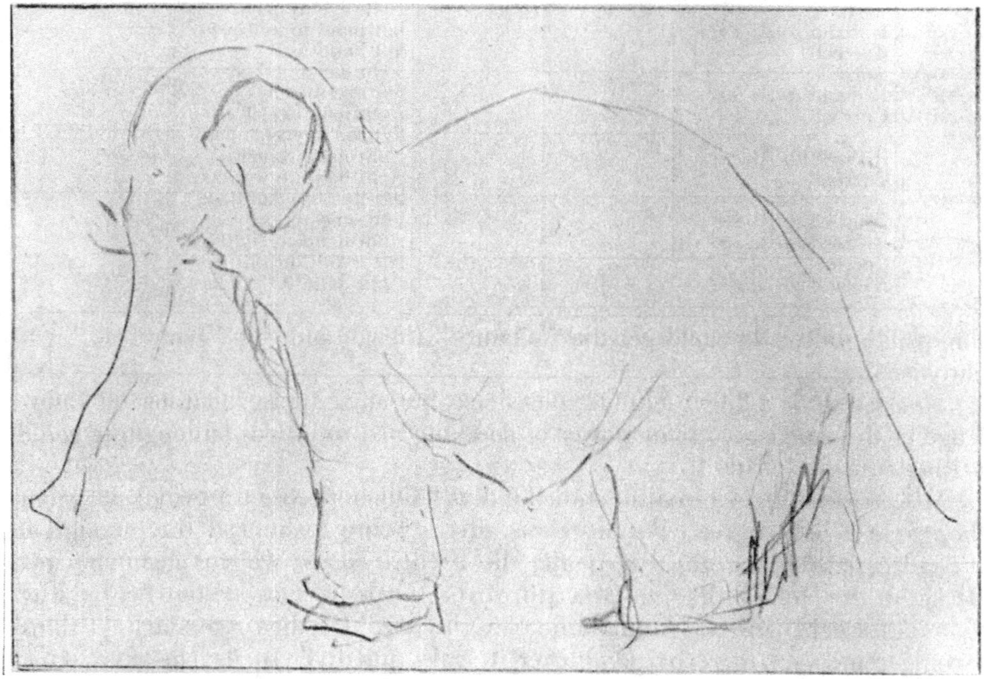

Fig. 19. Elephant drawn to command by No. 2 after he had recovered his powers of speech to a considerable degree (March 1921).

Serial Tests.

The actual records of the various tests corresponded so closely on the whole with those obtained five months before that it is unnecessary to give them in tabular form. Many of his comments, however, threw much light on his disabilities and these I shall produce under the heading of each particular test which evoked them.

(1) *Naming and recognition of common objects.* All these tests were executed correctly, but he named each object slowly and after considerable deliberation.

When making a choice to oral commands, he swept his finger along the row of objects on the table stopping at the one mentioned by me, for instance the "key." If I then said "pencil," which lay next to it, he again went back to the beginning and worked slowly along the series until he came to the pencil. He said in explanation, "I lose myself. The pencil now, I don't remember where it was...I think probably I had forgotten the name until I saw it (the pencil) again. Then I have to remember what the name of the thing is, when I *have* seen it." If the name was said to him, he had to pass in review the various articles on the table before the meaning of the word became clear from its correspondence with some concrete object. To printed commands he behaved in exactly the same manner. But, when a duplicate was placed in his hand out of sight, he pounced at once on the object he was seeking, without groping along the line of those on the table before him. "By feeling it," he said, "I don't have to say what it is; I just feel it like that and touch it without saying what it is. There is no strain on the brain, it's just a normal process."

Shown a familiar object, he could choose a printed card which bore its name, after some hesitation, but in the end correctly. When I held up a pencil he said, "I've seen it and I recollect it, but the name of it has gone until I concentrate again." He covered his eyes for a few moments and exclaiming, "Yes, I've got it... pencil," passed his hand over the cards to choose ultimately the one bearing the word "pencil." He added in explanation, "I have to see the picture of the pencil and then the picture from the writing of the pencil (printed card). It's the picture here (pointing to the pencil) and the picture there (pointing to the card). I want to get the picture of the pencil and the name to synchronise."

The name of each object in turn was written down correctly, but his spelling was defective. Thus, he wrote, "penney," "pencel" and "sissers," although all these words except the last were sometimes rightly spelt. He said that his spelling was "euphonic" (phonetic) and that "If I think too much about it, I lose the name of it or the picture of it. If I was going to drive (at golf) and someone showed me a penny I'd say the name at once; but if I concentrated on it I should lose the name."

(2) *Naming and recognition of colours*. All these tests were performed correctly, although he found the right names slowly and hesitated somewhat, when making a choice to printed commands.

(3) *The man, cat and dog tests*. He could read aloud correctly from print or pictures, repeated the words after me, chose a printed card corresponding to any two pictures he had seen and carried out the reverse operation without fail.

He wrote down these simple phrases slowly but accurately; but when writing to dictation twice substituted the word "dog" for man or cat. He copied perfectly from print in cursive script and said, "That's very easy, so much so that I don't think whether it's a man, or a dog, or a cat."

(4) *The clock tests.* As before he could tell the time and he executed oral and printed commands slowly with many corrections. He made two mistakes, when writing down the time, substituting 1 for 2 with "10 minutes to 2" and 5 for 6 with "20 minutes to 6."

(5) *The hand, eye and ear tests.* The records were almost identical with those given on Table 13, although oral and printed commands were somewhat better performed.

When attempting to write down the movements made by me, he frequently overcame his difficulty in deciding between eye and ear by drawing a picture of an eye instead of writing the word. This increased the number of right answers by obviating the necessity of formulating the name in written symbols. He explained, "The whole thing is whether I can spell 'eye,' and I can't; I can't remember if it is E A R or E Y E, and then I get exercised over it you see. When I'm trying to spell ear or eye I can't remember which is which."

CONDITION IN DECEMBER 1922 (*four years and ten months after the injury*).

Physically he was in superb health, alert, active and bright. In fact, to superficial observation he appeared as a normal man. The hemianopsia remained exactly as before and I could discover no other abnormal physical signs.

Symbolic Formulation and Expression.

His powers of speech had greatly improved; but, although the records were better than on any previous occasion, he was more conscious of his defects and difficulties. All the serial tests, with the exception of those with hand, eye and ear, were executed without mistakes; and yet his doubts as to the correctness of the answers and the hesitation with which he arrived at a final conclusion led him to suppose that his replies were "awfully bad." When I told him finally that he had never done so well, he expressed intense surprise; for increased capacity to perform these acts of speech was accompanied by greater consciousness of his want of ease and certainty.

He complained that a tendency to fusion of ideas led to perseveration of commands. In order that an answer might be given correctly, it was necessary that a formal break should be made between one question and the next. For instance, if I handed him a clock and, as soon as he had replied, gave him a second one set differently he was liable to become confused. If however I solemnly removed the clock after he had given his answer and some thirty seconds later placed it before him with the hands in a fresh position, he responded without mistakes. He was extremely particular in covering up each written answer before undertaking the next, a precaution I have always adopted throughout these investigations; but he insisted on it for his own comfort and carried it out unprompted.

He talked freely and, although he was frequently held up for want of the exact word to express his meaning, he was usually able to circumvent his difficulties. Sometimes, however, the use of the wrong word led to confusion that could only be resolved with the help of a sympathetic auditor. Articulation was good, intonation perfect and syntax was not primarily disturbed. He could repeat anything said to him, provided it was not embodied in a long and complicated sentence.

He seemed to have little difficulty in understanding general conversation provided the speaker expressed himself concisely. The majority of oral commands were executed promptly; but he hesitated over the choice of orange, violet and yellow and was somewhat slow in carrying out the complex hand, eye and ear tests.

All printed orders read silently were now performed without mistakes, though somewhat slowly. He could even set the clock to commands given in the ordinary nomenclature and executed the hand, eye and ear tests without fail. He still had some difficulty in gathering the exact meaning of all the words when reading to himself.

His writing had greatly improved in character and he now produced long and coherent letters after considerable effort. These he corrected and then re-copied, but even the final draft contained many errors in spelling, erasures and substitutions. He said, "In writing letters to my sister I don't mind about mistakes, I just go straight on and the letter is done in twenty minutes. When I am writing to you, I put down the mistakes and then cross them...put a tick on them...and what I thought was right you see...and then the question of an important letter, a business letter...I nearly always have it dictated by my sister. Another thing I might mention; I have a little dictionary...I can now look up the words that worried me a good deal a year ago."

He said the alphabet unprompted, repeated it after me and read it aloud perfectly. He wrote the letters spontaneously and to dictation and copied them from print in cursive script. Given the twenty-six block letters, he finally placed them in proper sequence, but worked slowly and had considerable difficulty in determining the position of H and R. He added, "I think this would have worried me sometime back...in fact at one time I didn't know one of them, I didn't know A."

He could now say the months in order, repeat them after me and read the names aloud without mistakes. Writing them spontaneously, he was somewhat slow and made two corrections; but he produced a perfect list to dictation, or if he was allowed to copy the words from print.

He produced a fair representation of an elephant to command naming its salient parts correctly.

All six problems in arithmetic were solved after much hesitation. He named coins accurately, but still had some difficulty in stating the relation between any two of them. Thus he gave the following answers:

Sixpence and a shilling—"There are three...oh! two."
One shilling and ten-shilling note—"Five."

One penny and sixpence—Correct.
Sixpence and half a crown—Correct.
One penny and two-shilling piece—Correct.
A sixpence and a ten-shilling note—Correct.
One penny and a shilling—Correct.
A sixpence and two-shilling piece—Correct.
A two-shilling piece and ten-shilling note—"Four."
One penny and half a crown—"Twenty-five" (instead of 30).

Monetary calculations still troubled him greatly in daily life and he became easily confused over change. He said, "If I buy something at say one and nine... I give the man a two-shilling piece...at the same time I say I can't be worried if it is two pennies, or three pennies, or four pennies...I look it up afterwards to see if he's an honest man...From Brentwood (his home) to Liverpool Street (the station at which he arrives in London) I know now it is going to be five shillings less twopence halfpenny...That's what I expect to get...to see...I figure it up beforehand."

Serial Tests.

He could now execute all these tests without fail, except those demanding movements of one or other hand to eye or ear. But it is interesting to find that he still showed greater hesitation and arrived at a correct answer more slowly with all those tasks that were originally grossly affected.

(1) *Naming and recognition of common objects.* Oral and printed commands were promptly executed. He was slower and more uncertain in naming and made several mistakes in spelling, when he wrote down the names of objects shown to him, particularly scissors and pencil.

(2) *Naming and recognition of colours.* Here again he hesitated somewhat over the names of colours, although they were written down correctly. To oral and printed commands his choice was made quickly and with greater certainty. But at the end of these tests he said, "When we've done about ten colours, I have to concentrate very hard to get the right colour and name. It's the names that bother me. I can see them, but when I have to say them I have to write in my mind the word Y E L L O W, etc....When I've done so many tests of colours...now this particular word (pointing to the orange coloured silk on the table)...now I'm not quite sure that there is an orange colour or whatever it is until I say it...I have to get something to catch hold of." "There's been no practice in this at all; but my ...I can call it focus...is quicker. I'm convinced that I can see these colours four times quicker than I used to be able to. I can now see what my mistakes are, whereas before I didn't know."

(3) *The man, cat and dog tests* were executed without mistakes and he wrote down the short phrases accurately from pictures, to dictation and when copying print.

(4) *The clock tests.* He set the hands to oral or printed commands, whichever nomenclature was employed, and both told the time and wrote it down without mistakes.

He insisted that I should carry out these tests slowly, saying, "It would be much easier if I waited twenty-five seconds before I said another one, because they...because the one you have just told me is still in my mind and the next one goes into that."

Any order given in railway time was easier than one in the ordinary nomenclature. "I can tell you why," he said, "because in seeing railway time I have only to concentrate on the ...on the time in figures...whereas in the other...I have to read it...read the words...not only the words...there are two processes...'five minutes' and then I have to turn my mind to see 'to two'...In the other one it's all figures...just like seeing Big Ben (the clock on the Houses of Parliament) from a distance."

(5) *The hand, eye and ear tests.*

Table 14.

	Imitation of movements made by the observer		Imitation of movements reflected in a mirror	Pictorial commands	Pictorial commands reflected in a mirror	Oral commands	Printed commands	Writing down movements made by the observer sitting face to face
	1st series	2nd series						
L. hand to L. eye	Correct	Correct	Correct and quick	Correct	Correct and quick	Correct	Correct	R. hand to L. eye
R. hand to R. ear	,,	,,	,,	,,	,,	Correct; slow	,,	R. hand to L. ear
R. hand to L. eye	Reversed	,,	,,	,,	,,	Correct	Corrected	Correct
L. hand to R. eye	L. hand to L. eye	,,	,,	,,	,,	,,	Correct	L. hand to L. eye
L. hand to L. ear	Reversed	,,	,,	,,	,,	,,	,,	Correct
R. hand to R. eye	,,	,,	,,	,,	,,	,,	,,	,,
L. hand to R. ear	,,	,,	,,	Corrected	,,	,,	Corrected	,,
R. hand to L. ear	,,	,,	,,	Correct	,,	,,	Correct	,,
L. hand to L. eye	,,	,,	,,	,,	,,	Corrected slowly	,,	,,
R. hand to R. ear	Correct	,,	,,	,,	,,	Correct	,,	,,
R. hand to L. eye	Reversed	,,	,,	,,	,,	,,	,,	R. hand to L. *ear*
L. hand to R. eye	Correct	,,	,,	,,	,,	,,	,,	Correct
L. hand to L. ear	,,	,,	,,	,,	,,	,,	,,	,,
R. hand to R. eye	,,	,,	,,	,,	,,	,,	,,	,,
L. hand to R. ear	L. hand to L. ear	Corrected	,,	,,	,,	,,	Corrected	,,
R. hand to L. ear	Correct	Correct	,,	,,	,,	,,	Correct	,,

This was the only group of tests in which he made any definite mistakes and yet the records showed profound improvement. Oral and printed commands were carried out slowly and with considerable hesitation, though without actual errors. When we sat face to face, he was slow to understand exactly what was required of him; but towards the end of the series he said, "Now I think I understand," and asked to be permitted to try again. He then imitated every one of my movements slowly and with deliberation. He made four mistakes only in writing them down on paper.

He then gave the following excellent analysis of the difficulties he found with these tests. "I have to see whether it's your right hand or your left hand moving first...because sometimes you use your right hand to your right eye...or your right hand to your left eye...sometimes it's a cross...sometimes there's no cross. At the same time it's sometimes...sometimes it's the word ear or eye...they're so alike...in the English language...in writing...and in speech."

During the period of these observations the patient showed profound improvement in his powers of symbolic formulation and expression. So great was this increase in capacity that, with the exception of a few trivial mistakes and some corrections, all the serial tests could be carried out four years and ten months after the injury. Yet, in spite of this recovery of function, the want of facility remained of the same character, though diminished greatly in degree. Simple oral and printed commands were executed perfectly, but those of greater complexity were performed slowly and with hesitation. Although he could name objects placed before him, he found considerable difficulty in discovering the exact word to fit his meaning. This was exaggerated in writing, which was laboriously carried out and abounded in corrections. Arithmetical problems were solved after considerable effort and he found difficulty in the monetary transactions of daily life.

His fundamental defects of speech still consisted of lack of appreciation of verbal significance and inability to discover the word which exactly expressed his meaning. This was clearly evident from the last set of records, although at that time he might have passed on superficial observation for a normal man.

No. 4

A case of slight Verbal Aphasia, due to a grave gun-shot injury of the skull and thrombosis of the superior longitudinal sinus followed by hernia cerebri.

There was profound right hemiplegia with some loss of power in the left lower extremity. Sensibility, especially to passive movement, was grossly affected on the right side and to a slighter degree in the left leg. Both plantar reflexes gave an upward response. The left upper extremity was in every way normal.

He talked fluently, but had difficulty in forming the longer words and could repeat anything said to him, provided the sentence was not long and complicated. He understood almost all that he heard and executed oral commands correctly. He could carry out printed orders without mistakes, but he complained that, when reading to himself, he had a tendency to miss some of the words. This want of verbal exactitude was liable to cause confusion, if he tried to recall what he had read. He wrote with the left hand comparatively fluently, but his spelling was faulty and he tended to omit some of the words. To dictation his writing showed the same kind of defects. Printed matter was copied with complete accuracy in cursive handwriting. Although he had been a bank-clerk, he found some difficulty in solving problems of simple arithmetic and in adding up long columns of figures. He drew perfectly, both spontaneously and to command. Orientation was not affected. He could play any form of game.

Lieut. Charles Henry H., aged 23, was wounded on May 16th, 1916, by a rifle bullet, probably fired from a machine gun. He fell, but did not become unconscious. As he lay on the ground, completely paralysed down the right side, he slowly lost his senses and did not recover them until several days later in the casualty clearing station. Here he was operated upon sometime before June 3rd; for a note made on that day, ran as follows: "Glancing gunshot wound of the skull. There was a large gutter-shaped fracture running along the left side of the superior longitudinal sinus; X-rays showed fragments of bone driven in, in a cone-shaped fashion, for about 2½ in. No other foreign body. The sinus was partially thrombosed and no serious bleeding occurred. Right hemiplegia and partial aphasia. All fragments were removed. A large flap was turned down and the edges of the bone chipped away and cleaned up."

He was admitted to the Empire Hospital under my care on June 11th, 1916.

He then showed a huge overhanging hernia cerebri, extending from 17 cm. to 24 cm. along the nasion-inion line and lying from 1 cm. to 5 cm. from the middle of the scalp. Fluid withdrawn from the swelling clotted, but did not contain pus cells; no organisms, aerobic or anaerobic, could be cultivated from it.

The surface of the hernia was carefully cleansed twice daily with hydrogen peroxide and dressed with absolute alcohol. But, as it seemed to remain stationary in size, we resorted to lumbar puncture; every week, between July 27th and

September 19th, from 10 to 25 c.c. of cerebro-spinal fluid were removed. The effect was remarkable; on each occasion the swelling diminished in size, although it tended to increase again about forty-eight hours later. Finally, by the beginning of September, it was reduced to two small button-shaped projections on a somewhat depressed surface, which pulsated. The wound healed completely on November 1st and resulted in a firm pulsating scar. Measurements taken at this time showed that the orifice in the skull measured 4 cm. in length by 1·5 cm. in breadth; it extended from a point 19 cm. to one 23 cm. along the nasion-inion line and the superior border of the opening was 1 cm. from the middle of the scalp.

When he arrived in England his mental condition was excellent. He was bright, cheerful and full of hope, in spite of the gravity of the injury.

His aphasia did not differ materially from that described below; in fact, from the beginning speech was not severely affected.

He had not suffered from convulsions and had little headache. The discs were normal and there was no limitation of the field of vision. The main feature of the case was a profound right hemiplegia with signs pointing to a slighter affection of the left pyramidal tract. In fact, he was a characteristic example of the consequences of thrombosis of the superior longitudinal sinus. The signs, as they appeared during the period when I could make more extensive observations on his defects of language, will be given later in full.

Condition between October 25th and November 1st, 1916 (*in the twenty-fourth week after he was wounded*).

During this week the wound healed finally, he was free from headache and could walk a quarter of a mile without excessive fatigue. I was able, therefore, to carry out an exhaustive set of observations on his powers of speech, followed by a complete physical examination; I shall describe the results in this order.

Symbolic Formulation and Expression.

To all who examined this man superficially with the usual clinical tests or listened to his conversation and watched his general behaviour, he seemed to be suffering from a pure anarthria. But more extensive observations showed that his defects of speech were not purely articulatory, even in the highest sense, but depended on faulty verbalisation, both external and internal.

Articulated speech. He talked fluently, but was liable to slur the longer words. "My voc-ab-lry (vocabulary) is still small," he said. "When I try to explain, I haven't got the words I want and when they say over a set of words I then say 'yes, that's the one.' I have to go over the roots; I trace the root back to the Latin or that, and get it e-ven-chaly (eventually)." He found difficulty with "ten-i-cal (technical) terms." "Yesterday I had diff-ulty (difficulty) in remembering what you do with the skull...tri...tre...trephine." "I find it easier," he said, "if there is some connection...if it seems to follow. I'm confine (confined) to the words I've got back...since my speech came back...I have to use the words I've got back...when they say 'what do you mean by so and so?' I haven't got a further example...of what I've said...to explain." He knew French and Spanish and sometimes was able to find the English word out of the French; but he had exactly the same difficulty in both of these foreign languages as in his native tongue. When he attempted to speak French, he was slow and hesitated over the words; moreover, he mixed up French and Spanish.

General intonation, apart from the tendency to elision and jerkiness of phrasing, was good. Syntax was unaffected and he did not talk jargon.

He could say the alphabet and the names of the months correctly; his pronunciation on the whole was good. He could repeat perfectly anything said to him provided the sentence was not very long and complicated; his enunciation was better than when he said the same words spontaneously.

Understanding of spoken words. To superficial observation he appeared to understand everything said to him and he was able to carry out even complex oral commands. But he confessed that "some words, when I listen to them, I can't collect the meaning. Nurse said quite a common thing, something about your coming this morning, but she said it too quickly, I couldn't collect it; she had to say it again."

He became very confused when spoken to in French. Asked, "Est-ce que vous pouvez parler Français?"; he said, "pouvez, what is that? I don't seem to know." Later in the afternoon, as I entered his room, he called out, "I've got it; pouvez... pouvoir, you know."

Reading. He could read correctly and understood what he read. Printed commands were carried out well, even those involving threefold choice, such as the hand, eye and ear tests. The results, yielded by the test-paragraphs given below, show how well he understood what he read silently or aloud; and yet he complained that he had difficulty in remembering a chapter he had read in a book. This was mainly due to a tendency to miss some of the words, when reading to himself, exactly as he did when he read aloud. This want of verbal exactitude was liable to cause confusion if he tried to recall what he had read.

Writing. He wrote his name and address, the alphabet and a short business letter perfectly. But his spelling tended to be faulty and the mistakes were such as could not have been made by any normal educated person. Moreover, he was liable to change the structure of the sentence so that the end did not correspond accurately with the beginning. He also tended to omit a word here and there and complained, "I can't carry many words at a time. If you give me a phrase containing four words, I can do three and then have to get you to dictate further or read it again. I find, on reading over, I leave the small words out, quite often." A good example of all these faults in writing is given by the following passage written to dictation, "The Somme battle must go on until it reaches its destined (military) conclusion and the politian (politician) who would cause it to have been fought in vain is one who (with whom) the public will reckon."

Reproducing the meaning of a printed paragraph.

(1) I gave him the following sentence in print, asked him to read it to himself and tell me what he had gathered from it. "The Westerners say: The flower of the German armies, led by all the Crown Princes, is on the French line. Defeat them, and the whole of the Prussian militarist cause is smashed." He replied, "That the flower of the German army is...are fighting against the French front. They were armies of Crown Prince...of the Crown Prince. It was the flower of the Crown Prince's armies."

He read this paragraph aloud correctly and wrote the following account of its significance: "The flower of the German Crown Princes armies were on the Western front and if they are smashed the flower of the Prussian armies are gone." When he had finished, he looked back over what he had written and said with a laugh, "I didn't know I had repeated myself. I didn't know I had mentioned the flower before. I can't trace anything back quickly. I say it as it comes to the head. If I get a pause and look back over what I have written or thought, it comes back slowly. It's the same in writing a letter...if someone comes in...I have to change the subjec (subject) because I can't remember what I have written."

Finally he copied the printed paragraph with complete accuracy in cursive handwriting.

(2) A few days later a prize fight, which had taken place nearly a year before, came up in conversation and I put together the following account as a test of his powers:

"Bombardier Wells fought Gunner Moore to a knock-out finish at the National Sporting Club on Wednesday evening, November the eighteenth, for a belt and a purse of £400."

This paragraph he read to himself and, when asked what he had gathered from it, gave a complete account of all the various facts it contained, although they were narrated in a different order. He added, "I didn't give the facts in the same order. I thought over what I had said and suddenly they came back."

He then read the story aloud without a mistake and again gave an account of what he had understood, which was complete in every way except for the omission of the knock-out. He then added in correction, "I should have said they fought to a knock-out. That should have been put in soon after mentioning Bombardier Wells and Gunner Moore."

Throughout this test there was none of that tendency to omit or substitute details so common in certain cases of aphasia belonging to a different order.

Numbers. He counted well, but sometimes slowly. The numbers, whether single or compound, were correctly pronounced, although enunciation was somewhat explosive and each word was separated from its fellows by a definite pause.

Addition.

231	859	687
526	324	856
757	1183	1543

Subtraction.

285	392	812
142	236	765
143	156	47

He complained that, although all these sums were solved correctly, he found difficulty in carrying over. This corresponded with the results of my observations; for he quickly gave the answer to the addition and the first subtraction sums, but was much slower over the last two. This is the more remarkable as he had worked in a bank before the war.

He said in explanation, "I had my banking book the other day. I couldn't do long columns of additions. I can't carry over. I was in a bank and used to do figures in my head. I know about it, it's not difficult, only the carrying over from one column to the top of the next column."

All coins were named perfectly and he had no hesitation in giving the exact relation of any two of them.

Drawing. He had acquired remarkable power of drawing with his left hand, whether from a model, from memory or to command. He drew an excellent picture of an elephant showing all its salient points with perfect accuracy.

Orientation and plan drawing. He could find his way without difficulty and described the various rooms in the hospital and their relation to one another easily and correctly. The ground-plan of his own room was accurate in every particular.

Games. He played all forms of card games, was fond of putting together jig-saw puzzles, and added, "I've found them very re-edjukate-ive" (re-educative).

Serial Tests.

(1) *Naming and recognition of objects.* The high intelligence of this patient and the fact that he was an officer in the artillery, led me to select a set of six simple geometrical figures for this test.

He had not the slightest difficulty in pointing to the one shown to him, or placed in his left hand out of sight, and he carried out correctly both oral and printed commands.

Table 1.

	Imitation of movements made by the observer	Imitation of movements reflected in a mirror	Pictorial commands	Pictorial commands reflected in a mirror
L. hand to L. eye	Correct	Correct	Reversed	Correct
R. hand to R. ear	L. hand; then correct	,,	L. hand to R. ear	,,
R, hand to L. eye	Correct	,,	L. hand to R. *ear*	,,
L. hand to R. eye	L. hand to L. eye	,,	Reversed	,,
L. hand to L. ear	Correct	,,	Correct	,,
R. hand to R. eye	,,	,,	Reversed	,,
L. hand to R. ear	L. hand to L. ear	,,	,,	,,
R. hand to L. ear	R. hand to R. ear	,,	,,	,,
L. hand to L. eye	Correct	,,	Correct	,,
R. hand to R. ear	,,	,,	Reversed	,,
R. hand to L. eye	R. hand to R. eye	,,	L. hand to R. *ear*	,,
L. hand to R. eye	R. hand to R. eye; then R. hand to L. eye	,,	Reversed	,,
L. hand to L. ear	Correct	,,	Correct	,,
R. hand to R. eye	,,	,,	,,	,,
L. hand to R. ear	,,	,,	Reversed	,,
R. hand to L. ear	L. hand to L. ear	,,	,,	,,

Asked to name the geometrical figures, he did so accurately; pronunciation of cylinder, pyramid and ovoid was, however, defective. His difficulty lay in articulation rather than in nomenclature.

He wrote slowly with his left hand, but made no mistake until he came to ovoid, which he spelt consistently "oboid." Pyramid was twice written correctly; the third time the word recurred he wrote "pre, pyri," erased both attempts and then became hopelessly confused. If, however, he was allowed to say the names aloud before writing them down, he made no faults in spelling and wrote more easily. To dictation he wrote hesitatingly, but without mistakes and he copied the printed words with remarkable fluency and correctness.

At the conclusion of these tests he said: "I have to give a pause. There is no fluency. I have to think and then I get it. If a person says a word, I can't connect it with what they are saying unless they give an instance—the use of it—a so and so, or what it is."

(2) *The man, cat and dog tests.* He could read these simple phrases correctly both from print and pictures and repeated them after me without error. He wrote them well to dictation and from pictures, showing no tendency to omit the articles or conjunctions.

(3) *The clock tests.* He set the hands of the clock with ease in direct imitation, or to oral and printed commands. He said, "This is very easy; if I don't get it straight, I can correct it at once."

Table 1 (*continued*).

Oral commands	Printed commands (not read aloud)	Printed commands read aloud and executed	Writing down movements made by the observer	Writing down movements reflected in a mirror
Correct	Correct	Correct	Left, left eye (correct)	Correct
,,	,,	,,	Correct	Left hand right ear
,,	,,	,,	,,	Correct
,,	,,	,,	,,	,,
,,	,,	,,	Left hand ("I forget which it was")	,,
,,	,,	,,	Correct	,,
,,	,,	,,	,,	Left hand right
,,	,,	,,	,,	Correct
,,	,,	,,	,,	,,
,,	,,	,,	Right hand ("I think it was the same side")	,,
,,	,,	,,	Correct	,,
,,	,,	,,	,,	Left hand left eye
,,	,,	,,	No response. ("I've forgotten")	Correct
,,	,,	,,	Correct	,,
,,	,,	,,	Left hand right *eye*	,,
,,	,,	,,	Correct	,,

When he told the time aloud, his enunciation was syncopated and staccato; but the words were accurate and he employed the usual nomenclature. There was no confusion between "past" and "to" the hour.

So long as he was allowed to see the clock throughout, he could write down the time accurately. He said, "I feel a difficulty in carrying the words in my head, whilst I am writing. I write the beginning and then I can't find the other words till I look at it again."

(4) *The hand, eye and ear tests.*

In spite of the paralysis of the right hand, I was able to carry out this test in its complete form; for he would seize the affected limb with the left hand and raise it to the eye or ear of one or other side. In this way he carried out correctly with quickness and certainty both oral and printed commands.

But, when he attempted to imitate my movements sitting face to face, he made many mistakes and complained, "I have to think and say 'left' or 'right' aksh-ly (actually) before I do it. I say 'eye,' 'ear'; as soon as I've done it, I think this is not right, I see my fault." Pictorial commands produced an even worse series of answers. He said, "This is the most difficult. I aks-ly (actually) do it with my mind with this side (left) and then I transfer it to the other side. I say it to myself."

As soon as he was allowed to imitate my movements or to see the pictures reflected in a mirror all doubt and difficulty disappeared; his replies became quick and accurate and he said, "It's easy that way; I go automatically."

When he attempted to write down my actions, he made many mistakes. The first words were usually written quickly; then he waited, puzzled, and not infrequently his lips moved silently before he wrote the second half of the statement. On three occasions he was unable to finish the sentence and complained that he had forgotten what I had done. Even when my movements were reflected in the mirror, he experienced extreme difficulty in describing them in writing; for in order to complete this task he was compelled to translate what he saw into verbal symbols.

At the close of these observations he said, "I have to remember which hand and then where that hand goes to. That's the difficulty. I can't always remember where the hand goes to. I can't contain the number of words required."

Physical Examination.

He was a right-handed man, who had acquired remarkable facility in the use of his left hand since his injury. There were no signs of apraxia.

He had been free from headache for more than a month, and had suffered from no fits, seizures or other similar attacks at any time.

Vision was normal and there was no hemianopsia or restriction of the visual field. He could hear well with both ears. Smell and taste were not grossly affected.

The pupils reacted well, there was no nystagmus and the eyes moved perfectly in all directions. The right angle of the mouth was slightly less mobile than the left, but the tongue did not deviate on protrusion.

On the right side of the body the arm-, knee- and ankle-jerks were greatly exaggerated and ankle clonus was easily obtained; the plantar reflex gave a characteristic upward movement of the great toe, but the abdominals were definitely present. On the left side the arm-jerks were normal; the knee- and ankle-jerks were, however, exaggerated, ankle clonus was obtained and the plantar reflex gave an upward response. On this half of the abdomen the reflex could also be readily elicited.

At first sight he appeared to be suffering from little more than a characteristic right hemiplegia. No isolated movements were possible in this hand, though he could close his fingers over mine in a grasp too feeble for measurement. The right upper limb usually lay flexed at elbow, wrist and fingers; but he could abduct and adduct the arm at the shoulder, flex and extend the elbow and slightly extend the wrist. When he abducted the arm and flexed the elbow, the index, middle and ring fingers became extended. The metacarpo-phalangeal joints remained flexed but the others were over-extended. This upper extremity was hypertonic although the fingers could be passively over-extended. It was not wasted and there were no organic contractures. There was much incoordination, associated with the profound loss of spacial sensibility.

The left arm and hand showed no loss of power, wasting or incoordination.

He stood unsteadily and the right leg was wildly ataxic, but he was able to walk a considerable distance on the level ground with help. He tended to fall, when his eyes were closed.

There was gross loss of power in the right lower extremity; dorsiflexion and plantar extension of the foot were just possible and movements at the knee were feeble. This leg was extremely incoordinate and became very ataxic, when his eyes were closed. The toes could be passively over-extended to a greater degree than those of the left foot.

The left lower extremity was obviously less affected than the right; but dorsiflexion and plantar extension were certainly diminished in range and force. Movements at the knee and hip were powerful. There appeared to be some incoordination of the left foot, but there was no definite alteration of tone.

Sensation was profoundly affected. He occasionally woke at night to find that he did not know the position of his right hand and sometimes it seemed to him as if he had lost the terminal joints of these fingers, but not of the thumb.

On systematic examination grave loss of appreciation of passive movement (measured) was discovered in the fingers of the right hand, wrist and elbow; the response from the right shoulder was slower than that from the left. There was also gross loss of discrimination to the compass points and defective localisation of the spot touched. Tactile (measured hairs) and thermal sensibility also revealed the characteristic defects found as the result of cerebral lesions. The left upper limb on the contrary was in every way normal.

On comparing the two lower extremities, both were found to show sensory changes; those on the right side were extremely severe and consisted of defective postural recognition, loss of discrimination of two points and of localisation. There was, however, no material change in tactile or thermal sensibility.

On the left side the changes were much slighter. Passive movement was defective in the toes and slightly diminished at the ankle; but at the knee and hip it was perfect. Discrimination of the compass points was possible at about 8 cm., a distance above normal and localisation was not materially affected.

No. 5

A case of Semantic Aphasia due to a wound in the right parietal region; a rifle bullet was removed from the brain beneath the inferior and posterior portion of the supra-marginal gyrus.

There was no disturbance of motion or sensation. The visual fields were not affected. All the reflexes were normal.

He had always been a strongly left-handed man.

Articulated speech was not directly affected and he named common objects and colours correctly. The most striking feature was his inability to formulate, to appreciate and to retain in his mind the general meaning or the exact intention of some act requiring symbolic representation. He understood simple statements and chose common objects to oral commands; but he made gross mistakes, when attempting to set the hands of a clock, or to carry out the hand, eye and ear tests. He failed more particularly to reproduce the sense of a simple narrative communicated to him by word of mouth. When he read to himself silently, his difficulty lay not so much in understanding a word or phrase as in gathering the general meaning of a group of statements; but he ultimately succeeded in executing all the tests to printed commands. He wrote spontaneously with remarkable ease. Yet the names of common objects and the time shown on a clock were written down badly; his handwriting deteriorated and his spelling was defective. To dictation he was inaccurate and even made mistakes in writing the phrases of the man, cat and dog tests. On the other hand, he could copy print excellently in cursive script. All these faults in reading and writing were particularly evident, when he was tested with a short account in printed characters of his life before the war. If he was asked to render the general meaning of a picture and its accompanying legend, he was liable to become confused and to invent some fantastic explanation. He failed to solve two out of the six problems in simple arithmetic and was frequently unable to express the relative value of two coins to one another. He failed completely to draw an elephant to order. Orientation was defective. He could not produce a ground-plan of the portion of the ward in the neighbourhood of his bed, although he recalled to mind the essential differences in the uniform of Sister and Nurse.

Corporal A. C. H., aged 19, was wounded by a rifle bullet in the right parietal region towards the end of August 1915. He was admitted to a Base Hospital at Boulogne on August 29th, without notes of any kind, and remained there until September 13th. I owe all my information regarding this period to a personal letter from the surgeon in charge at the time. On admission the patient was semi-comatose and very resistive. The wound was a minute punctured opening, from which exuded cerebro-spinal fluid mingled with minute quantities of disintegrated brain matter. On August 30th, the bullet was extracted from a point in the brain about $1\frac{1}{2}$ to 2 inches (4 to 5 cm.) in depth directly under the point of entry. It had bored a small circular hole in the skull and in the dura mater beneath it. This was enlarged sufficiently to admit the little finger up to the second joint. After this operation he made excellent progress and his mental condition improved rapidly.

He was admitted to the London Hospital on September 13th, 1915. At this time he showed a firmly healed semicircular incision and, in the centre of the large circular flap, the wound of entry was represented by a minute scabbed opening. This was situated 20·5 cm. backwards along the nasion-inion line and 11 cm. to the right of the middle of the scalp. The total nasion-inion measurement was 35 cm., and this was cut by the interaural line at a point 16 cm. from the root of the nose (Figs. 13 and 14, Vol. 1, pp. 461, 463).

I could obtain from him no account of how he was wounded nor what he was doing at the time. He was mentally confused and had difficulty in carrying out commands to put out his tongue or to touch his nose. Articulation was unaffected, speech was normal and there was no tendency to syntactical defects or jargon.

General examination of the central nervous system revealed no signs of gross organic injury. He had not suffered from convulsions or seizures of any kind and was entirely free from headache. Vision was normal; the fields were not restricted, but the discs showed some signs of previous optic neuritis. The pupils reacted well, movements of the eyes were carried out perfectly and there was no nystagmus. The face moved equally well on the two sides and the tongue was protruded in the middle line. All reflexes, including the abdominals and plantars, were normal. There was no paralysis, paresis or incoordination. Sensation was unaffected.

He had always been a strongly left-handed man, using even a chopper with the left hand.

Condition of Symbolic Formulation and Expression between October 21st and November 9th, 1915 (*about eight to ten weeks after he was wounded*).

He was a fairly well educated, country bred youth, who had reached the fifth standard in an elementary school at the age of thirteen. He had been gardener and handyman to an elderly lady.

He remembered joining the army, but could not tell the date. He said it was "August," but corrected himself, "No, I've not got that I can't remember that." He knew the name and number of his regiment and recollected that he was trained at Winchester. Asked how he got across, he answered, "From Southampton, sir. I can mind something about Boulogne; but that's all I can remember." He could not recall going on board the boat, landing in France or anything from that time onwards, except that he saw a dead German, "black and rotten, a horrible sight." He added, "I've been burying of them too."

He answered questions readily and during the examination was most anxious to help me in every way; but he was easily confused and ceased to talk, because he was unable to formulate exactly the information he wished to impart. Thus, asked what work he did he answered, "Miss D's, in the garden. I'd been there nearly two years. Then I left there and went to Miss D's... I said that first; I get muddled." I enquired where he went after Miss D's and he replied, "That's where I went into the army; left there and joined the army." I asked if he did any work other than looking after the garden. "I looked after a pony, Miss D's, a maiden lady; a little, rough pony." "Can you see the pony?" "Yes I can see him quite clearly. Sometimes stumbles, black tail, black mane. I get muddled, sir."

Throughout the examination the most striking feature was his inability to formulate, to appreciate and to retain in his mind the exact general intention of some action requiring symbolic representation. For instance, when testing his power of recognising passive movement, it was useless to insist on his adopting "down" or "up" or any similar nomenclature, even after he had agreed to do so as the result of a series of trial movements. As soon as his eyes were closed, he forgot his previous determination and said nothing. But, if he was told to imitate with one hand the direction of a passive movement made by me in the other, he usually responded correctly within normal limits.

Asked to compare two weights, placed on his hand one after the other, his answers were equally characteristic. He could not be persuaded to wait for the second application; as soon as 100 grms. rested on his palm he said, "That's heavy," and when it was followed by 70 grms. he added, "It's getting lighter." He did not express the relation in some such formula as "The first was heavier than the second."

When tested with the compasses, he would answer correctly for the first few applications and then remain silent or complain, "I forget what you told me to do." But our method of testing his power of localising the spot touched by indicating the situation on the hand of an assistant gave him no difficulty; each test was an isolated act of direct imitation.

Articulated speech. Articulation was perfect, words were produced without difficulty and the rhythm of the phrase was unaffected. His sole defect was shown in a tendency to forget the exact general intention of what he wanted to express. Sentences died away without reaching their formal conclusion.

He could name common objects correctly, except that he once spoke of a pencil as "pensum" and called a penny a "half-penny." In the same way he made no errors with the series of colours.

During these observations on articulated speech I tested him with the alphabet (vide infra) and then asked him to say the months of the year in sequence. He rattled them off up to May; then he paused and, beginning again with July, finished correctly with December. As he had omitted June I said to him, "Try again";

he immediately began to say the letters of the alphabet, remarking, "you told me to go right through the alphabet." I replied, "No, say the months of the year," and he then gave them in perfect order. This is another example of that peculiar inability to retain the intention of a command or the ultimate aim of an action so characteristic of this defect of language.

He had no difficulty in repeating single words or even phrases, provided they did not comprise many independent statements. Actual verbal reproduction might be perfect, but he tended to shorten the sentence by omitting some one or other of the facts. The first few phrases of a long paragraph might be repeated correctly; as the test proceeded he would lose touch and complain, "I didn't get that at all; I knew it as you were saying it and that's all."

Understanding of spoken words. On superficial examination he seemed to understand what was said to him and he chose all the common objects accurately to oral commands. He was not so exact in his choice of colours, although his errors usually took the form of selecting orange for red or violet for blue; once, however, he chose yellow for blue and black for white, and yet his colour-sense was undoubtedly normal. If, however, the words said by me contained some more complex order, as when setting the hands of a clock or carrying out the hand, eye and ear tests, he made many gross mistakes and the greatest defect appeared if he was asked to render the sense of some narrative statement communicated to him by word of mouth. After the first few remarks he would say, "I know there is some more to come, but I don't know what it is."

Reading. His difficulty lay not so much in understanding the meaning of a word or phrase, read silently to himself, as in comprehending the general significance of a group of statements. Thus, he chose common objects with ease to printed commands and made no gross errors in the selection of colours. The hands of the clock were ultimately set correctly in every instance and the hand, eye and ear tests were executed perfectly. Throughout all these observations the printed words remained in front of him for reference if he was in doubt, a fact which rendered the results better than those obtained with the more fleeting oral commands. But, when he attempted to read some story or series of consecutive sentences, he failed to comprehend the meaning and became confused. He complained, "I don't read a book because I can't remember it; as I read it I forget it."

His education had been restricted and many words used in books and newspapers were unfamiliar; this complicated all tests, which depended on reading aloud. He had no difficulty with the monosyllabic phrases of the man, cat and dog series and was able to read aloud correctly his own history, put together in simple printed words. But he failed badly with an extract, chosen by himself from the daily paper, which contained many expressions unknown to him in his normal condition.

Writing. He wrote his name and address rapidly and with ease and, when I told him to add that of his mother, he did so at once, saying, "That's the same."

The following letter was written spontaneously; handwriting and spelling were on the whole remarkably good: "London Hospital, Whitechapel, E. London. My Dear Mum and Father, Just a few lines to let you know that I am getting on alright and I shall will soon be home again. I must tell you that Uncle George and Aunt Ann cane (came) and see me yesterday and more so Bob Figgins so I am very Lucky for getting Friends. Now dear Mum I can't write a long letter yet but I will as," he then ceased, saying, "I can't pull it together very well, not yet."

He could translate any two pictures of the man, cat and dog series into cursive handwriting with ease and accuracy. But he had great difficulty in writing the names of common objects or of colours, when they were shown to him one by one; the words were badly spelt, although their nominal significance was correct. Thus pencil became "pecil," scissors "siccors," violet "wolet," and yellow "yewloo." Moreover, he tended to employ a curious letter half way between a cursive S and G. Shown the time on a clock, he wrote it down extremely badly; not only was he frequently wrong, but his handwriting deteriorated and at times became scarcely legible. Even when he was allowed to tell the time aloud, which he did accurately, he reproduced it just as badly in writing.

He could copy single words, or the simple phrases of the man, cat and dog tests, with ease and certainty transcribing the printed characters into cursive script without hesitation. With a more difficult task, such as the story of his life, he was equally successful and his handwriting was excellent; he held the copy in his left hand, wrote five or six words correctly and then consulted it again. He did not keep his eyes fixed slavishly upon it, whilst copying letter by letter.

On the other hand, when writing to dictation, he tended to shorten the sentence, to omit some part of its content, and to substitute words, which differed from those said by me. Thus the phrases of the man, cat and dog tests were well written and spelt, but he frequently failed to reproduce the correct pair of nouns; for instance, when I dictated the cat and the man, he wrote "the cat and the dog."

The alphabet. All the letters were perfectly pronounced, intonation was normal and the sequence correct. He tended, however, to run them off in groups, each of which was said with great rapidity as if he was afraid of forgetting how to continue, and between each series he occasionally dropped out a letter such as G and V.

Asked to write the alphabet he did so correctly, but looked back upon the result with doubt, although it was accurate. After writing T, he made a U, but said "It's supposed to be a V"; in spite of this remark he gave it the tail of a Y; he was much puzzled with how to form an X and ultimately constructed it correctly out of two crescents placed back to back.

He wrote correctly to dictation, but reversed the order of W and V.

A printed paragraph. I handed him the following simple history of his life before the war and told him to read it to himself silently. "My name is Charles H...and I live at Laurel Cottage, Pilley. Before I joined the army I worked for Miss D...

for nearly two years, I worked in the garden and looked after the pony. He was a forest pony, bay with a dark mane and tail."

Asked what he had gathered from his reading, he wrote, "I was worked for Mis D...and looked after a pony and Trap," adding, "That's all I remember."

I then made him read the story aloud; this he did with some little hesitation. But on attempting to reproduce what he remembered, he wrote, "I worked for Miss D...and I looked after a pony and trap and hilped in the garden," adding, "There's some more, but I don't know what it is."

He copied the account perfectly in perfect script; the handwriting was greatly improved and the spelling accurate. But, as soon as he attempted to reproduce the contents, his handwriting again deteriorated and he omitted many of the salient points. He wrote, "My name is Charles H...of Laurel Cottage. Pilley. nr (near) Lymington. Hants. and I worked for Miss D...and looked after a pony and trap and helped in the garden." After reading it over he said, "I don't think that's all. I haven't got the colour of his mane and tail; but I can't think of it to write it."

I read the story to him aloud sentence by sentence and he repeated each one after me. As far as his actual words were concerned, pronunciation and intonation were perfect; but he tended to shorten each phrase by omitting some detail. For instance, he left out "for nearly two years" at the end of the second sentence, saying, "I haven't got all of it," and the final one became, "He was a forest pony with dark mane and tail."

These faults were profoundly exaggerated, when he selected some printed paragraph from the newspaper containing many words that he did not fully understand. He would read it through with apparent interest, but was usually unable to reproduce much more than the catch-penny title which had arrested his attention.

Comprehension of the significance of a picture and its legend. He chose from a newspaper the picture of a man riding a cow over which stood the legend "Mayor's Curious Steed." After looking at it for some time he said, "That's a man riding on a colt...no, it isn't, sir, it looks more like a cow...or a young cow...no it isn't... heifer, sir." After he had read the legend I asked, "Who is the man?" and he replied, "A farmer, sir. No, Major...no, the Mayor curse sted...the Mayor curious stid. It's something you don't see every day...that stid...something very uncommon that animal. It's in a horse's place instead of where it is. I should think myself they are going to show that animal; it's uncommon, that stid, more so to see a man riding on it...You don't often see a man riding on a stid." When I asked, "What is a stid?" he replied, "It's something the same family as a cow."

Numbers and arithmetic. He counted perfectly up to the seventies or eighties; then he grew slower and occasionally dropped out a number, that should have come between the last of one group and the first of that which followed it. He would recognise that there had been some mistake, but made no attempt to correct it;

he seemed to have an idea that something was wrong without particular knowledge of where his error lay.

He was given the following sums in simple addition:

134	158	265
423	327	456
557	483 (wrong)	521 (wrong)

He then subtracted:

678	546	621
352	328	267
326	218	255 (wrong)

But after each of the two last subtraction sums he said, "I think I'm a little bit wrong; I didn't stop long enough to see it," although the answer to one of them was perfectly correct. It was obvious that he had some idea of rightness and wrongness apart from the actual condition of the answer.

Coins and their relative value. He had no difficulty in naming any coin or bank-note placed before him. But, when any two of them were laid on the table, he was frequently unable to express their relative value.

A sixpence and a two-shilling piece—"Two, I mean four."
A shilling and ten-shilling piece—"Ten."
A sixpence and a sovereign—"That's too much of a puzzle for me."
A sixpence and a ten-shilling piece—"I'll be able to tell you in a minute. I'm not good enough yet; I shall be in time."
A sixpence and a two-shilling piece—"Four."
A two-shilling piece and a ten-shilling piece—"Three. No, that would only make six shillings of it."
A two-shilling piece and a sovereign—"Ten."
A shilling and a sovereign—"Twenty."
A two-shilling piece and a ten-shilling piece—"I can't reckon up."
A shilling and a ten-shilling piece—"Ten."
A two-shilling piece and a ten-shilling piece—"Six."
A two-shilling piece and a sovereign—"Ten."
A sixpence and a two-shilling piece—"Four."
A sixpence and a ten-shilling piece—"That's too much of a puzzle. I don't think I can manage it; I shall in time."

Drawing. He drew the rough outline of a jug placed before him and reproduced it almost exactly, when the model was removed, adding, "I can see the picture in my mind, what I've drawn."

Told to draw an elephant he failed utterly and complained, "No, I've got it all wrong. I was going to try for an elephant, but I lost it somehow." After he had tried once more, again unsuccessfully, he said, "I think I've got two legs instead of four. Have I got the tusk? Have I got the tail? I've got the ears, haven't I? Yes, that's all."

Orientation. I took him into my room and asked him to point out the situation of the various objects he could see from his bed in the large ward. He indicated correctly the neighbouring beds, the door and the window behind his head; but he placed the bathroom wrongly and asserted that there was another window at the foot of his bed.

When I asked him to draw a plan of these things in relation to himself as he lay in bed, he was completely inaccurate, although he numbered the beds correctly, starting from his own. He said, "I can see all in my mind, but I can't put it down. I've got all in a picture in front of me," waving his hand in front of his eyes.

He described the situation of his next door neighbour's wounds and said that the Sister of the ward was "in a blue dress and I don't know what you call it, but a cap with a tail on behind it"; this was correct. I then asked how a Nurse was dressed; he replied, "Oh! yes, I know the difference between the Nurse and the Sister by the dress; Sister blue; Nurse, oh! I get muddled, just ordinary Nurse's clothes, white, blue..."

Serial Tests.

(1) *Naming and recognition of common objects.*

Table 1.

	Pointing to object shown	Oral commands	Printed commands	Duplicate in hand out of sight	Naming	Writing the name of an object indicated
Key	Correct	Correct	Correct	Correct	Correct	Peny
Pencil	,,	,,	,,	,,	"Pen...pensum"	Correct
Knife	,,	,,	,,	,,	Correct	,,
Penny	,,	,,	,,	,,	"Halfpenny"	,,
Match box	,,	,,	,,	,,	Correct	,,
Scissors	,,	,,	,,	,,	,,	Siccors
Penny	,,	,,	,,	,,	,,	Correct
Match box	,,	,,	,,	,,	,,	,,
Pencil	,,	,,	,,	,,	,,	pecil
Key	,,	,,	,,	,,	"Kay...key"	Chain
Scissors	,,	,,	,,	,,	Correct	Siccors
Knife	,,	,,	,,	,,	,,	Correct
Pencil	,,	,,	,,	,,	,,	pecil
Match box	,,	,,	,,	,,	,,	Correct
Knife	,,	,,	,,	,,	,,	,,
Key	,,	,,	,,	,,	"Kay"	Kiy
Penny	,,	,,	,,	,,	Correct	Correct
Scissors	,,	,,	,,	,,	,,	Sissors

From amongst a set of objects on the table he had no difficulty in selecting the one shown to him or placed in his hand out of sight. He also chose rapidly and with confidence to oral and printed commands.

His attempts at naming were sufficiently accurate to show that there was no loss of nominal capacity and he did not fall back on descriptive similitudes in order to communicate his meaning.

The words he wrote silently were badly spelt, and the handwriting was poor, but each one corresponded distinctly to the name of the object shown to him. For key he once wrote "chain," because a short chain was attached to the key he had actually seen.

(2) *Naming and recognition of colours.*

Table 2.

	Pointing to colour shown	Oral commands	Printed commands	Naming	Writing name of colour indicated	Printed command read aloud and executed		Copied from print
						He read	He chose	
Red	Correct	Orange	Correct	Correct	Correct	Correctly	Correctly	Correct
White	,,	Correct	,,	,,	,,	,,	,,	,,
Blue	,,	Yellow	Violet	,,	Bule	,,	Violet	,,
Black	,,	Correct	Correct	,,	Correct	,,	Correctly	,,
Orange	,,	Yellow	Yellow	,,	Salmon	,,	Yellow	,,
Violet	,,	Correct	Correct	"Blue"	Wolet	,,	Correctly	,,
Yellow	,,	,,	,,	Correct	Yewloo	,,	,,	,,
Green	,,	,,	,,	,,	Green	,,	,,	,,
Red	,,	,,	,,	,,	"I can't remember"	,,	,,	,,
White	,,	,,	,,	,,	Correct	,,	,,	,,
Blue	,,	Violet	Violet	,,	,,	,,	,,	,,
Black	,,	Correct	Correct	,,	,,	,,	,,	,,
Orange	,,	Yellow	Yellow	,,	,,	,,	Yellow; corrected	,,
Violet	,,	Correct	Correct	,,	Mauve	,,	Blue	,,
Yellow	,,	,,	,,	,,	Correct	,,	Correctly	,,
Green	,,	,,	,,	,,	Green	,,	,,	,,
Blue	,,	Violet	,,	,,	Correct	,,	,,	,,
Red	,,	Correct	,,	,,	,,	,,	,,	,,
Black	,,	,,	,,	,,	,,	,,	,,	,,
Green	,,	,,	,,	,,	,,	,,	,,	,,
Orange	,,	Yellow; corrected	Yellow	,,	,,	,,	Yellow	,,
Violet	,,	Correct	Correct	,,	Maved	,,	Correctly	,,
Yellow	,,	,,	,,	,,	Correct	,,	,,	,,
White	,,	Black	,,	,,	,,	,,	,,	,,

In every instance he was able to select from the colours on the table one corresponding to that he had been shown. He was much less accurate to oral and printed commands, although most of the errors were comparatively trivial, such as selecting yellow for orange and violet for blue. To oral command, however, he once chose yellow for blue and black for white; but, when the names were presented in print, serious mistakes of this kind did not occur, for he was able to look back if in doubt to the card in front of him.

On the whole he named all the colours correctly, but wrote and spelt the words badly. For the first letter of "Green" he employed a curious symbol half way between a cursive S and a G (S). He complained, "I get muddled up sometimes; I don't remember them sometimes." But all the words were copied perfectly in cursive script.

Although he read the printed names aloud without a single mistake, the choice he made was frequently erroneous, corresponding more or less to that which resulted from reading the words silently to himself.

Finally, I asked him to write down a list of the colours I had used in these tests; he made the following list, "blue, green, yellow, violet, white, black, salmon, mauve, red." All these names were perfectly spelt and the handwriting was better than when they were written to designate a colour shown to him. It is interesting to notice that he included both violet and mauve, words used indiscriminately by him for the same object.

(3) *The man, cat and dog tests.*

Table 3.

	Reading aloud	Reading from pictures	Writing from pictures	Writing from dictation	Reading aloud from print and writing what he had read		Copying from print
					He read	He wrote	
The cat and the man	Correct	Correct	Correct	The cat and the dog	Correctly	man cat	Correct
The man and the dog	"Man and the dog"	"The dog and the man; no, we'll have it the other way"	,,	The man and the cat	,,	Correctly	,,
The cat and the dog	"Cat and the dog"	Correct	,,	Correct	,,	the dog and the cat	,,
The man and the cat	"Man and cat"	,,	,,	The man and the dog	,,	the cat and the dog	,,
The dog and the man	Correct	,,	,,	Correct	,,	the dog and the cat	,,
The dog and the cat	,,	,,	,,	The cat and the dog	,,	Correctly	,,
The cat and the man	,,	,,	,,	The cat and the dog	,,	the cat and the dog	,,
The man and the dog	,,	,,	,,	The dog and the man	,,	Correctly	,,
The cat and the dog	,,	,,	,,	Correct	,,	,,	,,
The man and the cat	,,	,,	,,	,,	,,	and the cat and the man	,,
The dog and the man	,,	,,	,,	,,	,,	and the dog and the cat	,,
The dog and the cat	,,	,,	,,	,,	,,	and the dog and the cat	,,

All these simple phrases were read aloud correctly and he reproduced with ease the content of any pair of pictures, both by word of mouth or in writing. But, when the words were dictated to him, he became inaccurate, frequently substituting one noun for another in the combination. In the same way, if he was allowed to read them aloud, he did so perfectly; but, on attempting to write down what he had just said, he failed exactly as if the words had been dictated by me. Yet he copied all the phrases accurately from print in cursive handwriting.

(4) *The clock tests.*

Table 4.

	Direct imitation	Telling the time	Clock set to oral commands	Clock set to printed commands	Writing down the time shown on a clock	Telling the time and then writing it down	
						He said	He wrote
A quarter to 12	Correct	Correct	11.40	Correct	a quatr	Correctly	Quater to twelve
10 minutes to 1	,,	,,	1.30	,,	tin mintues to 1	,,	Correctly
20 minutes to 6	,,	,,	Correct	,,	Correct	,,	20 minites to 6 o'clock
10 minutes past 7	,,	,,	7.30	,,	tin minites past 7	,,	ten minutes past 6 o'clock
20 minutes past 4	,,	,,	Correct	,,	20 two, 20 minutes to 6	,,	20 minute past Six o'clock
half-past 1	,,	,,	12.30	,,	half past 6 o'clock	,,	half past 12 o'clock
5 minutes past 8	,,	,,	7.55	,,	Five minutes past 6	,,	five minutes past 6 o'clock
5 minutes to 2	,,	,,	12.5	1.5; then 2; then corrected	Five minute past 6 o'clock	,,	five minutes six
20 minutes past 9	,,	,,	8.40	8.40; corrected	20 minites past 9 o'clock	,,	20 minutes past 6
Half-past 2	,,	,,	Correct	Correct	1½ past	,,	½ past 2 o'clock
10 minutes past 8	,,	,,	7.50	,,	10 minuites past 8 o'clock	,,	ten minutes past 8 o'clock
A quarter to 9	,,	,,	Correct	8.40; corrected	¼ to 9 o'clock	,,	quater to... "eleven, but I've forgotten how to write it"
25 minutes to 3	,,	,,	"I didn't catch that"; 3.40; "No, that's wrong"	Correct	five and twenty	,,	20 mintues to 3 o'clock
20 minutes past 11	,,	,,	11.10	10.40; corrected	20 nintues past eleven	,,	20 minites past (undecipherable)
20 minutes to 6	,,	,,	Correct	Correct	20 mintues to six o'clock	,,	Correctly

He succeeded in setting the hands of a clock in direct imitation of one placed before him; but his actions were slow and he was obliged to keep his eyes fixed on the model. If he looked away, he forgot what he intended to do and became confused.

Oral commands evidently puzzled him and the results were inaccurate; amongst other errors he mistook "to" and "past" the hour. He succeeded somewhat better when the order was given in print, for he could look back at the card when in doubt.

He told the time perfectly and without hesitation. If, however, he attempted to write down what he had just said, he made many errors and he failed in the same way to record in writing the time shown on a clock set by me, even when he was not allowed to speak.

(5) *The hand, eye and ear tests.*

Asked to imitate my movements, sitting face to face, he failed grossly, but made one mistake only, when they were reflected in the glass. If the order was presented in a pictorial form, three quarters of the answers were wrong. These errors were greatly reduced in number, if the picture was seen in the mirror; but, even under these conditions, he tended to become puzzled and confused, unlike most patients suffering from other forms of defect of language.

Printed commands were carried out rapidly and with ease, but he made several mistakes to orders given by word of mouth. If he was permitted to read them aloud he succeeded somewhat better, although his actions did not always correspond to the words he said.

Table 5.

	Imitation of movements made by the observer	Imitation of movements reflected in a mirror	Pictorial commands	Pictorial commands reflected in a mirror	Oral commands	Printed commands	Reading aloud and executing printed commands: He read	Reading aloud and executing printed commands: Movement executed
R. hand to R. eye	Reversed	Correct	Correct; very slow	Correct	Correct	Correct	Correctly	Correct
L. hand to L. ear	Correct	,,	Reversed	R. hand to L. ear	,,	,,	"L. hand to L. eye"; corrected	,,
R. hand to L. eye	Reversed	,,	Correct	Correct	R. hand to R. eye	,,	Correctly	L. hand to L. eye
L. hand to R. ear	L. hand to L. ear	,,	Reversed	R. hand to R. ear	R. hand to L. *eye*	,,	"L. hand to R. eye"; corrected	L. hand to R. *eye*
L. hand to L. eye	Correct	,,	,,	Reversed	Correct	,,	Correctly	L. hand to R. eye
R. hand to R. ear	Reversed	,,	R. hand to L. ear; then L. hand to L. ear	Correct	,,	,,	,,	Correct
R. hand to L. ear	,,	,,	Reversed	,,	R. hand to R. ear	,,	,,	,,
L. hand to R. eye	L. hand to L. eye	,,	,,	,,	Reversed	,,	,,	,,
R. hand to R. eye	Correct	,,	Correct	,,	Correct	,,	,,	,,
L. hand to L. ear	Reversed	L. hand to R. *eye*	Reversed	R. hand to L. ear	R. hand to L. ear	,,	,,	,,
R. hand to L. eye	R. hand to R. eye	Correct	Reversed; then L. hand to L. eye	Correct	R. hand to R. eye	,,	,,	R. hand to R. eye
L. hand to R. ear	Correct	,,	Reversed	,,	Correct	,,	,,	Correct
L. hand to L. eye	,,	,,	,,	R. hand to L. eye	,,	,,	,,	,,
R. hand to R. ear	Reversed	,,	,,	Correct	R. hand to L. ear	,,	,,	,,
R. hand to L. ear	,,	,,	,,	,,	R. hand to R. ear	,,	,,	,,
L. hand to R. eye	R. hand to R. eye	,,	Correct	Reversed	L. hand to L. eye	,,	,,	,,

No. 6

A case of Verbal Aphasia, due to a gun-shot injury over the anterior portion of the left precentral gyrus, extending downwards on to the inferior frontal convolution.

There were no abnormal signs in the nervous system, except a transitory weakness of the right half of the lower portion of the face and some deviation of the tongue to the right. All the reflexes, including the abdominals and plantars, were normal. There was no affection of motion or sensation and the visual fields were not diminished.

When admitted to the London Hospital four days after he was wounded, he was speechless, but he soon began to say a few badly articulated words. He could neither say his name spontaneously nor repeat it after me. His power of finding words rapidly improved and throughout it was verbal structure and not nomenclature that formed his main difficulty. He could understand what was said to him and commands exacting a single choice were carried out accurately; but, as soon as two of these orders were combined, his response became slow and hesitating. His comprehension of printed phrases was obviously defective. Although he rapidly recovered the power of writing his name and address correctly, he could not write that of his mother with whom he lived. He was unable to count, but wrote the numbers up to twenty-one. He drew well spontaneously or to command.

Five months afterwards, he still had great difficulty in verbalisation. The words were badly formed and evoked with difficulty, although they corresponded in nominal significance to what he wanted to say. He did not employ wrong words and his power of naming was perfectly preserved. Asked to repeat what was said to him, the verbal content was accurately reproduced, but the words were badly pronounced. He now understood all that was said to him and carried out oral commands slowly but without mistakes. His power of comprehending the meaning of what he read to himself was undoubtedly good and he executed printed commands with several corrections, though few actual errors. As soon as he was permitted to read them aloud, his responses became perfect, for the sound of the words formed a self-given oral command. He could express himself in writing, but the form of the words was defective, tending to show the same faults as articulated speech. This was also the case when he wrote to dictation. He neither said nor wrote the alphabet correctly and was unable to place the block-letters in due order. He failed to solve simple arithmetical problems but played an excellent game of dominoes.

Seven years and eight months after he was wounded, he had regained his power of carrying out all the serial tests, except that his spelling was faulty; but he still remained a typical example of Verbal Aphasia. He hesitated in finding words to express his thoughts, the pauses were unduly frequent and prolonged, and enunciation was defective. He could read aloud intelligibly, but stumbled over the longer words and complained that, when reading to himself, he was obliged to go over the same passage twice before he could grasp its meaning. As he said the words to himself silently he was liable to mispronounce them and this confused him and destroyed his fluency. In the same way, although he could write an excellent letter unaided, he did so slowly. He still failed to say or write the alphabet perfectly and even hesitated in putting together the twenty-six block letters. But he could repeat the alphabet after me, read it aloud and write it correctly to dictation. He counted slowly without mistakes, though articulation was somewhat slurred. He succeeded in solving all the problems in arithmetic, except the most exacting of the subtraction sums. He had no difficulty with money. He drew excellently and produced a perfect ground-plan of the room in which we worked. He could play all games correctly, but with cards was somewhat slower than normal.

Private Thomas McB., aged 19, was wounded on March 12th, 1915. A piece of shrapnel struck him in the left temporal region, producing a long incised wound which penetrated the skull.

He did not become unconscious and remembers everything that happened. He was carried at once to a field ambulance, where no operation was performed. "At first," he said, "I couldn't speak at all...say oh!...only oh!"

He was admitted to the London Hospital on March 16th, 1915, and although he was not then under my care I was able to make a complete examination before his discharge on April 12th.

The wound, a suppurating cut like that of a knife, extended for 5 cm. almost vertically on the left side of the scalp. It penetrated all the tissues including the bone, and the dura mater could be seen laid bare in its deepest part. The upper end was about 5·5 cm. from the middle of the scalp, and 14 cm. back from the root of the nose. It lay 0·5 in front of the interaural line, whilst its extreme lowest point extended somewhat farther forwards (3 cm. in front). The whole nasion-inion measurement was 34·5, and this was intersected at 14·5 cm. by the interaural line. This wound closed rapidly and finally healed on April 12th (cf. Fig. 7, Vol. I, p. 445).

He was extremely bright and intelligent, amused at what went on around him and in no way emotional. He responded rapidly and well to commands.

He used his right hand in the normal manner and, on recovering his speech, asserted that he had always been strongly right-handed.

There were no convulsions or seizures and, although he suffered from a good deal of headache when first admitted, this passed away rapidly.

Vision was 5/15 in both the right and left eyes; but owing to his loss of speech this was difficult to test. The visual fields were in every way normal on perimetric examination. Hearing, smell and taste were intact.

The pupils reacted well and the eyes moved perfectly in all directions. The only abnormal signs were slightly defective movement of the lower half of the face on the right side and some deviation of the tongue to the right.

All the reflexes, including the abdominals and plantars, gave a normal response.

There was no paralysis, paresis, incoordination or difference in tone of the limbs on the two sides of the body.

Sensation was completely unaffected when tested within four weeks of the injury (April 7th). During these tests he showed his remarkable intelligence. When weights of 100 and 80 grm. were placed in succession on his right palm or fingers, he indicated correctly and without hesitation which was the heavier. Sometimes he said "erst" (first) or "hend" (second). If the heavier weight followed the lighter, he usually nodded his head and said "is" (this). Tested with the compass points he said "won" (one) and a guttural explosive sound, which I came to recognise as signifying two. Throughout the whole series he did not make a single mistake with the points at a distance of 1 cm. from one another. He was equally accurate with the vibration of a tuning fork, showing that no form of discriminative sensibility was affected.

Condition between March 16th and April 12th, 1915.

Symbolic Formulation and Expression.

At first he was speechless and silent, but shortly after his admission to the hospital he began to make articulate noises, which seemed to bear no obvious relation to the words he was striving to pronounce. Asked his name he said "Hō-nus," and told to repeat it after me, he again produced the same sound.

When a question put to him required an affirmative reply, he nodded, saying, "ep" or "ons"; on the other hand, to signify a negative he shook his head and uttered a nasal sound "ong," which closely approached a guttural rendering of "no."

His power of finding words rapidly improved, and less than a month after the date of the wound he could say the alphabet and days of the week, although both letters and words were extremely badly pronounced. An attempt to say the months of the year led to a series of incomprehensible sounds. When he repeated the alphabet, the days of the week, or the months, his pronunciation was equally defective.

He undoubtedly understood what was said to him, and commands demanding a single choice were carried out accurately. Thus, he had no difficulty in putting out his tongue, shutting his eyes, or giving his hand, when asked to do so. But, as soon as two of these orders were combined, his response became slow and hesitating, and he was liable to fall into error.

	Command.	*Movement executed.*
(1)	Give me your hand and put out your tongue	Correct
(2)	Shut your eyes and put out your tongue	Correct, but also gave the hand
(3)	Put out your tongue and give me your hand	Correct
(4)	Give me your hand and shut your eyes	Correct, but he opened his mouth though he did not protrude his tongue
(5)	Shut your eyes and put out your tongue	Correct
(6)	Give me your hand and shut your eyes	Correct
(7)	Put out your tongue and give me your hand	Correct
(8)	Give me your hand and put out your tongue	Correct
(9)	Give me your hand and shut your eyes	Correct; but lips were also parted
(10)	Shut your eyes and put out your tongue	Correct
(11)	Give me your hand and put out your tongue	Correct
(12)	Put out your tongue and give me your hand	Correct
(13)	Give me your hand and put out your tongue	Correct
(14)	Give me your hand and shut your eyes	Correct; but lips were also parted
(15)	Put out your tongue and give me your hand	Correct
(16)	Shut your eyes and put out your tongue	Correct

He could whistle perfectly any melody he happened to know, and sang "Tipperary" without the words in excellent time and tune. The musical phrases were superposed on many different articulated sounds, none of which were words; they consisted of various combinations of vowels and consonants, which might have been taken for words imperfectly heard.

Given a newspaper, he seemed as if he could read it, but his comprehension of printed phrases was obviously defective. He could reproduce accurately in writing the simple words of the man, cat and dog tests, after reading them silently, although the card was removed from his sight.

He could write his name and address correctly as "Thomas McBain, 44, Constable Street, Dundee"; but he directed a letter to his mother: "Mrs McBain, 44, Conbbse Street, Duddee." Thus he failed to write the same words correctly, if they were started in a less automatic manner.

I seated him at the window and asked him to write down what he saw, and he produced the following list: "Barrows, cars, shops, folowers (flowers), loan-office, artillery, four." The "loan-office" was a pawnbroker's shop, over which was the inscription "goldsmith and silversmith" and the usual three golden balls. Then some soldiers went by carrying their equipment; I asked how he knew they were artillery, and he pointed to his head in the position of the badge upon a military cap. "Four" was written as a funeral went by; but he could not explain himself further in writing, shook his head and gave up entirely.

Simple phrases were written badly to dictation, and he frequently failed to finish the sentence. He did not write wrong words; it was their formation that was faulty. He could, however, transcribe print into cursive handwriting.

Asked to count aloud, he began: "Ong, nud, ed, hon," and then stopped; but taking a pencil into his hand he rapidly wrote all the numbers up to twenty-one correctly.

He was particularly good at drawing, both spontaneously and to command. Asked to name the geometrical figures, he drew them rapidly, and occasionally appended some word such as "square," "ovel," or "marble," to represent the cube, ovoid and sphere.

He had no difficulty in finding his way, and there was no reason to suspect any defect of orientation.

CONDITION IN OCTOBER 1915 (*seven months after the injury*).

He was in excellent general health. The wound was a longitudinal painless scar with a deep fissure in the centre extending through the skull. No pulsation could be felt, and he did not suffer from headache or other local symptoms. There were no abnormal physical signs; even the lagging of the lower half of face on the right side and the slight deviation of the tongue had passed away.

He was extremely bright and intelligent. He could give a good account of what he wanted to express, in spite of his defective speech, and I was able to carry out a more exacting series of tests than was possible during the acute and severe stage of his disorder.

Articulated speech. He talked slowly, and had evident difficulty in forming his words. The phrases, and even the longer words, were split up into groups of syllables separated by pauses. He explained to me as follows the meaning of a picture selected from one of the illustrated papers: "It's the...North...um-land ...Fūs-leers...fighting fifth...met attack...on their first line of trenches" (How the Northumberland Fusiliers, the Fighting Fifth, met an attack on their first line trenches). In attempting to describe his condition on first entering the hospital he said: "When I come...I knew what you said...wanted answer back...knew what...couldn't get speshe right."

He did not employ wrong words, and his power of naming was perfectly preserved, although verbal structure was defective.

He did not change the content or significance of words or phrases he was asked to repeat; the words, however, were badly pronounced.

Understanding of spoken words. He could understand all that was said to him, selecting common objects and setting the clock correctly to oral commands. He was also able to carry out the hand, eye, and ear tests slowly, but without mistakes, when the order was given in spoken words.

Reading. He undoubtedly understood what he read silently and gave an excellent account of the information conveyed in a paragraph chosen from the newspaper. He selected the following: "The period of grace given to Bulgaria by

Russia in her ultimatum requiring Bulgaria to break with Germany and dismiss her German officers appears to have expired, but no reply had become known late last evening. In the meantime the Allies' proposals to hold a portion of Greek and Serbian Macedonia in trust for Bulgaria have lapsed as no answer has been returned to them." After reading this through to himself he said: "There was a message...sent from Russia to Bulgaria...to clear...out...all the German officers...art their country...They've got no response...to their message...so it means...the claration of war by the Ollies."

Writing. He now wrote well but the form of the words tended to show the same faults as those of articulated speech. Thus, the months written spontaneously became "Junuray, Febury, March, april, june, July, august, september, Otuober, november, december."

He could write down the movements I made when sitting opposite to him, although he complained that "It takes a lot of thinking."

Asked to write down the meaning of the passage he had read to himself (vide supra) on the ultimatum to Bulgaria, he produced the following account: "Russia sent a message to Bulgaria telling them to clear out all the german Officers out their country, but they got no response to their message, so that means the declaration of war by the Allies."

The same paragraph was then dictated and he wrote as follows, very slowly and with great effort: "the period of grace given to Bulgari by Russia in her altimatum requiring Bulgaria to break with Germany, and dismiss her German Officers apperes to have expired but no reply had become known leate last evening." He made several corrections which were all in the right direction.

The alphabet. Asked to say the alphabet, many of the letters, though recognisable, were grossly mispronounced. The first half was given in the correct order but he ended: "p q e u s t v double v x y and z." He said, "I don't know whether n comes before them" (the m), although he had placed it correctly.

He wrote the alphabet spontaneously in the following sequence, sometimes in capitals and sometimes in small cursive letters. *A b C d E F G H I J k l n m o p Q u r s t v w x y z.*

He was then given block letters and told to construct an alphabet from them. He quickly put together the first eleven in sequence and continued L N M O P Q W V W; he then removed V W, replacing them by R S T, so that the sequence ran P Q U R S T V W Z Y. After pondering over this for a time and shifting the last four letters, he produced A B C D E F G H I J K L N M O P Q U R S T V W X Y Z.

Thus obviously more than articulation was at fault in this case. Internal verbalisation, necessary for the production of a perfect alphabetical series, had also suffered; and indeed, when asked to think of the alphabet, most persons say the letters to themselves silently.

Arithmetic. He was an intelligent young Scotchman, who told me he had reached the fifth standard at 13 years of age, and said, "I was...pretty good... sums." But he failed to solve correctly the third addition and all the subtraction sums.

Addition.

123	356	287
243	235	376
366	591	653 (wrong)

Subtraction.

568	862	621
234	546	258
302 (wrong)	311 (wrong)	313 (wrong)

Games. He played an excellent game of dominoes and corrected me when I was wrong; he never hesitated or made a mistake.

Serial Tests.

(1) *Naming and recognition of common objects.* He had no difficulty in pointing to the object shown to him, named orally and in print, or placed in his hand out of sight. Asked to give their names he answered slowly but correctly although the words were poorly pronounced; he complained: "That's very slow, though I can make people understand what I mean." Each word could be repeated, but here his articulation showed the same kind of faults as voluntary speech. Told to write the names, as each object was shown to him, he wrote as follows: "knife, key, pencile, sissiors, matches, penny, sissiors, key, knife, penny, matches, pincile, sissiors, matches, key, pincile, knife, penny." He added: "How is it about scissors? ...Only time I write...write home...very difficult...still gittin better...every day."

(2) *Naming and recognition of colours.* He chose the colour shown to him, named orally or in print, without the slightest difficulty. Told to name the colours one by one, his nomenclature was perfect, but violet was liable to be called "voilet" and orange "orage." Except "voilet" they were written correctly, but very slowly. He explained "Slow in writing...I think I'm right...In Lon-on Hospedl I couldn't spell...my own name." This alludes to his previous stay in the hospital, when his power of writing was very defective.

(3) *The man, cat and dog tests.* He could read these sentences aloud from print, and both read and wrote correctly from pictures. He reproduced the different phrases exactly to dictation, and throughout these tests showed no hesitation. The difficulty was solely one of pronunciation.

(4) *The clock tests.* He had no difficulty in setting the hands in imitation and to oral or printed commands. He told the time slowly but correctly, pausing between each word. Many were badly pronounced; he spoke of "er-levn" (eleven), minutes became "mints," but he always employed the common nomenclature. When he wrote down the time, without saying it aloud, he made one mistake, which he ultimately corrected after two attempts; he wrote first 20 to 2 (for 8.20), then 20 to 8 and finally said, "That's wrong, ten past eight." He usually wrote in numbers, but never used railway time. He had evident difficulty in retaining the words in his memory and repeatedly looked back at the clock during the act of writing.

(5) *The hand, eye and ear tests.*

Table 1.

	Imitation of movements made by the observer	Imitation of movements reflected in a mirror	Pictorial commands	Pictorial commands reflected in a mirror	Oral commands	Printed commands (silently)	Reading aloud and executing printed commands: He said	Reading aloud and executing printed commands: Movements executed	Writing down movements made by the observer
L. hand to L. ear	Correct	Correct	Slow; correct	Correct	Correct	Correct	Correctly	Correct	Correct
R. hand to R. eye	,,	,,	Reversed	,,	,,	,,	,,	,,	,,
L. hand to R. ear	R. hand; then correct	,,	Correct	,,	,,	,,	,,	,,	L. hand to R. *eye*
R. hand to R. ear	Correct	,,	,,	,,	,,	R. hand to L. ear	,,	,,	Correct
R. hand to L. eye	,,	,,	,,	,,	,,	Slow; correct	,,	,,	,,
L. hand to R. eye	R. hand; then correct	,,	,,	,,	,,	R. hand; then correct	,,	,,	,,
R. hand to L. ear	Correct	,,	,,	,,	,,	Correct	,,	,,	,,
L. hand to L. eye	Reversed	,,	R. hand; then correct	,,	,,	L. hand to R. eye; then correct	,,	,,	,,
L. hand to R. ear	Correct	,,	Correct	,,	,,	Correct	,,	,,	,,
R. hand to L. eye	,,	,,	,,	,,	,,	,,	,,	,,	Very slow; correct
L. hand to L. ear	,,	,,	,,	,,	,,	Slow; correct	,,	,,	Correct
R. hand to R. eye	,,	,,	R. hand to R. *ear*	,,	,,	R. hand to L. eye	,,	,,	,,
R. hand to L. ear	,,		Correct	,,	,,	Correct	,,	,,	,,
L. hand to R. ear	,,		L. hand to R. *eye*	,,	,,	,,	,,	,,	,,
L. hand to R. eye	R. hand; then correct		Correct	,,	,,	,,	,,	,,	,,

When he attempted to imitate my movements sitting face to face, or when carrying out pictorial commands, he made several errors; but as soon as either my hands or the pictures were reflected in the mirror, he had not a moment's hesitation in performing the desired actions correctly. He said, "Do 'em right...you at back of me." He was somewhat slower in executing oral commands and made several errors in answer to printed phrases read silently. But, when he was permitted to say them aloud, all his answers became correct and he explained, "All the time I'm telling myself what to do." He wrote down my movements sitting face to face with one mistake only; but he said, "It takes a lot of thinking."

On the conclusion of these tests he explained, "I do the think...I think about it...after-wds...to see right or wrong...often try to make it right...it's gone...most cases...Afterwards...when I think about the thing...I've got to spell the word...every letter."

CONDITION IN NOVEMBER 1922 (*seven years and eight months after he was wounded*).

The wound was represented by a firm scar running somewhat obliquely upwards in the left temporal region; the opening in the bone, just over 3 cm. in length and 0·75 cm. in breadth, formed a long gutter-shaped slit, exactly as if it had been cut away with a gouge. It did not pulsate, and throughout the period of five days during which he was under observation the scalp was not tender and he was free from headache. He could lift bales of cotton and stoop to do up his boots without discomfort; but violent changes in posture, and the intellectual effort of reading, were liable to produce pain over the forehead, particularly on the left side, associated with tenderness in the neighbourhood of the wound.

He had not suffered from any form of fits or seizures and was free from nausea or vomiting. On examination I could find no signs whatever pointing to any abnormality in the central nervous system. Face and tongue moved well, the reflexes were normal and there was no paresis, or affection of even the highest forms of sensibility.

His general condition was excellent and he was in full work as an unskilled labourer. His intelligence was extremely good; willing and anxious to help, he was easy to examine and his answers often showed remarkable powers of introspection.

Communication with his fellows was hampered by his difficulties of speech and this tended to make him reticent, except with those who took the trouble to understand him. On this he laid great stress; for, when people did not grasp what he said, he was liable to become confused. "It seems this has left me more simple-like than I should be...There seems to be some weak part about me that I can't understand...I don't seem to be like the other men...I can't seem to go and be hearty...I go quietly...I enjoy myself, when I go quietly."

Articulated speech. He talked slowly and with obvious difficulty; the words, especially the longer ones, were badly formed. When he pronounced a word badly, he went back over it again, recognising that it was wrong; but his efforts to correct it frequently ended in confusion. He did not omit or seek to avoid some difficult word required to express his thoughts, but made an attempt to employ it and, if he failed, would try until he either succeeded or became confused. He spoke in a sing-song manner, breaking up his sentences into short blocks of words; but their grammatical sequence was usually perfect and he showed no tendency to omit conjunctions, prepositions and articles. For instance, "My mother says...I moan terribly...when I sleep." The rhythm was, however, disturbed, because his phrases were broken up into abnormally short groups of words in consequence of difficulty in verbal expression.

He repeated accurately single words, such as the names of familiar objects, colours, or the days of the week, and found no difficulty with the simple phrases of the man, cat and dog tests. But articulation and rhythm were affected in exactly the same manner as with voluntary speech, though to a somewhat less degree.

Understanding of spoken words. There could not be the slightest doubt that he comprehended the meaning of simple language. Thus he said, "I quite understand what they say...It's difficult sometimes...I can't exactly explain...At home ...on important business...I always have someone with me...They don't understand me...I don't understand them if they speak too quick for my thinking. ...It's quite alright if one understands you...but if I've got to explain my position ...I'm fixed."

Orders given by word of mouth, even the complex hand, eye and ear tests, were quickly and accurately executed.

Reading. He read little to himself and, when I asked for the reason, replied, "I've no desire to...I need to read the same thing over twice...before I could explain...what I've been reading about." All printed commands were, however, carried out perfectly.

Writing. He could now write an excellent letter, provided he was allowed "plenty of time." The only defects appeared as occasional doubt with regard to the position of the letters in some word, often of the simplest character.

The alphabet. In spite of the fact that his only faults appeared to be articulatory, he failed to say the alphabet spontaneously. He gave the letters correctly up to L, then paused and continued, "N M O P Q V...wrong there...Q R S T E W X Y Z."

He repeated the whole series correctly after me and read them somewhat slowly from print, adding, "It's the Q's and U's I get mixed up."

Asked to write the alphabet, he produced with obvious difficulty an accurate sequence up to *p*; then he continued, *q u v w x y z*. On a second attempt he wrote *q u r s t v w x y z*, adding "That's hard." All the letters were written perfectly to dictation; but, when transcribing capitals into cursive script, he made two mistakes, which he finally corrected.

Given the twenty-six block letters he had difficulty in recognising the A because it was upside down; I reversed it and he at once started to put together A B C D E F G (upside down) H I J K L M N O P R S T U V W X Y. He then discovered the Q, and, after much hesitation, placed it correctly and added the Z. This, he said, was easier than writing, "because of course there is no spelling attached to it...Q's and U's mostly get mixed up."

A printed paragraph. I used for this series of tests the following short account of his own history: "I was a private in the 4th Battalion of the Black Watch, Royal Highlanders. I was trained in Dudup Castle, and went to France in February, 1915.

Nineteen days later I was wounded by the explosion of a shrapnel shell. Within a few days after being wounded I was taken to the London Hospital."

This he read silently and when asked what he had gathered, replied, "I've been a private in the 4th Black Watch and training at Dudup Castle. I went to France in 1915. I was wounded by the explosion of a shell nineteen days later. I was taken to the London Hospital. I don't forget that."

After again reading the paragraph through silently, he wrote, "I was a privat in the 4th Battalion royal highlanders and trained at Dudup castle. I went to France in February 1915 I was wounded, in a few days later I was taken to London Hospital." Then he said, "I've missed out some word, I think...I was wounded by the explosion of a shell...shap...shapnal...That's what I left out."

He read these sentences aloud from print as follows: "I was a private in the fourth Bē-taln of the Black Watch, Royal Highlanders...I was train in Dudup Castle, Dundee and went to France...in Feb-ūrie...1915...Nineteen days later ...I was wounded by an explosion of...a sher-ap-nel shell...Within a few days after...being wounded...I was taken to the London Ors-pedl." He added, "The words...seem to...stand still...I can't go further...as if I were in a deep thought...When I'm like that...I have to draw away my head from the print and look back again...By that time I may have lost my place...and have to start over again."

To dictation he wrote: "I was a privite in the 4th. Battalion of the Black Watch Royal Highlanders. I was trained in Dudup Castle Dundee and went to France in Feburary 1915 ninteen later I wounded by the expload of a s shell within a few days after being wounded I was taken to the London hospital." Then he wrote spontaneously in amplification of the sentence where he had failed, "ninten days later I was wounded by the esplocdion of a — shrapnel."

He then copied the whole paragraph correctly from print, adding, "That's a great piece of work for me doctor...It's the forgetting...I know what's to be done...and yet I can't do it...Just the same as your speaking to me...I understand what you say...but later on I would forget...quite a lot that you would be speaking about...I don't forget what I'm...talking about...It seems that words that are spoken...have a better impression...on my mind."

Finally I asked him to tell me what it was all about, and he replied, "About being a private in the Black Watch...and being nineteen days in France...I'm trained at Dudup Castle, Dundee...nineteen days in France...I was wounded... a few days after being wounded I was taken to the London Hospital...wounded by explosion of a shell...a shar-a-nel shell. I quite remember in France what I did...and then I don't remember any more...I knew the pre-dick-ment (predicament) I was in...I saw the flare of the shell...and I felt the burning sensation in my head...When I tried to speak...I'd no speech...The right thumb was dead...I couldn't feel with it for about three days."

Numbers and arithmetic. He counted slowly and deliberately without mistakes up to 100. Articulation was somewhat slurred, especially when he came to the seventies; he said "Seven-y-one" instead of seventy-one and "hun-dert two" for a hundred and two. All the numbers were written in sequence without error of any kind.

Given the following exercises in simple arithmetic, he failed to solve the last subtraction sum, saying, in conclusion, "The diff-ulty...I can hardly explain...it's the thinking...a kind of...hesitation...If I'd be getting plenty of time to do it... I'd be doing it perfectly...The num-mers (numbers)...you see I must move my lips...I had to say...different figures...and different methods...I must find the smallest of the words...because I can't speak much."

Addition.

123	356	287
243	235	376
366	591	663

Subtraction.

568	862	621
234	546	258
334	316 (corrected)	263 (wrong)

Coins and their relative value. All the pieces of money from a halfpenny to a pound note were named accurately, and their relative value was explained with ease. He experienced no difficulty with change and managed his money affairs with considerable ability; thus, he took his own ticket from Scotland with the money I sent him, and gave me an exact statement of his expenditure.

Drawing. He had no difficulty in drawing either from a model or from memory. He produced an excellent outline of an elephant, naming each salient part correctly as he filled it in.

Orientation and a ground-plan. He found his way with ease even in London and was entirely free from confusion with regard to the objects in a familiar room. He drew an excellent ground-plan, saying, "I just imagined...for a moment...I was in that room...I could see the room." I then asked, "Can you see the colour of the things in the room?" He replied, "The cupboards are white...the table where we were sitting was square...it was brown"; all of which statements were correct.

Games. He played a good game of draughts and was fond of cards; but he added, "I play in the slow style...I've got to think."

Serial Tests.

(1) *Naming and recognition of common objects* was performed accurately, but he said, "If I didn't pay strict attention I'd be wrong." All the names were written

correctly except scissors, which became "cissors" or "sissors," and he complained "That's the diff-ult (difficult) one." To dictation the words were somewhat better written, and he copied them correctly from print.

(2) He named and recognised *colours* perfectly, and carried out—

(3) The *man, cat, and dog tests* without difficulty.

(4) The *clock* was set to oral or printed commands given either in the usual nomenclature or in railway time, and he told the time correctly, though his articulation was somewhat defective; thus, five minutes past eight became "Fi min-uts pass eight," though in every case the hour was given without hesitation. Asked to write down the time, he found great difficulty in spelling minutes (written "munites," "ninutes," or sometimes correctly); but the hour was never in doubt.

(5) All the *hand, eye and ear tests* were now executed correctly. To oral and printed commands the movements were made with quickness and precision, but imitation face to face was carried out more slowly, and when executing pictorial orders he corrected himself on several occasions. He showed remarkable accuracy in writing down movements made by me, although he was slow and deliberate.

No. 7

A case of Nominal Aphasia, due to gun-shot injury of the brain within the limits of the left angular gyrus.

There were no signs pointing to gross injury of the deeper structures. He suffered from no convulsions or seizures. Vision was normal. Movements of face and tongue were unaffected and he showed no changes in motion or sensation. The reflexes, including the abdominals and plantars, were equal on the two sides.

When he first came under my care six weeks after he was wounded, he was so grossly aphasic that it was impossible to obtain from him any coherent information. The few words he uttered were, however, comprehensible, and, if he succeeded in producing a short phrase, the syntax was perfect and the syllables were touched off correctly. But he could not express himself either in speech or in writing, and had obvious difficulty in discovering a method of formulating his meaning. Throughout, the character of his disabilities remained the same, although he rapidly gained sufficient facility to allow of more extensive observations.

He then failed to say his name and address or the days of the week and the months correctly. He could not name familiar objects and colours and was unable to tell the time shown on the face of a clock. His power of repetition was gravely affected, though the sounds he uttered usually bore some remote resemblance to the words said by me.

He showed obvious defects in comprehending the significance of spoken words and phrases. Oral commands were badly executed; he chose common objects or colours after great hesitation, and frequently gave up the attempt altogether. He failed to set the hands of a clock, carried out the coin-bowl tests badly, and made many mistakes in the more complex choice between hand, eye and ear. Simpler commands of the same kind were performed with one exception correctly, showing that he still retained some power of appreciating verbal significance.

He had considerable difficulty in understanding the meaning of single words put before him in print and selected familiar objects and colours slowly with obvious effort. He set the clock badly to printed commands, confusing "past" and "to" the hour. In the same way he failed to place the proper coin into the right bowl and made many mistakes with the more complex hand, eye and ear tests. Even simple orders, such as "Shut your eyes," "Put out your tongue," were misunderstood when given in print.

Shown any two pictures of the man, cat and dog, he found difficulty in evoking the names correctly. If he attempted to read these monosyllabic phrases from print, the results were even worse and he struggled ineffectually to find the correct expressions. Asked to read aloud the orders of the coin-bowl test, he converted them all into numbers and "the second into the third" became "two into three"; but even this simplification did not materially improve his answers.

With great effort he succeeded in writing his name imperfectly, but he could not add his address and failed entirely to compose a letter. He was unable to write down the name of any of the colours shown to him and transcribed the time badly, although he employed numbers only. Writing to dictation was almost impossible; but he was able to copy correctly, using cursive script, interrupted occasionally by irrelevant capitals.

Asked to say the letters of the alphabet in order he was unable to go beyond H; he repeated them after me slowly with obvious effort, but read them aloud almost correctly. He was unable to write them spontaneously, had great difficulty when they were dictated, but could copy them in capitals.

He found it almost impossible to state the relative value of any two coins placed before him. Yet in spite of his confused replies, he undoubtedly recognised their monetary value, provided he was not compelled to express the relation of the one to the other in words; for he was able to put together the equivalent of any one of them from amongst a heap of money on the table.

Drawing to order was grossly affected. He drew an elephant without trunk, tusks, eye or ear, and was unable to produce a ground-plan of the ward in which he lay; and yet he could indicate one by one the position of the various objects visible from his bed.

He played dominoes and draughts slowly but correctly.

He could sing in perfect tune and time, provided he did not attempt to pronounce the words. Although a professional singer, he had never learnt to read musical notation and sang by ear.

Four years and nine months after he was wounded, his power to use all forms of language had improved profoundly; but, although he could speak, read and write, he remained as definite an example of Nominal Aphasia as before. He managed to execute correctly all the serial tasks in which he had previously failed. But his powers of speech were obviously defective and he confessed that he had difficulty in finding names and that this confused him. Although he could carry out oral and printed commands, closer examination showed that any test, which demanded prompt recognition or formulation of differences in meaning between two or more words or phrases, was performed slowly and with difficulty. Above all he found trouble in writing; spelling was defective and capitals were interspersed amongst ordinary cursive script in an arbitrary manner. But he wrote well to dictation and copied excellently. The alphabet showed the same kind of defects as before and he failed completely to place the twenty-six block letters in due order. He counted slowly but correctly and solved all but one of the simple arithmetical problems. He could name coins and state their relative value with some hesitation. He had recovered his power of drawing an elephant to command, but could not construct a ground-plan of the room in which we worked. Orientation was not affected. He could play draughts and billiards, but not card games. He sang well without words; as soon as he tried to add them he fell out of tune, the volume of his voice decreased and a bad tremolo made its appearance.

Gunner Aloysius McN., aged 22, was wounded in the head by a fragment of a high-explosive shell, on October 15, 1917. He was admitted on the same day to the 3rd Australian Casualty Clearing Station, where an operation was performed and the following notes made. "Shell wound of the left parietal bone. Large compound depressed fracture. Laceration of the dura. Protrusion of brain substance. Loose bits of bone were removed including the margins of the fracture, but no foreign body."

On October 18 he was admitted to No. 12 General Hospital, where he remained until November 23. The field card bore the following record of this period:

"October 29. Wound in the parietal region discharging pus profusely. Speech impaired.

"October 30. Disc edges are both less sharply outlined than at the previous examination, but no definite choking can be made out. Patient is more stuporous this morning and headache more pronounced and more sharply localised.

"November 1. Small operation to increase drainage. Anterior margin of the wound incised. Free discharge of pus began this morning. Almost complete recovery of use in the right arm. Speech also returned.

"November 3. Wound draining well. Speech improving. Talks a good deal; still unable to say certain words. Movements of the right arm good, but there is still some weakness.

"November 9. Draining freely through three rubber tubes. Speech gradually improving.

"November 21. Discharge considerably abated. Speech fairly good. No complications."

Throughout his stay in this hospital his temperature did not rise above normal limits.

He was admitted to the London Hospital under my care on November 24, 1917, with a superficial granulating stellate wound in the left parietal region, which pulsated heavily. The anterior limit was level with a point 19·5 cm. along the nasion-inion line; posteriorly the wound extended further backwards for 7·5 cm. In front it was 7 cm., behind 9 cm. from the middle of the scalp. The total nasion-inion measurement was 34 cm., and this was transected by the interaural line at a point 14 cm. from the root of the nose. (Cf. Figs. 10 and 11, Vol. 1, pp. 456 and 457.)

An X-ray photograph showed an area of removal of bone in the anterior parietal region measuring 4 cm. by 2 cm. at its broadest part, with a fissured fracture running directly forwards.

Pure cultures of staphylococcus only were obtained from the wound. It was firmly healed by December 10th, 1917.

On admission he was so grossly aphasic that it was impossible to obtain from him any information with regard to his injury or subsequent events. The words he uttered were comprehensible, but he could not find the means to express himself in speech or writing. Throughout, the character of his disabilities remained the same, although he rapidly regained sufficient facility in utterance to make more extensive observations possible.

He had not been the victim of convulsions or seizures of any kind, and although he still suffered from considerable headache, he had not vomited since October 20th.

His vision was $\frac{6}{6}$ and the optic discs and fundi were in every way normal. Hearing, smell and taste were unaffected.

The pupils reacted well. There was no ocular paralysis or nystagmus. Movements of the face and tongue were normal.

All the deep reflexes were equal on the two sides, the abdominals were brisk and the plantars gave a downward response.

There was no paralysis or paresis; tone was not affected and the movements of the limbs were neither incoordinate nor ataxic.

At this stage it was impossible to test sensation or to map out the visual fields; but subsequent examination showed that they were normal and that sensibility, even to measured tests for recognition of passive movement, discrimination of the compass points, localisation of the spot touched, and appreciation of differences in form, was not affected.

Condition between December 10th, 1917, and February 11th, 1918 (*eight to seventeen weeks after he was wounded*).

He was a well-built healthy young Scotchman, who had lived all his life in Yorkshire. He had been originally employed in the steel works, but, finding he possessed a powerful baritone voice, he had taken to the music hall stage, where he sang sentimental songs. When first admitted, he was puzzled and frightened by his lack of power to express his thoughts. But he soon settled down and became a contented and popular patient, most helpful in the daily life of the ward.

Symbolic Formulation and Expression.

Articulated speech. He had little power of spontaneous speech; but if a question was put to him, he answered intelligently, so far as the paucity of words at his disposal permitted. For instance, asked his age, he replied, "Twenty...twenty... two."

Q. "What did you do before enlisting?"

A. "I was in...Middle...Middle...boro...stale...steel...yes, steel...walk ...work...I can't bring it out." I suggested "steel-works?" and he said, "Yes, yes...that's it."

Q. "You used to sing, didn't you?"

A. "Yes...yes...when I was young...about ni...about twelve...when I was about twelve...but then I went to the steel...I can't get it."

Q. "Can you remember any of the songs you used to sing?"

A. "I've always tried...to see if I could think of them...but I've never been able to think of any of them. I used to think of them...before I went over" (waving his hand to show that he meant over the top) "...I used to say them...but now...since" (putting his hand to his wound) "...since that...I can't even think."

Throughout this last answer intonation and expression were almost normal and his gestures showed that he had been vividly excited by my question. When in doubt he moved his lips silently, as if seeking for a word in which to express himself. If he could find the phrase he required, the syntax was perfect and the syllables were touched off correctly.

Asked his name he said "MacNally" correctly, but could not precede it by the somewhat difficult "Aloysius"; for his address he simply repeated several times in succession, "Middle, Middle-boro" (Middlesbrough).

He was entirely unable to say the months or days of the week spontaneously in order.

He could not repeat the names of common objects or colours exactly, although the sounds he uttered usually bore a distinct relation to the words said by me. Thus for scissors he said "Sis" or "Sit, sitty, sizz": knife became "Nike" or "Night, nie, a nie"; black was "Blat, berlat, blad" and orange "Od-je, od-inge, orridge." In the same way attempts to repeat the months after me produced the following results:

January: "Jan-jer-ley, Jan, Jan."
February: "Fenchurch, Jan-jey, Jan-jey."
March: "Mart, Mar, Mar, Marts."
April: "What was it? Aper, Aperl."
May: "Mage, Made, Mage."
June: "Ju, June."
July: "June, June, Jun-eye."
August: "Orgeons, Or-just."
September: "Eps-ten, Ex-pent, Ex-penst."
October: "Ex, Ox, Ox, Ox-toe, Ox-tove."
November: "No-vendl, New-vender."
December: "Ex. What was it? Ex-pend. Ex-cembr."

When he attempted to repeat the simple phrases of the man, cat and dog tests, he succeeded after much hesitation; once, however, he made the characteristic mistake of responding with a wrong combination, substituting "the cat and the man" for the dog and the cat.

Comprehension of spoken words. He showed obvious defects in comprehending spoken words and phrases; choice of a common object or colour was slow and he frequently gave up the attempt altogether. He set the clock and carried out the coin-bowl tests badly to oral commands. He made many mistakes in executing the complex choice between hand, eye and ear, although simpler commands of a similar kind were carried out, with one exception, correctly.

Reading. He had considerable difficulty in comprehending the significance of single words put before him in print, selecting common objects or colours slowly and with obvious effort; often he gave up all attempt to make a choice. He set the clock badly to printed commands and confused "past" and "to" the hour. In the same way he frequently failed after several attempts to place the proper coin into the right bowl. Simple orders, such as "Shut your eyes," "Put out your tongue," presented to him in print, were poorly executed and he failed grossly to perform the more complex choice demanded by the hand, eye and ear tests.

He read aloud the names of the colours with difficulty and his pronunciation was extremely defective. But the words, badly formed as they were, evidently conveyed their proper significance; for the choice he made was more accurate than when he was not permitted to utter them aloud.

Even such simple words as the man and the dog were defective, when evoked in response to pictures. The man became "mand, mant," the dog was called "got, god, gone," whereas the cat was always pronounced perfectly. When he attempted to read these simple phrases from print, the results were even worse and he struggled ineffectively to find the correct expressions.

Asked to read the orders of the coin-bowl test aloud, he converted them into simple numbers; for example "the second into the third" became "two into three"; but this did not materially improve the way in which he executed the task set him in print.

Simple commands, such as "touch your nose," etc., were read aloud extremely badly and the movements made in response were no better than if he executed them in silence.

Writing. With great effort he succeeded in writing spontaneously "McNally A." and "A McNally, mid," but could get no further in his address. Wishing to write to his mother he began "Mothr, I" and then ceased altogether.

To dictation he wrote "Aloi——McNally, 22. Ba——Steer, Middes"; he was unable to finish either his Christian name or any part of his address. But, in response to a printed copy, he produced the following, in cursive handwriting, with interjected capitals:

"Aloysius McNally,
28 Balekow street [t's uncrossed]
MiddleBoRough."

He was unable to write down the name of any one of the colours shown to him, although he copied them from print without a mistake. Here again he employed cursive script, interspersed with irrelevant capitals.

The words, corresponding to any two pictures of the man, cat and dog tests, were written correctly and in most instances he inserted the definite articles. He copied these phrases from print in perfect handwriting, slowly and without error of any kind.

Although he employed numbers only, he expressed the time extremely badly in writing. Frequently he wrote the hour, but failed altogether to indicate the minutes shown on the clock-face.

Writing to dictation was almost impossible, as can be seen from his attempts to write his name and address. When the simple phrases of the man, cat and dog tests were dictated to him, his written response was in every instance incomplete.

The alphabet. Asked to say the alphabet, he began very slowly "A B C"; then after a pause he continued "E F F Jay (evidently intended for G) H F did I say F? I forget the next one." He made several more attempts without further success.

He could repeat the alphabet after me slowly, but I was compelled to say each letter several times. On the first occasion his lips would move, although he uttered no sound, not even a whisper; when I again said the same letter, he pronounced it accurately, though with some effort.

Separate letters were read aloud correctly, bearing in mind his Scotch accent.

He could copy the alphabet in capitals; but, when he attempted to write it spontaneously, he was only able to produce with great effort the following sequence: A E C D *f* J.

To dictation he wrote extremely slowly and, in almost every instance, it was necessary to say the letter more than once. During this test his lips moved although he uttered no sound.

Numbers. Asked to count, he started quickly and correctly, but rapidly slowed down and ended in confusion, "Five, six, seven, nine, seven, eight, nine, nine, ten, ten, twelve, fourteen." He then began again with the following result: "One, two, three, four, four, five, six, seven, ny, nine, ten, eleven, ten, twelve, four, four, twelve, four-teen, seven, seven, seven-teen." I suggested he should begin at twenty and he said "Twenty, one, two, three, four, five, seven, eight, eight, ten"; throughout he never repeated the word twenty, but counted the decade as if he was starting from one. I asked "What is twenty and ten?" and he replied "Twenty ten, twenty ten, thirty." He then started to count at thirty, saying "Thirty, twenty-one, thirty, thirty-two, twenty-two, twenty-thirty, twenty, no, thirty-two, twenty-three, thirty-four, twenty-six, twenty-five, twenty-seven, thirty, thirty, thirty-eight, thirty-seven, thirty-six, no, thirty-nine."

Arithmetic.

Addition.

123	228		345	
214	734		868	
337	9 5 12	He said "twelve," "five," "nine," and wrote them down independently.	11 10 12	Again he said "twelve," "ten," "eleven," writing them down independently.

Subtraction.

685	752	821
342	536	467
342 (wrong)	224 (wrong)	446 (wrong)

Throughout he subtracted the lower from the higher number, oblivious of whether it was in the top or bottom line.

Coins and their relative value. A series of coins were laid upon the table and he named them as follows:

Penny—"Penny."
Sixpence—"Six...six...six-pence."
Two-shilling piece—"Shill-un...no, two...two shill-un."
Shilling—"Shill-un."
Threepenny piece—"Six...no, three...shill-un...three penny."
Shilling—"Shell...shill-un, shill-un."
Sixpence—"Six...six-pence."
Two-shilling piece—"Shill-un...two...two shillun."
Threepenny piece—"Six...three six...thrup...threp...threp-pence."
Penny—"Pen-nuth...penny...pen...penny."

Two coins were then placed before him and he was asked how many of the one went to make the value of the other. He answered as follows:

One penny and sixpence—"Six."
One penny and threepence—"Four...penny...four...fourpence." (He evidently added the two coins.)
A sixpence and a shilling—"Six...sixpence...shillun...six...sixpence."
A shilling and a two-shilling piece—"Three shillun" (I then asked the question again and he replied "Shillun").
A penny and a sixpence—"Six...six."
A penny and a shilling—"Shillun...six...sixpence" (question repeated) "Six."
A penny and a threepenny piece—"Three...three pennies."
A threepenny piece and a sixpence—"Sixpence" (question repeated) "Six...two...two ..sixpence."
A sixpence and a two-shilling piece—"Two...two...two shillun" (question repeated) "Four...no...four six...sixpence."

But, in spite of these confused replies, he undoubtedly recognised the monetary value of each of these coins, provided he was not compelled to express their relation to one another in words. For he was able to put together the equivalent of any one of them from amongst a heap of money on the table in front of him. Thus, when given a shilling, he picked out a sixpence, added a threepenny piece and then piled three coppers (pennies) one on the other, making in all a shilling; with a two-shilling piece, he chose a sixpence, a threepenny bit, a shilling and then slowly added three coppers to complete the correct sum.

Drawing. He made a poor outline drawing of a spirit-lamp placed before him and did not attempt to represent the mechanism of the burner and wick. This, with all its faults, he reproduced from memory after removal of the model.

But, when I drew a picture of the same object, he made a faithful copy not only with my drawing in front of him, but also from memory, although he tended to detach the lower part of the wick from the burner.

Asked to draw an elephant, he produced an absurd figure. I asked if he would like "to put in anything" he had omitted; he replied, "Yes, doctor, but I don't know where to put it." To the question "What is it?" he placed his forefinger on the head, but said nothing.

I then drew the outline of an elephant without trunk, tusks, eye or ear. Giving him the pencil, I asked him if there was anything he would like to add; he marked in crudely the parts I had omitted. Told to name them, he said, "Near" (ear), "Eye," and for trunk, "I know what it is, but I forget what they call it." *Q.* "What does he do with it?" *A.* "His mouth" (placing his right hand to his own mouth). When I pointed to his drawing of a tusk, he replied, "I know what it is, but I can't say what it's called...trunt, trunce...I forget that." *Q.* "What does he do with it?" *A.* "Eat it...your mouth," touching his teeth with his hand.

Orientation and plan drawing. He found his way about the hospital with ease and, when taken into a room apart, evidently had an accurate conception of the relation of his bed to the other objects in the ward. But he failed to draw a satisfactory ground-plan, although he made marks on the paper indicating the true position of the cupboard, windows, door and the neighbouring unoccupied bed.

In the middle of a sheet of paper I drew a rectangle, to represent his bed, with a human figure lying upon it. He was able to point out accurately the relative situation of the surrounding objects, adding the following explanatory remarks. "There's a bed, no one there now"; on the other side, "No other bed, there's only my bed"; he pointed below the foot saying, "The war (wall), the rawd, the door, yes the door." Asked what was above the head of the bed, he struck with his hand the wall of the room in which he was being examined, saying, "The, the, war." He indicated the cupboard in its correct position, exclaiming, "I never can say that...form close...clothes."

Games. With dominoes he was slow in fitting the numbers together in series, although he made no actual mistakes. His conception of the task was perfect, but he kept looking backwards and forwards from the last domino to the heap on the table, evidently unable to keep in his head the number he required. When he picked out the right one from the pool, he brought it close to the piece already in place in order to be certain that it bore the number he required. He worked on silently and steadily with no uncertainty of aim.

He played a game of draughts correctly, making the moves necessary to avoid the loss of his pieces; he had little power of playing for position. He cleverly avoided the traps I set him and never missed taking one of my pieces that fell his way, although he did not see how to force me to give him two for one.

Singing. Before he joined the army he was on the music hall stage as a singer of serious and sentimental songs. He had never been able to read music quickly from notes and was accustomed to learn mainly by ear. At the time he was under my care, he seemed to be completely unable to read musical notation. But, if he was given the opening notes of a song he had known, he sang it through accurately without words. Time, tune and modulation were perfect and his voice had the full volume of a powerful high baritone. He could not, however, sing any song, if he attempted to pronounce the words.

Serial Tests.

(1) *Naming and recognition of common objects.*

Table 1.

	Pointing to object shown	Oral commands	Printed commands	Naming an object indicated	Duplicate placed in hand out of sight	Repetition	Copying from print
Key	Correct	Correct	No response	Impossible	Correct	"K...chay"	In capitals only
Knife	,,	"I missed that. Say it again." Correct on repetition	Correct	,,	,,	"Nike...nike"	,,
Match box	,,	Correct	Correct; great hesitation	,,	,,	"Mat...mats... mert"	,,
Penny	,,	"I don't think I heard that"	"Can-na"; gave up	,,	,,	"Pen...penny ...palty"	,,
Scissors	,,	Correct	Gave up	,,	,,	"Sis"	,,
Pencil	,,	,,	Correct	,,	,,	"Pen...pent"	,,
Key	,,	Gave up	"Can't"; gave up	,,	,,	"Kay"	,,
Knife	,,	Correct	Correct	,,	,,	"Night...nie... a nie"	,,
Match box	,,	,,	Correct; very slow	,,	,,	"Matze...mat... mack...mat"	,,
Penny	,,	,,	Gave up	,,	,,	"Pen...penny"	,,
Scissors	,,	No reply	"Don't think I know it"	,,	,,	"Sit...sitty... sizz"	,,
Pencil	,,	Correct	Correct, but uncertain	,,	,,	"Pen...pentil... pint-ua"	,,

He was completely unable to name a single object presented to him; he did not even make imperfect attempts to do so, but ejaculated some such expression as "It's a...I know if I could say it," "I think I would know it, but I couldn't...," "I ken, but I can't say it."

He had great difficulty in repeating the names said by me, although his utterances usually bore some relation to the correct word.

He chose the right object quickly, when a duplicate was shown to him or placed in his hand out of sight.

But selection to oral or printed commands was very imperfect.

When I gave any one of these common objects into his hand and asked "What is it for?" he used it correctly with singularly appropriate gestures.

(2) *Naming and recognition of colours.* (See Table 2.)

He could not give names to the colours and fell into such errors as calling black blue, or orange red. But his greatest difficulty was to find the appropriate words and in several instances he gave up the attempt. Repetition was extremely defective.

Choice to oral and printed commands was also imperfect; but he responded better if he was allowed to read the names aloud.

He could not write any one of them completely in response to a colour shown to him. All the names were, however, copied correctly from print in cursive handwriting, broken by irrelevant capital letters.

(3) *The man, cat and dog tests.* (See Table 3.)

He read aloud these simple phrases in an extremely imperfect manner; the sounds showed that he was striving to render the correct content, but the words were scarcely recognisable. Reading from pictures was executed somewhat better and, when he repeated the words said by me, he made one serious mistake only. This was however characteristic, for he substituted "the cat and the man" for the dog and the cat.

He wrote almost equally badly from dictation and from pictures; but every phrase was perfectly transcribed from print into cursive handwriting.

(4) *The clock tests.* (See Table 4.)

He set the hands of one clock in direct imitation of those of another without a mistake of any kind. His lips did not move, but he looked backwards and forwards frequently from the model to the clock he held in his hand.

Both to oral and printed commands he made many errors, obviously misunderstanding the order given and occasionally setting both hands at the same point.

There were many gross defects, when he attempted to tell the time aloud, and he frequently failed altogether. Occasionally, instead of the number of minutes indicated by the long hand, he would give the hour at which it stood; for instance, 9.15 was called "nine three," 8.5 "eight one." He also wrote the time shown on the clock extremely badly.

Here it was not the power of forming words that was at fault, but comprehension of their full significance for internal use and when they were presented to him orally or in print.

(5) *The coin-bowl tests.* (See Table 5.)

Oral and printed commands, whether read silently or aloud, were badly executed. This test showed clearly that he found the same kind of difficulty in using numbers as we have already noticed with words.

Table 2.

	Pointing to colour shown	Oral commands	Printed commands	Naming	Repeating the names of the colours	Writing name of colour indicated	Copying names from print	Printed names read aloud and colour chosen	
								He said	He chose
Black	Correct	Correct	Correct	"Blue...no, blay...lack...ack...luff"	"Bŭ-lack"	ba	Black	"Be-lack"	Correctly
Red	,,	Doubtful, finally correct	,,	"I don't know whether I could say it"	"Lead...ret...red"	Ke	Red	"Led...red"	,,
Yellow	,,	"I don't know"	"I don't know"	"I could only think of what it was"	"Leller...lead-o...li-go"	gn	YeLLow	"Bell-a"	,,
Blue	,,	Correct	No choice	"Loo...loo...loo"	"Ber-loo"	B	BluE	"Berew...brew"	"I don't know which one it is"
White	,,	,,	Doubtful, finally correct	"Why...white"	"Why...white"	hwi	WHiTE	"Why"	Correctly
Orange	,,	Yellow	Yellow	"Ride...rite"	"Oag-inge...ollidge"	—	Orange	"Orrig"	,,
Violet	,,	"I don't think I know"	"I don't know"	"I forget that"	"Valley...val-edge...vi-et-chek"	wi	Violet	"Wy...wall...wall-et"	,,
Green	,,	No choice	Blue	"I don't get them right"	"Glee...glee...green"	ge	green	"Reed"	,,
Black	,,	Correct	Correct	"Lad...blad"	"Blat...berlat...blat"	Ba	Black	"Brack"	,,
Red	,,	,,	Orange	"Rite...I can't say what I think"	"Gred...ger-ed"	w	Red	"Ru...red"	,,
Yellow	,,	Doubtful, finally correct	Correct	"Ref...rite"	"Gerons...gerletchy...kellow"	ge	Yellow	"Ledder...redder"	,,
Blue	,,	No choice	Green	"Blute...blue"	"Ber-loo"	gule	Blue	"Loo"	,,
White	,,	Correct	Very slow, correct	"Will...wit...will...light"	"Whīde"	wh	white	"Wy...wide"	,,
Orange	,,	Doubtful, finally correct	"I forget which one"	"Red"	"Od-je...ed-inge...orridge"	r	ORange	"Rod-ji"	,,
Violet	,,	Correct	Blue	"Was it blowit...blute?"	"White"	bu	Violet	"Wy-el-et"	,,
Green	,,	Doubtful, finally correct	Correct	"I think I know it"	"Ger-ee...keree...gree"	gee	green	"Ree"	,,

Table 3.

	Reading aloud	Writing from dictation	Writing from pictures	Reading from pictures	Repetition	Copying
The cat and the man	"Dē...carnt...art ...that...mart"	tat the Man	the Cat the Man	"A cat...the mand, man, mant"	Correct	Correct
The dog and the cat	"Dē...god...and the...cat"	the dog the cat	dog cat	"Got...a god... cat"	"The cat...the cad and the man"	,,
The man and the dog	"The...māt...and ...these, the... gone, gone, got"	the ca	the man the dog	"Mand...got, the gone, dog, dog"	Correct	,,
The cat and the dog	"Dē...gāt, gone, cat ...and...ee...dot"	the cat and the god	the cat the dog	"Cat...god, dog"	,,	,,
The man and the cat	"Thēte...mat, mant, mand...and...then ...cad, cat"	the man and the cat	the man the cat	"Man...cat"	"The man...the man and the... cat" (correct)	,,
The dog and the man	"The...gond...and ...the...mem, man"	the god and the man	the dog the man	"Dog...mant, mand, a man"	"The dog...the dog...the dog and the...and the man" (correct)	,,

Table 4.

	Direct imitation	Oral commands	Printed commands	Telling the time	Writing down the time
A quarter to 9	Correct	Correct	Correct	"I could get it, if I could say it"	9
10 minutes to 1	,,	,,	Both hands at 1	"I can't say it"	12.10
20 minutes past 11	,,	Both hands at 11	Correct	No reply	11
Half-past 1	,,	Both hands at 1	,,	"Yes, one"	1.30 (correct)
5 minutes to 2	,,	Both hands at 2	,,	"Two, two"	1 "I've lost that one"
10 minutes past 8	,,	Short hand at 8; long hand at 12	,,	"Aye, ayte"	8.10 (correct)
20 minutes to 6	,,	Both hands at 6	Set 6.20	"Fye, isn't it?"	5
Half-past 2	,,	Correct	Set 2.15. "I don't think I got that one"	"Two, six; is that six?" pointing to long hand	2.30 (correct)
20 minutes past 9	,,	,,	Correct	"Nine is it? and four was it?"	9 "I don't know what that is," pointing to long hand
10 minutes past 7	,,	Short hand at 7; long hand at 12	,,	"Seven...two," pointing to long hand	7.10 (correct)
20 minutes to 4	,,	Short hand at 4; long hand at 10	Set 4.20	"Four...ayte," pointing to long hand	3
10 minutes to 7	,,	Correct	Set 7.10	"Seven...ten"	6.10
A quarter past 9	,,	Short hand at 9; long hand at 12	Short hand at 9; then completely puzzled	"Nine...three"	9.15 (correct)
20 minutes to 3	,,	Correct	Short hand at 3; then puzzled	"Two...ayte"	2 "I can't get that"
5 minutes past 8	,,	,,	Correct	"Ayte...one"	8.5 (correct)

Table 5.

	Oral commands	Printed commands (not read aloud)	Printed commands read aloud	
			He said	Movement executed
2nd into 3rd	Correct; slow	Correct	"Two, three"	Correct
1st into 3rd	,,	Correct; slow	"Won, tree"	,,
2nd into 1st	2nd coin..."I forget which one" (repeated) correct	1st coin...2nd coin...No further action	"Two, won"	1st into 1st
3rd into 2nd	3rd coin..."I forget" (repeated) correct	2nd into 3rd	"Ree, tree, two"	3rd into 3rd
1st into 4th	1st coin; (repeated) correct	Correct; slow	"Won, four, four"	1st coin "Was it four?"; did nothing
4th into 3rd	3rd into 2nd	3rd into 4th	"Four...one, ree, tree"	3rd into 3rd
2nd into 4th	Correct	Correct	"Two, four"	Correct
4th into 1st	4th coin..."I forget" (repeated) correct	,,	"Four, won, won"	1st into 4th
3rd into 1st	Correct	3rd coin..."I forget which one I've got"	"Tree, won, tree"	Correct
1st into 2nd	2nd into 1st	Correct	"One, two, two"	,,
3rd into 4th	Correct; slow	3rd coin..."I forget which one to put it in"	"Three, four"	3rd into 3rd
4th into 2nd	"I forget which it was" (repeated), 4th into 1st	Correct	"Four, taw"	Correct

(6) *Simple movements requiring no choice of right or left.*

Table 6.

	Printed commands	Oral commands	Reading aloud and executing printed commands		Copying and then executing printed commands	
			He said	Movement executed	He wrote	Movement executed
Shut your eyes	Touched R. eye with R. hand	Correct	"Shine...you...eye, eye.""Show...eyes"	Did nothing	Shut youR eyes	Touched eye with hand
Give me your hand	Pointed with R. hand to L. hand. "This isn't it"	,,	"Gee...me...you... ann"	Touched L. hand with R.	Give Me youR hand.	Touched L. hand with R.
Touch your nose	"I think I know that word," pointing to nose. Did nothing	,,	"Too, too...you...no, now, new. New no"	Correct	touch youR nose	Correct
Put out your tongue	Did nothing	,,	"Pew...two...you.. toe." "I don't know what this is"	Did nothing	Put out youR tonGue	Did nothing
Give me your hand	Touched L. hand with R.	,,	"Gee...me...you... ann, fan, ann"	Touched L. hand with R.	Give me me youR hand	Touched L. hand with R.
Touch your nose	Correct; very slow	,,	"Chew...you...no, nose"	Correct	touch youR nose	Correct
Put out your tongue	"Was it toe?" Did nothing	,,	"Pew...no, no...you ...tow"	Did nothing	Put out youR TonGue	Did nothing
Shut your eyes	Touched R. eye with R. hand	Touched R. eye with R. hand	"Show, shoud, shout... you...eye, eye"	Touched R. eye with R. hand	Shut youR eyes	Touched R. eye

I gave him a series of simple commands, such as "Touch your nose," "Put out your tongue," etc.; these he carried out almost perfectly in response to words said by me. When, however, the order was given in print, which he read silently, his responses were faulty. Instead of closing his eyes he would touch one of them with his hand; told to give me his hand, he pointed with one of them to the other and rarely executed correctly the movement required. He read these orders aloud extremely badly and carried them out even worse than when he remained silent.

Asked to copy the printed sentences, their content was correctly given, but the writing was a curious mixture of cursive script interspersed with irrelevant capitals. Although the actual words as written contained the correct commands, they were carried out extremely badly.

(7) *Hand, eye and ear tests.*

This series of tests brought out the same difficulties in an exaggerated form. He could not imitate my movements when we sat face to face, nor could he carry them out correctly from pictures. When either my movements or the diagrams were reflected in a mirror, his responses were not only much quicker, but he made four mistakes only in the double series of thirty-two observations.

As with all tests of this order, he found great difficulty in executing oral and printed commands and occasionally failed to complete the movement or mistook ear and eye.

Table 7.

	Imitation of movements made by the observer	Imitation of movements reflected in a mirror	Pictorial commands	Pictorial commands reflected in a mirror	Oral commands	Printed commands
L. hand to R. eye	R. hand to R. eye	Correct	Reversed	Correct	Lifted L. hand	R. hand to R. eye
R. hand to R. ear	Reversed	,,	,,	,,	Correct	R. hand...
R. hand to L. eye	R. hand to R. eye	,,	,,	,,	L. hand to L. *ear*	R. hand to R. eye
L. hand to R. ear	L. hand to L. ear	,,	L. hand to L. ear	,,	L. hand to L. ear	R. hand...
R. hand to R. eye	Correct	,,	Reversed	,,	Correct	Reversed
L. hand to L. ear	Reversed	,,	,,	,,	L. hand to R. ear	No response
L. hand to L. eye	,,	,,	,,	Reversed	L. hand to L. *ear*	Reversed
R. hand to L. ear	,,	,,	,,	Correct	R. hand to R. *eye*	L. hand to L. *eye*
L. hand to R. eye	R. hand to R. eye	,,	,,	,,	R. hand to R. eye	R. hand to R. eye
R. hand to R. ear	Reversed	,,	,,	,,	R. hand to R. *eye*	Reversed
R. hand to L. eye	R. hand to R. eye	L. hand to L. eye	,,	,,	L. hand to L. eye	L. hand to L. eye
L. hand to R. ear	L. hand to L. ear	Correct	L. hand, then R. to L. ear	R hand to R. ear	L. hand to L. ear	L. hand to L. ear
R. hand to R. eye	Correct	,,	Reversed	Correct	L. hand to R. eye	L. hand to R. eye
L. hand to L. ear	L. hand to R. ear	,,	,,	,,	Correct	L. hand to R. ear
L. hand to L. eye	Reversed	,,	,,	,,	Reversed	L. hand...
R. hand to L. ear	,,	,,	R. hand, then L. to R. ear	R. hand to R. ear; then L. to R. ear	R. hand to L. *eye*	Reversed

CONDITION IN JULY 1922 (*four years and nine months after he was wounded*).

The wound was represented by a tough arrow-shaped scar, lying over a triangular opening in the bone; this was depressed and in normal circumstances did not pulsate. But if he lowered his head towards his knees, the surface came up flush with the scalp and pulsation occurred. The skin did not seem to be tender in the true sense of the word, although he intensely disliked anything to touch this part of his head and was evidently frightened at the prospect of contact.

He complained of occasional "headaches" in the morning, which disappeared an hour or so after getting up. Stooping or lifting brought on this feeling, which was more a discomfort and sensation of "dizziness" than an actual pain. It could also be induced by reading or intellectual concentration. He had suffered from no fits or other attacks. The discs were normal; vision was perfect and there was no limitation of the field. All reflexes, including the abdominals and plantars, were normal. There was no paresis, incoordination, or change in tone, and sensibility was in no way affected. In fact, I could discover no abnormal physical signs of any kind. His general health was excellent.

Symbolic Formulation and Expression.

He had returned to his occupation as a music hall singer, but recently lost his engagement because his voice had deteriorated, and he was about to return to manual work.

Articulated speech. He was somewhat nervous and anxious, speaking little except when in quiet and familiar surroundings. He said, "I'll tell you what I'm most afraid of...I can't speak much in company...I get nervous and it stops me from speaking...I get confused...the words." To my question whether he knew what he wanted to say, he replied, "Yes, Doctor...but if they speak quickly I get taken off what I wanted to say."

He said the months correctly in order and had regained his power of naming common objects or colours, although he occasionally hesitated before replying. He had no difficulty in word-formation, once he knew what he wanted to say; if he failed to find the correct expression, he did not stutter and make repeated attempts at articulation, but paused as if lost. Syntax was entirely unaffected and he showed no tendency to employ true jargon.

He could repeat everything said to him accurately and without verbal distortion.

Understanding of spoken words. Common objects or colours were chosen rapidly without error to oral commands and he set the hands of the clock correctly. He made no mistakes even with the complex hand, eye and ear tests, although his choice was somewhat slow and hesitating. His appreciation of the significance of general conversation was excellent, provided I did not speak too rapidly, or talk of some entirely unfamiliar subject.

Reading. He evidently understood what he read to himself, choosing common objects or colours and setting the clock correctly to printed commands. Even the hand, eye and ear tests were executed without mistakes to orders given in print.

He read aloud the phrases of the man, cat and dog tests with ease. But, when reading from a book, he occasionally hesitated at some unusual word, saying, "I can say the names...unless they might be...big words...big names...or I can say them all if I have a good look at them...read them over...have a good look at them and say them over."

Writing. He wrote his name and address perfectly and produced the following excellent letter, marred only by the insertion of irrelevant capitals.

"Dear Sir, I feel much better than I was, four years ago. In fact I feel Better in every way, of course I feel a Little Depressed at times, but it is nothing. Well I cannot write much, and it also takes me a Long time to do it

Yours faithfully

A. McN."

Designation in writing was still somewhat slow, although he could execute all the serial tests with few if any faults. Thus he found some difficulty with the names of common objects, but made no mistakes except with the spelling of knife and scissors. Colours were given correctly, he wrote the phrases of the man, cat and dog tests accurately, and even put on to paper the complex hand, eye and ear movements without mistakes. The months were written in due order and February alone was wrongly spelt (Febuary), a trivial fault.

He wrote well to dictation and copied excellently keeping his eyes fixed on the printed matter before him.

The alphabet. In spite of his extensive recovery of speech he experienced profound difficulty with this test. He had reached a high standard at an elementary school, and said, "I was a good scholar before I was wounded." Asked to say the alphabet he began "A B C D E F G..."; he ceased and started again, "A B C D E F G H..." Then he said, "I can say the end of it, I L M N O P Q W X Y Z...there is one or two...letters...there...I'm not sure of." Yet he repeated the letters after me and read them aloud perfectly.

Told to write the alphabet spontaneously, he produced the following: *a b* C D E F G H L O P Q R S T U V W X Z; and to dictation he wrote *a b* C D ℰ ℱ 𝒢 H I J K L ℳ 𝒩 *o p q* R S T 𝒰 V W *x v z* (y troubled him greatly and was left unfinished). Given a series of capitals and asked to copy them in ordinary handwriting, he did so as follows: *a b c* 𝒟 ℰ ℱ 𝒢 H ℐ 𝒥 K ℒ *m n o p q* ℛ S *t u v w x y z*.

I then placed on the table the twenty-six block letters and asked him to make an alphabet; he completely failed to do so. He first ranged in order A B C D E F G I; then exclaiming, "I think I've done it wrong," he removed the I and added H I. After much hesitation he continued L M N O P U R S T and then gave up altogether.

Thus, in spite of the profound recovery of speech, this test still revealed gross lack of power to manipulate verbal symbols.

Numbers and arithmetic. He counted perfectly up to 69, but hesitated at 70; he then continued, "71, 72, 73, 74...70, 71, 72, 73, 74, 75," and so on correctly up to 100. Each number was considered separately and uttered individually, and not as part of a series.

Addition.

123	228	345
214	734	868
337	962	1213

Subtraction.

685	752	821
342	536	467
343	236 (wrong)	474 corrected spontaneously to—
		354

Coins and their relative value. All forms of money from a pound note downwards were correctly named and the relative value of any two of them was given slowly but accurately. He added, "I used to be awful...I couldn't count the change... not correctly...It is much better...now and again I make mistakes...if I try to do it quick I make mistakes."

Drawing. He drew a spirit-lamp excellently from a model and reproduced it fairly well from memory. He was also able to draw an elephant with all its salient points, naming them correctly as he added each one to his drawing.

Pictures and images. He showed perfect recognition of the full significance of pictures and carried out pictorial commands without fail.

When drawing the elephant, he insisted that he could see it "in my mind." Asked what colours I had shown him on the previous day, he gave them all correctly and added, "I can see them...see them all."

Orientation and plan drawing. During his stay in London he found his way about alone, came to my house from the hospital unattended, and showed no signs of defective orientation.

Asked to draw a plan of the room in which we worked, he was much puzzled as to the relative position of the various objects and tended to draw them in elevation instead of indicating them on the flat. When, however, I drew a four-sided outline figure to represent the room and asked him to point to each object in turn as I named it, he did so with complete accuracy. It was the power of formulating the relation of the various pieces of furniture to one another which was at fault.

Games. He could play billiards and draughts, but not cards; they had always given him trouble, since he was wounded, and he had not attempted to re-learn these games.

Singing. He could never read musical notation sufficiently to help him with his songs and learnt them all by ear. He still sang well without words; his voice had its full volume and showed no unsteadiness. But as soon as he attempted to sing the words of a song, he fell out of tune, the volume of his voice decreased and a bad tremolo made its appearance. Evidently the words hindered him, and he complained, "It's the words that worry me...better without words."

Serial Tests.

(1) *Naming and recognition of common objects.*

Table 8.

	Pointing to object shown	Naming an object indicated	Oral commands	Printed commands	Duplicate placed in hand out of sight	Writing name of object indicated
Knife	Correct	Correct	Correct	Correct	Correct	Knike
Key	"	"	"	"	"	Correct
Penny	"	"	"	"	"	"
Matches	"	"	"	"	"	"
Scissors	"	"	"	"	"	Siccors
Pencil	"	"	"	"	"	Correct
Key	"	"	"	"	"	"
Scissors	"	"	"	"	"	Siccors
Matches	"	"	"	"	"	Correct
Knife	"	"	"	"	"	"
Penny	"	"	"	"	"	"
Matches	"	"	"	"	"	"
Scissors	"	"	"	"	"	Siccors
Pencil	"	"	"	"	"	Correct
Penny	"	"	"	"	"	"
Knife	"	"	"	"	"	Nife
Key	"	"	"	"	"	Correct
Pencil	"	"	"	"	"	"

Oral and printed commands were executed without the slightest difficulty, and he named the various objects correctly, although with occasional hesitation; but his lips did not move, even during the moments of doubt. Told to write down the name as each object was shown to him, the nomenclature was correct, but the spelling of scissors and knife defective.

(2) *Naming and recognition of colours*. All these tests were carried out perfectly and the names were even written without mistakes. This shows the profound extent to which he had recovered power to use language in its various forms.

(3) *The man, cat and dog tests*. He read aloud from print or pictures and repeated these phrases perfectly. He could write them from pictures or to dictation and copied print in ordinary handwriting without mistakes of any kind. In fact, he said that these tests gave him no trouble.

(4) *The clock tests*. He set the clock to oral and printed commands, placing the short hand throughout in a position proportionate to the minutes indicated. He told the time perfectly and wrote it down without mistakes, adding, "It seemed to come to me all of a sudden, when I got home first...I seemed to read the clock."

(5) *The coin-bowl tests* gave him no difficulty and were executed rapidly and well.

(6) *Hand, eye and ear tests*. These showed in a striking manner the profound recovery of power which had occurred since he first came under my care. He not only imitated my movements sitting face to face, but carried out oral, printed or pictorial commands correctly, though somewhat slowly. When my movements or the pictures were reflected in a mirror, his response was much quicker. He could even write down without mistakes my movements sitting face to face, or those indicated in the diagrams, a task of considerable difficulty even for a normal person.

During the course of these tests he volunteered the following statements: "I looks at your arms...then I...well I looked at your right arm or your left...and that kind of tells me...I say it." "It's difficult if it's quick...when I do it quick...I don't think I'll do it correctly."

At first this patient showed profound loss of power to find names and the indicative words he required to express his thoughts. He could not carry out oral or printed commands and was unable to write although he could copy. In the course of somewhat over four years, he recovered his power of speaking, reading and writing sufficiently to carry out all the serial tests, excepting only those set by the alphabet. But it was obvious that he still had difficulty in naming, and the more complex oral and printed commands were executed with abnormal deliberation. In fact, he still remained an example of nominal aphasia, in spite of the remarkable restoration of the power of speech in all its forms.

No. 8

A young officer was struck in the left parieto-occipital region by a fragment of shell casing. The missile travelled across the brain and was removed thirteen days later through a minute trephine opening on the opposite side. The effective wound, that of entry, consisted of an opening in the bone measuring 4 by 2·75 cm. on the left side, lying over the supra-marginal gyrus and part of the superior parietal lobule. No symptoms accompanied the comparatively slight injury to the right of the middle line.

At first he suffered from occasional headaches on the left side of the head unaccompanied by epileptiform attacks. Seizures appeared, however, four months after he was wounded and recurred at varying intervals dependent on whether he was worried or not. They usually consisted of loss of consciousness with or without slight convulsions; each attack was preceded by a period of confusion and "loss of memory."

There was definite right hemianopsia, which assumed a form occasionally found with lesions of the cortex. The loss of vision over the defective half of the field was not absolute and he could appreciate moving objects. Moreover, if with both eyes open two similar objects were exposed at exactly the same distance from the fixation point, that to the right was frequently not appreciated, although it might be recognised if shown alone. This was due to defective and fluctuating attention within the affected parts of the field of vision.

Reflexes, motion and sensation were unaffected, but the optic discs showed signs of previous swelling.

The disorders of symbolic formulation and expression were of the Semantic type. He frequently failed to recognise the intention of what he was told to do and was unable to combine details, duly appreciated, into a coherent whole. This was associated with difficulty in grasping a general idea. Articulated speech was unaffected and he could name objects correctly. He chose them to oral and printed commands and had no difficulty in comprehending the meaning of single words or short phrases. Yet he could not set the hands of a clock and frequently failed to gather the full meaning of general conversation. Reading aloud was unaffected, but he gave an imperfect account of what he had read to himself. Writing as such was perfect, although he had the same difficulty in putting down on paper exactly what he had gathered from conversation or reading. He could not solve problems in arithmetic and became confused over money. Drawing was defective. He could not find his way alone or plan where he wanted to go. Games, such as billiards and jigsaw puzzles, were impossible.

He recovered to a great extent and six years after he was wounded could carry out all the serial tests without a mistake. But he still showed in a minor degree those disabilities which made him so characteristic an example of Semantic Aphasia.

Second Lieut. R. E. C. M. was wounded on June 4th, 1916, with a fragment of a high explosive missile, probably a rifle grenade. He was standing at the time and dropped to the ground; he can remember being helped to walk by his men, but lost consciousness on reaching the dressing station.

He was admitted to a hospital in Rouen on June 14th, where he arrived without medical records of any kind. He had evidently been trephined over the left parieto-occipital region and the flap had healed except for a small septic sinus, presumably the site of a drainage tube. He was drowsy and talked in a disconnected manner. Optic neuritis was present in both eyes and, on the day after admission, he developed a divergent squint with ptosis of the left eye.

A foreign body, which had traversed the brain from side to side, was localised close to the surface beneath the right half of the skull. On June 17th this was removed through a small trephine opening directly over the spot; it turned out to be a fragment of shell casing about 1 by 0·75 cm. which lay immediately beneath the surface of the cortex.

His mental condition rapidly improved and all signs of ocular paralysis disappeared. There was no fit or seizure at any time and motor power was unaffected.

He was admitted to the Empire Hospital under my care on July 3rd, 1916. At that time there was a small pouting wound lying in the centre of a trephined area, which measured 4 by 2·75 cm. in the left parieto-occipital region. This was situated from 26 to 29 cm. along the nasion-inion and 8 cm. from the middle line of the scalp as seen from behind (Figs. 12 and 13, Vol. 1, pp. 460 and 461).

On the right side of the head was a minute opening in the bone 1·25 cm. in diameter, which lay 17 cm. back from the root of the nose and 8 cm. from the middle line; this was the sole evidence of the second operation, which had produced little or no destruction of brain tissue.

The total nasion-inion measurement was 35 cm. and this was cut by the inter-aural line 15 cm. back from the root of the nose.

By July 19th, 1916, the wound on the left side had entirely healed, but the area from which bone had been removed pulsated heavily.

During the two months he remained in the Empire Hospital, he was intelligent and cheerful, but easily fatigued. His memory was extremely poor; thus, he would ring the bell and, when the nurse arrived, had forgotten what he wanted. He complained that he could not "reason things out" or recall dates and "reckon out" how long he had been in hospital. He could not keep his mind on what he read, although his attention was fairly good under examination.

He suffered from occasional headaches, which lasted for two or three days, usually confined to the left half of the head. Before admission they had been associated with nausea and vomiting, which ceased whilst he was under my care. There were no convulsions or seizures.

The most striking physical abnormality consisted of defective vision over the right half of the field. This was worked out repeatedly on many occasions and, as it did not alter materially, I shall combine in one account the results obtained up to the end of October 1916. His visual acuity was $\frac{6}{5}$ both with the right and the left eye; but he tended to miss letters towards the right of any line he was reading, unless his attention was concentrated directly upon them. Over the right half of the field a moving object could be appreciated up to the periphery, but a stationary white square 1 cm. in size was frequently unrecognised. I placed him at a distance of 45 cm. from a large white screen in a darkened room, and, by means of an electrical key, projected upon it from behind a circular patch of light 1 cm. in diameter; sometimes it fell to the right, sometimes to the left and occasionally at an equal distance on both sides of the middle line simultaneously. He never failed to appreciate the luminous object on the left half of the field, whilst he was frequently uncertain to the right. He complained, "I detect the left-hand one quicker than the right. Sometimes I think there is only one on the left and immediately afterwards I discover one on the right."

The field for the appreciation of colours was greatly diminished, but not completely abolished to the right of the middle line.

On admission (July 3rd) the edges of the optic discs were ragged and blurred, showing distinct traces of previous swelling which had subsided.

Hearing was normal; smell and taste were poorly developed, but not otherwise affected.

The pupils reacted well. The movements of eyes, face and tongue were normal. The reflexes including the abdominals and plantars were unaffected. Careful examination failed to reveal any disturbance of motion or sensibility and his answers to the latter tests were remarkably trustworthy and accurate.

From the Empire Hospital he passed on to a Convalescent Home, where he greatly improved in general health, and, at the end of September 1916, returned to London for further examination. His physical condition was excellent and I could discover no abnormal signs beyond the condition of his visual fields and the disorder of speech.

He was an intelligent young man of twenty-four, who had been a student at Oxford when the war broke out. He joined the regular army and easily passed into Sandhurst, where he obtained his commission; at that time his mental capacity was of a high order. Throughout he was a most willing and attentive patient, always anxious to do his best, but peculiarly liable to become confused if pressed to perform some difficult task.

Simple orders were carried out perfectly. He could shave himself, blow his nose or brush his hair, when told to do so. He tied a knot, lit a match and blew it out or lit a cigarette to command. He went through the act of drinking in pantomime without a cup and of blowing his nose without a handkerchief.

Condition of Symbolic Formulation and Expression during the first week of October 1916 (*seventeen weeks after he was wounded*).

Articulated speech was unaffected; the words were well formed, intonation was normal and the grammatical structure of the sentences perfect. He could count and say the alphabet, the days of the week and the months in due order. Nothing abnormal was noticeable in ordinary conversation beyond a tendency to become confused if the subject was complex. He could repeat exactly what was said to him and the words were perfectly articulated.

Understanding of spoken words. He had no difficulty in comprehending the meaning of single words or short phrases and chose common objects to oral commands. He could even perform the hand, eye and ear tests, but failed to set the clock correctly to orders given by word of mouth. But he did not always understand the full significance of what he was told and frequently failed to gather a general idea from conversation.

Reading. He carried out even the complex printed commands of the hand, eye and ear tests without reading them aloud; but he had considerable difficulty in setting the clock to orders given in a mixture of words and figures.

Asked to retail the meaning of a paragraph he had read to himself from a book or a newspaper, he shortened down the contents, saying, "I find difficulty in grasping the general idea of the thing. In reading the newspaper I have to letter out each thing and it does not convey so much to me as it should." The following passage was selected as a test: "The summer day was splendid and the world, as he looked at it from the terrace was a vault of airy blue arching over a lap of solid green. The wide still trees in the park appeared to be waiting for some daily inspection and the rich fields with their frill of hedges to rejoice in the light." Asked what this meant he replied, "It doesn't convey much; it seems to go out of my mind; he is looking out from a terrace onto a park."

He read these words aloud with scarcely more than the slightest hesitation and replied to my question as to the significance of the passage, "It conveys to me a man looking out onto a park with a fringe of beautiful trees and then I can't remember the rest. These trees resembled a lot of people waiting to be inspected." He added, "I had to letter these words out as I read it. The meaning did not come to me at once. I had to look at it very carefully before I could read it so to speak."

Writing. He wrote his name, his address and the letters of the alphabet with ease spontaneously and composed an account of the events of his last Medical Board, which was coherent and contained no verbal errors. Shown any two pictures of the man, cat and dog tests, he wrote down the contents correctly in phrases properly constructed.

But, when he was asked to reproduce in writing some passage he had read silently to himself, he shortened it considerably, complaining that he had difficulty in "grasping the general idea of the thing." I gave him a short description of the room of a man, who collected furniture and other objects of artistic value. After reproducing a couple of phrases, he said, "The main impression is the room of a collector, but I can't get the general idea. I can see the room, but I have to conjure my brain to get the picture and then I get an imperfect picture."

He wrote easily to dictation and the same passage I used for testing his powers of reading was written down without mistake. But he complained, "If I am writing I am apt to write on and then to wonder if I have put two l's or one. I can't be sure if I've written it rightly or not."

He could copy printed matter in cursive handwriting accurately and without the slightest difficulty.

Numbers and arithmetic. He counted perfectly and appreciated the direct significance of a number without reaching it through a sequence.

Even simple arithmetical operations gave him considerable trouble; he complained, "I don't find that easy; I easily get muddled over it."

Addition.

231	648	856
356	326	275
587	970 (wrong)	1131

Subtraction.

865	782	912
432	258	386
433	534 (wrong)	836 (wrong)

Coins and their relative value. He had no difficulty in naming any coin shown to him; but, when any two of them were placed on the table, he hesitated and showed great uncertainty in expressing their relation. Thus, with a sixpence and a half-crown (two and sixpence) he said, "Let's see...two, four, six"; given a penny and a two-shilling piece, he replied, "A penny...twenty, twenty-four pence in two shillings." To a halfpenny and a sixpence he responded as follows: "Well, supposing they were pennies...oh! twelve, yes twelve," adding, "I get muddled up especially with the halfpenny." He said he found the task easier and he certainly answered more quickly, when he was asked these questions without the coins on the table before him.

In ordinary intercourse he was extremely careful with money and found considerable difficulty with change.

Drawing. He had always been unusually fond of drawing and possessed a considerable reputation in his family for his sketches. But, since he was wounded, most of this facility had deserted him. He drew a poor representation of a wineglass from a model and reproduced this drawing almost exactly from memory. He complained, however, "I have difficulty in reasoning out how the lines go. I see, but I can't get a clear impression in my mind how this (the stem) goes in and how the bottom comes."

Asked to draw an elephant, he moved his pencil about aimlessly, saying, "I can't get the idea." Then he suddenly drew the outline of the head, back and belly, adding the four legs and an eye; the tusks were indicated, but he omitted the trunk. I asked, "What is the characteristic of an elephant?" to this he replied, "It's trunk; I see I've omitted to put in his trunk."

Orientation. He complained, "I never had a good head for finding my way, but I now have no sense of direction. I can find my way about in the house, how one room opens into another and that sort of thing." This was borne out by the difficulty he experienced in finding his way and at this time he always chose a companion, when he left the hospital.

Games. He was unable to play games of any kind. "I can't reason out the various strokes at billiards; I can't cannon off the cushion. I have to get someone to tell me. I can make a direct shot. In fact I've rather funked playing it."

He failed completely in his attempts to put together puzzles; "I tried working out jigsaw puzzles, but I was very bad at them. I could see the bits, but I could not see any relation between them. I could not get the general idea."

The general significance of pictures. Simple straightforward pictures, such as a woman acting as a shepherd and one in charge of a rabbit farm, he appreciated at once, adding, "War-work and women I should think." But, as soon as the picture carried a command, he failed to appreciate its significance. "Somehow or another I don't seem able to get the right part of the picture; sometimes I seemed to look at one, sometimes at the other. I had to reason out the meaning of the whole picture."

He found it extremely difficult to understand a joke. "Some jokes," he said, "are too intricate for me; I can see simple plain ones. That is as bad when I'm told it as when I see the picture." This was borne out by closer examination; so long as the point of the joke lay entirely within the limits of a simple picture, it could be appreciated. But, if in order to gather its full significance, he was compelled to combine picture and legend, he always failed to recognise its meaning completely.

The general intention of an act. He complained that "when at table, I am very slow in picking out the object, say the milk-jug, which I want. I don't spot it at once. When I'm going to shave, I can't collect my things; I have to look hard at them all and then I am sure to miss some of them. In the same way I have to look at the things on the breakfast table; I see them all, but I don't spot them. When I want the salt or the pepper or a spoon, I suddenly tumble to its presence."

He also complained that, when his servant had cleaned his belt, the runners had been displaced and "I could not for the life of me think how to bring them into place."

Serial Tests.

(1) *Naming and recognition of common objects.* None of these tests presented any difficulty. He could name an object indicated and choose correctly to oral or printed commands. He was even able to write the names without mistake or hesitation.

(2) *The man, cat and dog tests.* The simple phrases of this test were read aloud from print or from pictures, written to dictation, copied and transcribed from pictures without the slightest difficulty.

(3) *The clock tests.*

Table 1.

	Direct imitation	Oral commands	Printed commands	Telling the time	Writing down the time shown on a clock-face
5 minutes to 2	Set 11.55; corrected	Set 2.5	Set 2.5	Correct	Correct
Half-past 1	Correct	Correct	Correct	"	"
5 minutes past 8	"	"	"	"	"
20 minutes to 4	Set 4.40; "No, that's 20 to 5"	Correct; slow	Set 4.40	"	"
10 minutes past 7	Correct	Correct	Correct	"	"
20 minutes to 6	"	Set 6.20	Set 6.20	"	"
10 minutes to 1	"	Set 1.10	Correct; hesitated	"	"
A quarter to 9	Finally correct	Correct; slow	Set 9.15; corrected	"	"
20 minutes past 11	Set 10.40	"	Correct	"	"
25 minutes to 3	Set 1.35	Set 3.20	"	"	"

Like all the patients of this group, he experienced considerable difficulty in carrying out these tests. He could tell the time correctly and write down silently the position of the hands of a clock set by me. But he made many mistakes in his attempt to set a clock to oral and printed commands. When I said "a quarter to nine," he placed the hour hand at nine and then explained, "I don't know from which side to approach it," and with "twenty-five minutes to three," he set 3.20 and added, "I don't know whether what I've set is to or past." To printed commands he also had difficulty in knowing if he was wrong or right and had the same tendency to confuse "to" and "past." For instance, for "twenty minutes to six" he set 6.20 and said, "I can't make out the difference between past and to six; I haven't got it right, I think."

The most curious defect appeared when he had imitated on one clock the position of the hands on another set by me. This is usually an easy task; but he was evidently puzzled. He looked at my clock intently and after a pause said "yes"; then he proceeded to move the hands and, even if he set them correctly, he was evidently uncertain whether he was right. He failed to understand exactly what he was expected to do.

(4) *The hand, eye and ear tests.*

Table 2.

	Imitation of movements made by the observer	Imitation of movements reflected in a mirror	Pictorial commands	Pictorial commands reflected in a mirror	Oral commands	Printed commands	Printed commands read aloud and executed	
							He said	Movement executed
L. hand to R. ear	L. hand to L. *eye*	Correct; slow	L. hand to L. ear; corrected	Correct	Correct	Correct	Correctly	Correct
R. hand to L. eye	R. hand to R. eye	Correct	L. hand to R. *ear*	,,	,,	,,	,,	,,
R. hand to L. ear	Reversed	Correct; slow	R. hand to R. ear	L. hand to R. *eye*	,,	,,	,,	,,
L. hand to L. eye	Correct	Reversed	L. hand to L. *ear*	"I can't make it out"; no reply	,,	,,	,,	,,
R. hand to R. ear	,,	Correct	Correct	Correct	,,	,,	,,	,,
L. hand to R. eye	L. hand to R. *ear*	L. hand to R. *ear*; corrected	L. hand to L. eye; corrected	L. hand to L. eye	,,	,,	,,	,,
L. hand to L. ear	Correct	Correct	Correct	Correct	,,	,,	,,	,,
R. hand to R. eye	,,	,,	,,	,,	,,	,,	,,	,,
L. hand to R. ear	,,	,,	,,	,,	,,	,,	,,	,,
R. hand to L. eye	Correct; slow	,,	Reversed	Reversed	,,	,,	,,	,,
L. hand to R. eye	Correct	L. hand to L. *ear*; corrected	L. hand to L. eye	R. hand to R. eye; L. hand to L. eye	,,	,,	,,	,,
R. hand to L. ear	,,	Correct	Reversed	Correct	,,	,,	,,	,,

He made many mistakes, when he attempted to imitate my movements or to carry out the same actions to pictorial commands. But his failure to carry out the task, when they were reflected in a mirror, is unusual in most other forms of speech defect. He explained his difficulties as follows. "I never could work the semaphore (in army signalling) without thinking right and left. When I imitated you, I had to think 'Is that his right or his left?' When I'm looking in the glass, it is easier because the sides are the same; but then I begin to think it out and get puzzled. I then revert to what we were doing before."

Oral and printed commands were, however, carried out perfectly. He thought the former were somewhat easier and said of the printed orders, "I read it over to myself; the words are meaningless at first, then suddenly I've got hold of it." Reading the command aloud made its execution somewhat more easy.

He returned home to the country in excellent spirits and splendid general health. But on the evening of October 16th, 1916, whilst kneeling to pack a box, he lost consciousness and fell, striking his forehead. He returned to London, but I could discover no physical signs other than those described above. He did not suffer from headache, his fields of vision were exactly as before, and the optic discs were unchanged.

A second attack occurred on November 14th whilst he was in a theatre. He became unconscious in his seat, was slightly convulsed, but was able to walk out and returned in a cab.

He went back to his quiet home in the country and was free from attacks for seventy-six days. Unfortunately, towards the end of this period, a Medical Board sent him into a hospital in a large and noisy provincial town. This he felt to be a "tremendous strain"; the movement of the streets "troubled and bothered" him. There were twelve officers at dinner every night and, as he could not take part in the conversation, he became shy, anxious and ill at ease. Moreover, he was disappointed that he was not permitted to return to our care.

Shortly after his admission, on April 26th, 1917, he had another attack, followed by others on the 27th, the 30th, May 10th and June 3rd. Finally, at our urgent request, he was sent home again and had no further fit for six months (December 9th, 1917).

Throughout 1918 and up to July 1919, they recurred about every three months, generally in pairs with an interval of a few days between the two seizures; but after July he remained free until December 23rd.

During 1920, he had one attack only (November 21st) and they have steadily decreased since that date.

He described a seizure as preceded by "a feeling like going under an anaesthetic." "Just before I have an attack a quiet period comes on from which I seem to wake up with a jerk. I then go out of the room and the fit comes on." On one occasion he was going to the bathroom and lost his way; on another he became incoherent so that he could not express himself. Once in the streets he "became dazed" and lost his memory. He thought he sometimes had this "quiet period, a feeling of not being aware of what is going on around you," without its culminating in a fit.

In a severe attack he fell and was generally convulsed; but as a rule he did not bite his tongue and never passed urine involuntarily. It was not preceded or followed by any change in vision.

Worry or long concentration on some troublesome task, such as his income tax return, was liable to induce an attack.

During this period of five years I made many observations on his physical and mental condition. He did not suffer from headache and was not conscious of the opening in his head except after a long and rough railway journey. The orifice remained depressed, even in the horizontal position, and did not pulsate unless he stooped profoundly.

Concentration and intellectual effort did not evoke a headache; but, when he tried to make a calculation, his mind went "blurred" and he did not feel "safe" that he was not about to have a fit.

Throughout, the fields of vision were determined repeatedly, but invariably showed the characters described above. He suffered from an incomplete hemianopsia and over the right half of the visual field tended to miss objects such as letters, unless his attention was concentrated directly upon them. All the observations made with a large screen in a darkened room were confirmed on many occasions (see p. 110).

I was able to carry out several complete sets of observations on the condition of symbolic formulation and expression, but shall give as an example those made in March 1920.

Symbolic Formulation and Expression in March 1920 (*three years and nine months after he was wounded*).

He had had no epileptiform attack for three months and was in excellent mental condition.

Articulated speech was perfect; the words were well pronounced, intonation was unaffected and the grammatical structure of the phrases was complete. He did not, however, employ complicated expressions or elaborate turns of speech, but reduced what he had to say to the simplest form sufficient to convey his meaning. The alphabet, the days of the week and the months were said in due order and without hesitation. He could repeat anything said to him with ease, provided it did not consist of many unconnected details.

Understanding of spoken words. He understood all that was said to him and could carry out the complex commands of the hand, eye and ear tests. But he did not always appreciate the full general significance of what he was told. "If a long direction is given me, 'go up to such and such a room and fetch such and such,' it's annoying and I can't get it. I can't anticipate it in my mind; I have to listen right through. I don't always get it, I get impatient. If the thing were put more cut and dried it would be easier."

Reading. He had no difficulty in reading words or short phrases to himself and carried out printed commands perfectly. But he became confused over a passage of any considerable length and had little power of summarising its meaning or shortening it by the omission of its less significant details. I gave him the following passage from Landor's letters and asked him to read it to himself and to narrate to me what he had gathered from it:

"To his sisters, 1830—But my country now is Italy where I have a residence for life and literally may sit under my own vine and my own fig-tree. I have some thousands of the one and some scores of the other, with myrtles, pomegranates, oranges, lemons, gageas and mimosas in great quantity. I intend to make a garden not very unlike yours at Warwick; but only time is wanting. I may live another ten years, but do not expect it. In a few days, whenever the weather will allow it,

I have four mimosas ready to place round my intended tomb and a friend who is coming to plant them."

After long study of this passage, he responded as follows: "He is writing to his sisters. Tells them that he is literally living under his own vine and fig-trees...yes, the former in hundreds, the latter in scores. His garden is...oh! yes...is full of mimosa and gageas and I forget the others. I hope to make my garden at Warwick similar to this or to plant them with such and such a thing. At my age I suppose this is too much. I have had a friend planting mimosas, which are to be on my tomb, when I die."

In many ways this was a remarkably complete reproduction of the passage he had just read, in spite of certain subtle deviations from its general significance. For instance, Landor was obviously writing from Italy about a garden there, which he wished to make "not very unlike yours at Warwick"; but he was made to say that he was anxious to "make my garden at Warwick similar to this." In the same way the friend, whose visit was anticipated, was said to have already completed his task of planting mimosas on the tomb. This was the sort of error that disturbed his comprehension of the contents of the newspaper or of the books he read to himself.

He read aloud perfectly, though rather slowly, and did not stumble over the words or make prolonged pauses between them.

Writing. He found no difficulty in writing his name, address or short phrases, such as those of the man, cat and dog series, correctly. He also composed with considerable labour an amusing letter on the servant problem; here it was not lack of ideas which troubled him, but the composition and method of expressing what he wanted to say. He wrote: "The servant problem at home continues to be rather a bore. If we only had a reasonable number of maids one could spend one's time in a more profitably, e.g. there would be no duties to think of before starting on some fishing expedition, etc. In my opinion and in that of others who are more 'au courant' it is essential on hearing of a possible maid to write immediately, or preferably to wire and thus lessen the chance of her being snapped up by a greater opportunist than oneself." When I laughed, he said, "By opportunist I mean people who are quicker than those at home; they always delay until it is too late."

Slowness in formulating the nature of an act carried out before him led to many errors, when he attempted to write down silently movements made by me; not only was he wrong over right and left, but occasionally mistook eye and ear.

He could write a long passage to dictation without fault and copied it perfectly; but he did not always comprehend the exact general significance of what he had written.

Numbers, arithmetic and the relative value of coins. He counted perfectly and on the occasion of this examination carried out all the simple arithmetical exercises correctly. But he complained, "I find things hard to understand; I'm thick. If I try to do any business, it is difficult to do any arithmetical calculation."

He made no actual mistakes in the relative value of two coins placed before him, although he was occasionally remarkably slow. This did not always depend on the apparent severity of the task; for although he took ten seconds to determine that five sixpences made up half-a-crown, he required three seconds only to give the answer "sixty," when a halfpenny and half-a-crown were laid before him.

During these tests he made the following remarks: "The calculation does not bother me. I suppose it's the in-between ones that are difficult, sixpence into two and six. But a penny into a shilling is easy; it's one calculation, twelve pence into a shilling. But the other is like this; sixpence into a shilling goes twice and into two shillings four times. Then, if it is two and six, there is one sixpence over, that's five." Obviously some of his answers are calculated by one step, others by two, and it is these which give him difficulty.

Drawing. He again produced the figure of an elephant without a trunk and did not recognise the omission until he was questioned.

He then said, "I'd like to draw a landscape. You wouldn't think it, but I've got a reputation for painting, an eye for colour; but I'm living on my old reputation." After making a few meaningless scrawls on the paper he explained his difficulty as follows: "I want the thing in front of me. I don't know how to build it up, to build up the foreground. I can see it in my mind, but I can't put it down."

I placed a tall glass in front of him and he made a fair drawing of its outlines. But ten minutes later, when he was asked to reproduce it from memory, he became confused and, after several alterations, said, "There's something I've forgotten about the bottom, something square; whether the glass went out at this part, I can't remember."

I took him into another room and asked him to draw a plan of the one in which we had so often worked; he produced a poor diagram in which the windows and doors were omitted, although he marked in details such as my typewriter and ophthalmoscope lamp.

I then placed a sheet of paper before him and, after indicating the usual position of our two chairs and the table at which we worked, I desired him to point to the relative situation of the various objects in my consulting room. This he did one by one with astonishing accuracy and fulness; he even described the colour of the paint and said, "I can see it in my mind."

General significance of pictures. He recognised perfectly the meaning of simple pictures and could describe them in detail; but he tended to miss their general significance, especially if the legend was necessary for their complete comprehension.

He still complained that he was "thick at jokes" and found it difficult to see the point however they were presented.

The general intention of an act. Throughout all the tests, he showed a combination of remarkable accuracy with absurd and unexpected lapses. He not uncommonly seemed to be puzzled with regard to the nature of the task he was to perform. Thus, before starting the coin-bowl tests, he counted the four bowls and the four coins from left to right; but, when I showed him the first printed order to place "the first coin into the third bowl," he took the first bowl and placed it into the third. Once this misunderstanding was corrected, he carried out all the subsequent commands, both oral and printed, correctly. It was errors of this kind which gave him trouble in the affairs of daily life.

He was an ardent and expert fly-fisher and tied his own flies and fishing knots. These he demonstrated to me, saying, "I've done them ever since I was a child." But he was not familiar with a reef knot and, after I showed him how it was tied, he failed time after time to reproduce it; finally on the sixth attempt he succeeded. It was startling to notice the ease, rapidity and precision with which he tied the familiar fishing knots compared with the slowness in making a reef knot, which he was not in the habit of using.

Serial Tests.

(1) He could name *common objects* and choose them correctly to oral and printed commands and he wrote the names silently without mistake. But he was easily puzzled with regard to the task he was expected to carry out; thus he would say, "Am I to point? oh yes!" "You want me to write the name do you?" When I answered "Yes" or repeated the order, he set to work rapidly and executed it without error.

(2) As before, *the man, cat and dog tests* were carried out perfectly throughout. He said, "I found no difficulty at all; there is no thinking about it."

(3) *The coin-bowl tests.* Before he began these tests I explained their nature to him and told him he was expected to place one of the coins into a certain bowl. He counted the coins and then the bowls from left to right. When, however, he was shown the first printed order to place "the first coin into the third bowl" he took the first bowl and placed it into the third. Asked if this was right he exclaimed, "Oh no!" and from that time onwards carried out all these tests correctly. This was a characteristic lapse in understanding.

(4) *The clock tests.*

He had improved considerably to this test, but still showed some uncertainty in direct imitation. He found oral commands the easiest to fulfil and he not only carried them out with great rapidity, but set the hour hand at a point proportionate to the minutes. This was not the case with direct imitation.

Table 3.

	Direct imitation	Oral commands	Printed commands: Railway time	Printed commands: Printed words	Telling the time	Writing down the time shown on a clock face	Telling the time aloud and writing it down: He said	Telling the time aloud and writing it down: He wrote
5 minutes to 2	Correct; very slow	Correct	Correct; slow	Correct	Correct	Correct	Correctly	Correctly
Half-past 1	Correct	,,	Correct	,,	,,	,,	,,	,,
5 minutes past 8	Correct; slow	,,	,,	,,	,,	,,	,,	,,
20 minutes to 4	Correct	,,	,,	,,	,,	,,	"Twenty five to four"	Twenty five to four
10 minutes past 7	,,	,,	,,	,,	,,	,,	Correctly	Correctly
20 minutes to 6	,,	,,	,,	,,	,,	,,	,,	,,
10 minutes to 1	,,	,,	,,	,,	,,	,,	,,	,,
A quarter to 9	A quarter to 3	,,	,,	,,	"A quarter to 3"	quarter to 3	"A quarter to three"	Quarter to three
20 minutes past 11	Correct	,,	,,	,,	Correct	Correct	Correctly	Correctly
25 minutes to 3	,,	,,	,,	,,	,,	,,	,,	,,

(5) *The hand, eye and ear tests.*

Table 4.

	Imitation of movements made by the observer	Imitation of movements reflected in a mirror	Pictorial commands	Pictorial commands reflected in a mirror	Oral commands	Printed commands	Writing down movements made by the observer
L. hand to R. ear	Correct	Correct	Reversed	R. hand to R. ear	Correct	Correct	Correct
R. hand to L. eye	,,	,,	,,	R. hand to R. eye	,,	,,	Right to left *ear*
R. hand to L. ear	Correct; very slow	,,	Correct	R. hand to L. *eye*	,,	,,	Correct
L. hand to L. eye	L. hand to R. eye	,,	,,	Correct	,,	,,	,,
R. hand to R. ear	Correct	,,	,,	,,	,,	,,	Left fto left *eye*
L. hand to R. eye	L. hand to L. eye	L. hand to R. *ear*	,,	,,	,,	,,	Correct
L. hand to L. ear	Correct	Correct	,,	,,	,,	,,	,,
R. hand to R. eye	,,	,,	,,	,,	,,	,,	Left to left eye
L. hand to R. ear	,,	,,	L. hand to L. ear; corrected	,,	,,	,,	Correct
R. hand to L. eye	R. hand to nose; corrected	,,	Correct	,,	,,	,,	Left to right eye
L. hand to R. eye	Correct	,,	,,	,,	,,	,,	Correct
R. hand to R. ear	,,	,,	R. hand to R. *eye*	,,	,,	,,	,,
L. hand to L. eye	,,	,,	Correct	Correct; very slow	,,	,,	,,
R. hand to L. ear	,,	,,	R. hand to L. *eye*	Correct	,,	,,	Right to right ear
L. hand to L. ear	,,	,,	Correct	,,	,,	,,	Correct
R. hand to R. eye	,,	,,	,,	,,	,,	,,	,,

Here he had also improved; as before oral and printed commands were properly executed and he was better able to imitate movements or pictorial commands reflected in the mirror. As might be expected he found somewhat greater difficulty in writing down than imitating movements made by me, sitting face to face.

I made another complete set of observations in July 1921, five years and one month after he was wounded. These bore out exactly the results detailed above and the records obtained with the clock and with the hand, eye and ear tests were on the whole identical. He carried out accurately oral and printed commands; but my movements or pictorial orders, even when reflected in a mirror, were imperfectly executed. He still showed the same lapses of general comprehension.

The act he performed did not of necessity follow his reasoning and his conclusions were often logically faulty.

I had the opportunity at this time of testing his power of playing billiards; this brought out in a striking manner his inability to formulate the intention or aim of an act he was about to perform. He could hit a second ball directly and could pocket it with ease. But, if he attempted to put the ball into the pocket off another, he not infrequently struck it on the wrong side. For the same reason he was unable to make a simple cannon and was quite incapable of bringing off any stroke from the cushion. He complained, "I can't think out which side to hit it. I have so much difficulty in thinking out the scheme of it."

CONDITION IN OCTOBER 1922 (*six years and four months after he was wounded*).

On October 5th, 1921, he started for a tour round the world in the company of a doctor and I did not see him again until twelve months later. Throughout the whole of this year he had three slight epileptiform attacks only, the last of which occurred on August 21st, 1922.

When he returned to my care, he had obviously improved greatly. He did not suffer from headaches and was much less easily fatigued.

He was completely unconscious that his vision was in any way defective, except for the fact that at times he "loses somebody" in an unaccountable manner. As he looked around him with both eyes open, he was entirely unable to recognise that his field was restricted; and yet the hemianopsia was unchanged.

Symbolic Formulation and Expression.

He was extremely bright and cheerful and had greatly enjoyed the journey. But he found he was unable to look out trains or plan the route to be taken, which was settled for him by his companion. He still had difficulty in coordinating details to form a general conception.

Articulated speech was in every way normal and he could repeat anything said to him.

Understanding of spoken words. He understood ordinary conversation and carried out all the tests correctly to oral commands, even setting the hands of the clock without mistakes. But he was still liable to be puzzled by some general suggestion that he should behave in some particular manner, or by a logical statement of the reasons for such action. Thus, when dealing with his plans for the future, he wrote down a series of questions he wanted to put to me, but could not combine my answers into a coherent whole. I was compelled to let him lay his questions before me one by one and then to frame my reply as a single direct statement.

Reading. He could read to himself with pleasure and read aloud with perfect ease. The improvement in power to grasp the meaning of what he read was profound; but he was still liable to become confused, if the subject matter was complex or difficult to understand.

Writing. His writing had greatly improved and he was able to set down without error the time shown on a clock and the movements made by me in the hand, eye and ear tests.

Arithmetic. On his travels he kept accurate accounts of his private expenditure and managed his own money, paying all the smaller bills in hotels and restaurants. But he could not estimate the larger expenditure of a projected journey; this he left to his companion.

He carried out all the arithmetical tests correctly, without that doubt and hesitation so obvious on previous occasions. Moreover, he could now state the relative value of two coins with ease and certainty.

Visual images. There is no doubt that he normally employed visual images, when attempting to recall some place or scene. He described to me in detail the various features of my waiting room; but his power of evoking a mental picture of any definite object to command was uncertain. Thus, after he had described my waiting room, I asked him if there were any pictures; he replied, "I don't remember seeing your father's picture to-day, but I know it was there before." Although he recollected the existence of the portrait, he could not recall it to order.

Serial Tests.

In view of the fact that he had long been able to name and choose common objects with ease, to execute the man, cat and dog tests correctly and to place a numbered coin into one of the bowls to order, I concentrated my attention more particularly on the following tests:

(1) *The clock tests*. He set the hands without a single mistake in direct imitation and carried out oral and printed commands whether they were given in ordinary nomenclature or in railway time. He tended to place the hour hand opposite the number on the face of the clock and then sometimes shifted it forwards or backwards to correspond to the number of minutes; this was, however, the only fault. He also told the time aloud or wrote it down in silence without a single error. Thus, these tests, which caused him the greatest difficulty at first, were now executed without mistakes.

(2) *The hand, eye and ear tests*. Here again there was profound improvement. He imitated movements made by me or represented in pictures, carried out oral or printed commands and wrote down my movements exactly. In explanation he said, "I look at you and then I say 'he's got his hand on my left therefore it's on the right.' I have to translate it, to transfer it in my mind." When my movements or the pictures were reflected in a mirror, his responses were quick and certain for, as he explained, "There was no translation there." Printed commands were somewhat less easily executed than those given orally and he said, "I had to read it and go carefully"; but he made no mistakes throughout the series.

No. 9

A case of Verbal Aphasia, due to a severe and extensive gun-shot injury in the left parieto-occipital region.

This produced profound right hemiplegia, both motor and sensory, with gross hemianopsia which included half central vision.

His speech was reduced to little more than the use of "yes" and "no" and he could not even pronounce his own name correctly. He had extreme difficulty in finding the names of common objects and colours, but the sounds he uttered bore a distinct relation to the words he was seeking. When he attempted to repeat what was said to him, articulation was extremely defective. His comprehension of single spoken words was good and he executed oral commands, provided they did not necessitate elaborate choice. He could select a familiar object in response to its name in print, but was slower and less certain with colours and failed grossly with the more complex tests. He wrote his name, but could not add his rank, regiment or address, and was unable to write down the names of common objects. He could copy printed matter in capitals only. These defects in writing were not due to mechanical inability to form the letters, but rather to a difficulty in using them as appropriate symbols; for, if he were shown an object and asked to compose its name from a set of block letters, he was unable to do so. He counted up to ten, but could go no further and failed to solve simple problems in arithmetic. He succeeded in naming coins, although the words were badly pronounced, and in every case recognised their relative value. He showed a vivid appreciation of pictures and could draw on the whole correctly even to command. He produced a ground-plan of his corner of the ward, but tended to draw some of the objects in elevation. Orientation was in no way affected. He played an excellent game of draughts.

Examined three years and nine months after he was wounded, he was still somewhat hemiplegic. The loss of power in the right arm and leg was mainly afferent in origin; although the deep reflexes on this half of the body were exaggerated, the plantar gave an upward response and the abdominals were not obtained. There was still complete right hemianopsia.

The defects of speech, though less severe, retained the same character, consisting mainly of loss of power to evoke words in a correct form and still greater difficulty in translating them into written symbols. His improved condition allowed me to carry out all the tests with greater elaboration and the records exhibit on the whole a good example of a somewhat severe case of Verbal Aphasia.

Sergeant John M., aged 27, was wounded in the left parieto-occipital region on August 14th, 1918. A note made in the field ambulance on the same day ran as follows: "On admission he was deeply unconscious. Pupils dilated and inactive to light; conjunctival reflex almost gone. Pulse rapid and irregular, in force and

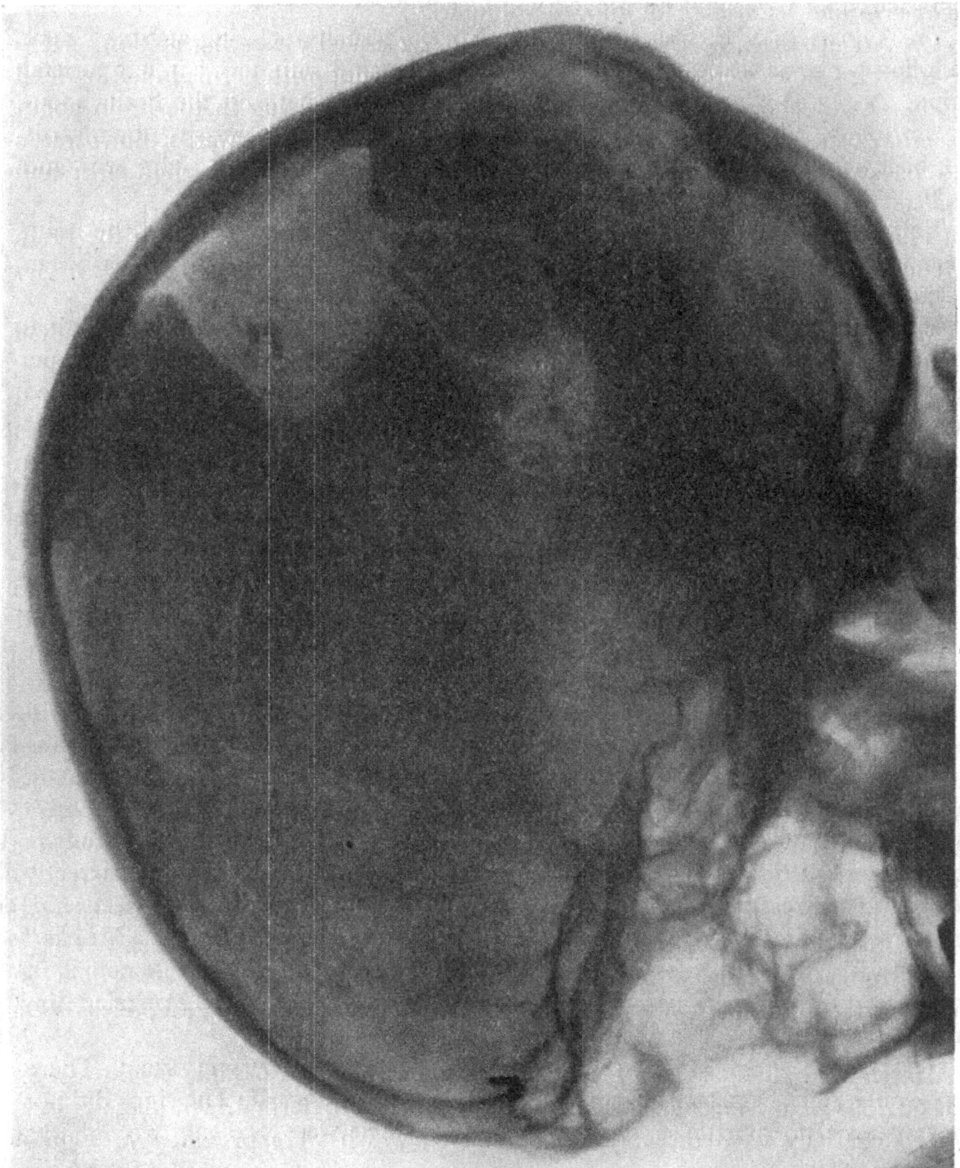

Fig. 20. To show the injury to the skull in No. 9, a case of Verbal Aphasia.

rhythm, but full in volume. After two hours he recovered consciousness and was able to make signs and respond to simple requests (as 'put out your tongue'). Right arm and leg cannot be moved voluntarily."

On August 15th, he was admitted to No. 22 casualty clearing station. Here the following notes were added: "Lacerated scalp wound with hernia in left parietal region. X-ray showed a foreign body of circular shape lying in the brain about 2·5 cm. deep. There were widespread fractures extending forwards, downwards and backwards. Aphasia; face normal. Complete paralysis of right arm and leg."

The wound was excised and fragments of bone were removed from the brain by suction. By September 9th, the incisions in the scalp had healed. Power began to return to the leg by August 28th, and to the arm two days later.

When he was admitted to the London Hospital on September 19th, the original wound was represented by a granulating patch, roughly triangular in shape, measuring about 1 cm. horizontally, and 2 cm. in a vertical direction; this occupied the centre of a pulsating area from which the bone had been removed. It was situated in the parieto-occipital region, 21·5 to 26·5 cm. along the nasion-inion line and extended from 1 to 3 cm. to the left of the middle of the scalp. The total nasion-inion measurement was 34 cm. and this was transected by the interaural line at a point 14 cm. backwards from the root of the nose.

An X-ray photograph showed a roughly quadrilateral area, from which bone had been removed, with several fissured fractures extending downwards and forwards (Fig. 20).

The wound healed completely by September 30th.

On admission he could say "yes" and "no" and employ them correctly in answer to questions; but he was otherwise completely aphasic. Although he was unable to say the alphabet spontaneously or to repeat it after me, he succeeded in counting up to ten with some difficulty. When I said his name he repeated "John," uttered an incomprehensible sound for "Munks," but failed altogether to reproduce the name of his home. He was unable to carry out printed commands correctly and could not read even single words aloud. His right hand was paralysed and, when I asked him to write his name with the left, he produced "Juck Munks" (Jack Munks), but failed altogether with his address. Simple words were copied in capital letters, but not in cursive script. Dictation was impossible and puzzled him completely.

He showed all the signs of a right hemiplegia of gross organic origin. There was obvious right hemianopsia, but the optic discs were normal. The signs did not differ materially from those described below, which were present two months later.

CONDITION BETWEEN NOVEMBER 9TH AND DECEMBER 9TH, 1918 (*twelve to sixteen weeks after he was wounded*).

He was a bright, intelligent man twenty-seven years of age, who had risen to the rank of sergeant in the new army. He was gay and happy, a willing witness, amused and interested in the tests I set him He performed many useful tasks in the ward in spite of his hemiplegia.

Symbolic Formulation and Expression.

Articulated speech. He could use "yes" and "no" correctly but employed no automatic expressions except "No, sir." Asked his name, he answered "John Muns," but he could not give the name of his regiment, his rank, or the address of his home. When he attempted to find the word "Currie," the name of the ward of which he was an inmate, he said "Mor-rock-ĕ," "Mor-ay," "Mol-kie."

He could not give the days of the week or the months of the year in sequence or as isolated words. He had extreme difficulty in finding the names of common objects and with colours he frequently failed entirely. But the sounds he uttered in his attempts bore a distinct relation to the form of the words he was seeking and once he called a knife "dinner" correcting it later to "naive."

The number of words at his disposal were too few to test his syntactical powers; but, when translating pictures of the man, the cat and the dog into words, he uttered sounds obviously intended to represent the articles and the conjunction. Moreover, the structure of these phrases was not broken up, as in cases of disordered syntax.

He frequently failed altogether to find words in which to tell the time; occasionally he overcame this difficulty by expressing the minutes in terms of the hour-number to which the long hand was pointing. Thus, for twenty-five minutes to six, he said "six, seven."

When he tried to repeat a series of simple phrases, the words were extremely badly formed; and yet they obviously represented correctly the content of what I had said.

Understanding of spoken words. His comprehension of single words was good and he carried out oral commands perfectly, provided they did not necessitate elaborate choice. Thus he selected the common object or colour mentioned by me, and set the clock correctly to my orders. But he was slow in executing the more complex hand, eye and ear tests, making three mistakes in sixteen attempts.

Reading. He understood the meaning of single words, selecting without difficulty the right object in answer to printed commands. But his choice of colours was slower and less certain; he twice fell into error in the course of eighteen serial tests.

He set the clock without difficulty to orders given in a mixture of printed words and numbers. He made many mistakes over the hand, eye and ear tests, on four occasions mistaking eye and ear.

But when these printed commands were simplified to a single act of some definite part the results were as follows:

Shut your eyes—He said, "Aye, aye," and touched his eye with his hand.
Give me your hand—He said, "And," holding up his right hand and moving the fingers.
Touch your nose—He said, "Do-do," and pinched his nose.
Put out your tongue—He said, "Tongue," and touched his toe; then he shook his head but made no further movement.
Give me your hand—He said, "Hand, hand," and moved the fingers of the left hand.
Put out your tongue—He said, "Gone," and touched the tip of the tongue with the left hand.
Shut your eyes—He said, "Aye," and touched his eye with his left hand.
Touch your nose—He said, "Nose," and pinched it.
Put out your tongue—He said, "Tong, tang," and touched his tongue.
Shut your eyes—He said, "Eyes," and touched them with his left hand.
Give me your hand—He said, "And, hand," and clenched his left fist.
Touch your nose—He said, "Noise, noise," and touched his nose.

He read aloud the names of common objects and colours extremely badly, although the sounds he uttered bore a definite relation to the word he was striving to pronounce. In the same way, the simple phrases of the man, cat and dog tests were almost as poorly articulated as if they were produced spontaneously in response to pictorial combinations.

Writing. He wrote "John Munks," but not his rank, regiment or address and he could not write down the name of a common object. When, however, he was shown any two pictures of the man, cat and dog tests, he succeeded in printing with the left hand an imperfect series of capital letters, sufficient to indicate the words he was striving to reproduce.

He could copy printed matter in capitals only, and was unable to transcribe it into cursive print.

He failed completely to write to dictation, producing a few isolated letters only. In response to pictures he wrote somewhat better, although the words were for the most part badly spelt or incomplete.

These defects in writing were not due to mechanical inability to form the letters, but rather to a difficulty in using them as appropriate symbols. For if he was given a set of block letters and asked to compose the name of an object shown to him, he was entirely unable to do so. A series of twelve observations produced the following result:

Object shown.

Key—He chose K N, and said, "No."
Penny—He chose N, and said, "No."

Match-box—He shook his head and said, "No."
Knife—He chose K E, and shook his head.
Pencil—He made no choice and said, "No, sir."
Scissors—He made no choice and said, "No."
Key—He chose K.
Penny—He chose N.
Match-box—He made no choice and said, "No, sir."
Knife—He made no choice and said, "No, sir."
Pencil—He chose N, and said, "No, sir."
Scissors—He made no choice and said, "No, sir."

And yet when he was shown the name of each of these objects in turn, printed on a card, he rapidly selected the block letters necessary to compose them. He then pointed correctly to the corresponding object on the table, showing that he understood fully the significance of what he had done.

But he had more difficulty in putting together in block letters words expressing the pictures of the man, cat and dog tests, although he finally reached the correct answer in every instance.

The alphabet. He could not say the letters in spontaneous sequence. He started with "A D C," then again "A D C G, don't know," and finally "A D C A C, no, sir."

He wrote the alphabet as follows: A B C E, but could get no further.

I dictated letter by letter and he wrote A × C D E F G × I J K L M N O T Q L S T × × × X Y Z. The crosses represent the letters he was unable to reproduce. It was noticeable that when he could say a letter clearly he could as a rule write it; for B, he perpetually said "D" or "C" and "H" he could not say at all. For P, he insisted on saying "T" and he could not articulate U V W correctly.

He had no difficulty in copying the alphabet in capitals, but could not transcribe the letters into cursive script.

Given a quantity of block letters and asked to compose an alphabet, he put together the following sequence: A B C D E G H I L; he then removed the L, and continued, M N J L U W V Y O, to which he slowly added X and Z. I then asked him if there was anything wrong and he placed the J between the I and the M, shaking his head as he did so.

I then removed all the letters from the table, except those contained in his alphabet and the additional ones necessary to complete it. After many trials and changes he produced the following: A B C D E G F H K O I J M N L P U S R T W V Y Q X Z.

I asked him to read the letters aloud as they lay on the table. The first seven were pronounced correctly; H and K became "Aitch" and "Kai" probably due to his provincial accent, O was "Oi," I "One" and "Ae," J "Gee," M "Am, an," N correctly, L "Lai, ell," P correctly, U "O-you," S "Ezz," R "don't know," T "Dee," W "Dol-two," V "don't know," Y "I, lai; no," Q "Qu-er," and then correctly, X "Zuzz," Z "Zizz, zuzz."

Numbers. He counted correctly up to ten and the words were fairly well pronounced. He continued, "eleven, twenty," and stopped; then after a pause he began again, "eleven, twelve, ten, twelve, no sir."

Asked to write the numbers, he produced a perfect series of Roman figures up to VIII and then ceased. When I suggested that he should write the ordinary (arabic) numerals he did nothing and finally said, "no, no."

But he copied the numbers up to 10 fluently and I then asked him to write them without a copy. He at once reproduced them perfectly, stopping at 10.

In spite of his inability to evoke with certainty in sequence numbers higher than 10, he used 20, 30 and 40 correctly to express the minutes, when writing down the time shown on the clock.

Arithmetic. He was fairly well educated and his intelligence had carried him to the rank of sergeant; but he was greatly puzzled by simple sums.

Addition.

```
325        458
432        122
---        ---
757         10
            0  He wrote 10 then changed the 1 into 6, added an o below and
                  became confused.

567
358
---
  5 He wrote 5 at once. Then he became puzzled and stopped, saying, "no, no."
```

Subtraction.

```
586          653                        422
242          215                        148
---          ---                        ---
344          "No," shaking his head       0
                                        "No"
```

Coins and their relative value. He named the difference in coins as follows:

	1st series	*2nd series*	*3rd series*
Penny	"Punny"	Correct	Correct
Two-shilling piece	"Two...shi"	"Two shields"	"Two shilns"
Sixpence	"Sixes"	"Sixes"	"Arf-a-shiln"
Halfpenny	"Ae-punny"	Correct	"Arf-a-deddy"
Two and sixpence (half a crown)	"Arf-sixes" (then correct)	Correct ("arf a crown")	Correct
Shilling	"Shiln"	"One shiln"	"One shiln"

In every instance the name was correct.

Moreover, he invariably stated their relative value accurately; even when given a penny and a two-shilling piece, he answered, "Twelve, twenty-six, four, twenty-four," repeating the last number. In the earlier days of his stay in hospital, when he could not name a single coin, he indicated their relative value correctly by raising the requisite number of fingers.

Drawing. He made a good drawing with his left hand of a spirit lamp, placed before him, and reproduced it with fair accuracy from memory, after removal of the model.

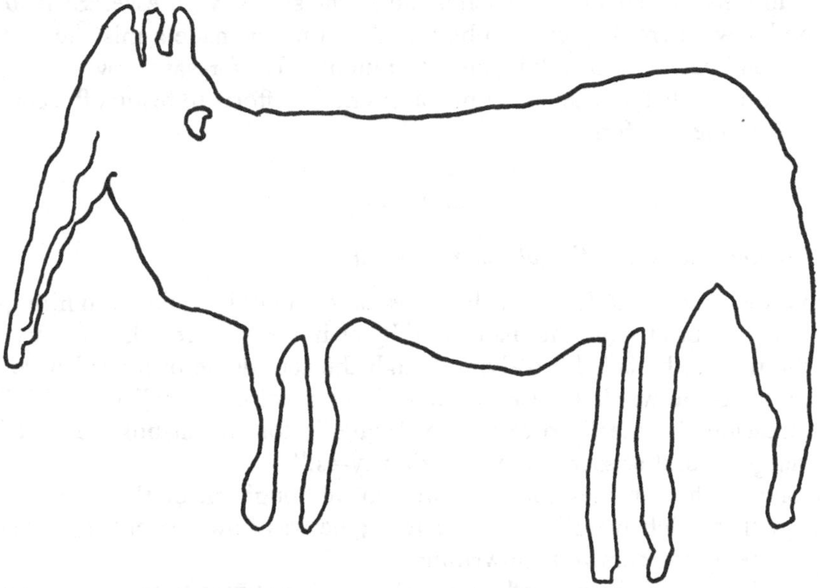

Fig. 21. Attempt by No. 9 to draw an elephant to command.

Asked to draw an elephant, he produced the figure given above and proceeded to point out its various parts as follows. The projection in front, obviously intended for the trunk, was called "Crank, crack, grat." Then he drew the irregular line along the trunk, evidently representing a tusk, and called it "Teet." The curious projections on the top of the head were "His ears."

I then requested him to draw anything he liked and, saying "Man, man." he sketched an excellent diagram of a face. He named the eyes correctly; the mouth was called "Mouse, mout," the nose "Morse, mose." When he came to the ears he said "Eye, lay"; then he caught hold of his own ear repeating "Lie." The neck was called "Seph."

Thus he could draw from a model or from his memory of it and also fairly well if allowed to choose his subject; but an obligatory task, like that of drawing an elephant, was executed less successfully although he inserted all its salient features.

He showed a vivid appreciation of the significance of pictures. I drew a teapot and said, "What would you do with this?" he made a motion of drinking. But when I said, "Would you drink out of that?" he replied, "No, no," and, seizing a pencil, drew the picture of a cup.

Plan and orientation. He was able to indicate correctly the relative position of the beds, tables and windows in that part of the ward which he occupied. He tended, however, to draw the windows, cupboard and other objects in elevation, although the three beds were represented in plan.

He found his way about the hospital and in the streets with ease. Sent to fetch things, he knew where they were to be found and never made a mistake.

Games. He played a splendid game of draughts. He foresaw moves long ahead and, when I neglected to take one of his pieces in my efforts to bring off a combination, he made me pay forfeit at once.

Serial Tests.

(1) *Naming and recognition of common objects.*

He pointed out correctly and without hesitation an object shown to him, placed in his left hand out of sight, and named orally or in print. But, when he attempted to find the names, he failed grossly, although the sounds he produced bore a distinct relation to the words he was seeking. Thus a knife was called "naide" and on one occasion "dinner" corrected to "naive"; for match-box he said "box, buxes, marges," and scissors became "ziz-zuy-es."

Not one of these names could be written, although all of them were copied correctly with the left hand in capital letters; he was however entirely unable to transcribe them into cursive handwriting.

He could not read the printed names aloud. Sometimes the sounds resembled those produced, when he attempted to name these common objects spontaneously; but on the whole the results were worse and on two occasions he gave up altogether.

(2) *Naming and recognition of colours.*

He selected without hesitation the colour on the table which corresponded to that shown to him. But, on attempting to indicate the one named orally or in print, his choice was made more slowly and with less certainty; he fell into few actual errors, but was doubtful about such colours as yellow, violet and pink.

He named the colours extremely badly and on several occasions gave up the attempt to do so altogether. Asked to read the printed names aloud, he was almost equally at fault; but the choice he made, though slow, was correct except in one instance, when orange was chosen for blue.

Table 1.

	Pointing to object shown	Oral commands	Printed commands	Duplicate placed in left hand out of sight	Naming object indicated	Writing name of object indicated	Copying from print	Reading aloud from print
Key	Correct	Correct	Correct	Correct	"Queer, quiz, way"	Impossible	In print only	"Chin, chin"
Scissors	„	„	„	„	"Suz-zers"	„	„	"Siz-zers"
Match box	„	„	„	„	"Box, buxes, marges"	„	„	"Maxes, masses, baxes"
Pencil	„	„	„	„	"Per-zes"	„	„	"Tier-cel, lĕr-cel, ser-sel, lĕr-sel"
Knife	„	„	„	„	"Nide"	„	„	"Night"
Penny	„	„	„	„	"Punny" (almost perfect)	„	„	"Pun-ny"
Match box	„	„	„	„	"Batches, burges"	„	„	"Batches"
Knife	„	„	„	„	"Dinner; no, naive"	„	„	"No, no." Shaking his head "No, sir"
Key	„	„	„	„	"Wee, nize"	„	„	"Tchin"
Penny	„	„	„	„	"Pun-ny"	„	„	"Pun-ny"
Pencil	„	„	„	„	"Pesh-il, pesh-wl"	„	„	"Woz-il, woz-it, no"
Scissors	„	„	„	„	"Ziz-zuz-es"	„	„	"Ziz-zors"

Table 2.

	Pointing to colour shown	Oral commands	Printed commands	Naming colour shown	Printed name read aloud and colour chosen	
					He said	He chose
Red	Correct	Correct	Correct	"Wex, green"	Correctly	Correctly
White	„	„	„	"Whey, wed, wait"	"Wide"	„
Yellow	„	„	Orange	"No, sir"	"Wully"	Correctly; very slow
Green	„	„	Correct	"Greel, gree"	"Grin"	Correctly
Orange	„	„	„	"Wullies, wullis; no, sir"	"Orāze"	„
Pink	„	„	„	"No, sir"	"Plink"	„
Blue	„	Correct; slow	Correct; slow	Correct	Correctly	Correctly; very slow
Black	„	„	„	"Blike, blake"	"Blax"	Correctly
Violet	„	Correct; slow	Correct; slow	"Gruze, gruce; no, sir"	"Wo-ruz"	„
Green	„	Correct	Correct	"Breen, breem"	"Brin"	„
White	„	„	„	"Wide"	"Wer-ight"	„
Violet	„	„	Yellow	"Greeze, green"	"Or-er-er"	„
Black	„	„	Correct	Correct	"Blike"	„
Orange	„	„	„	"No, sir"	"Rogers, rogers"	„
Red	„	„	„	"No"	Correctly	„
Blue	„	Correct; slow	„	"No"	„	Orange
Pink	„	Yellow	„	"Ping"	"Ping"	Correctly
Yellow	„	Correct; slow	„	"No, sir"	"Lowly, lol-o-la, low-o-ly"	„

(3) *The man, cat and dog tests.*

Table 3.

	Reading aloud	Reading from pictures	Repetition	Copying	Writing from dictation	Writing from pictures	Words composed of block letters to correspond with pictures
The man and the dog	"Mon, mun an dug"	"Man...gad, jag, gad"	"The man and the dug"	Correct in printed capitals only	D	MON GON	Correct
The dog and the cat	"Thos dug of dut, dat, cat"	"Uzz gad...cat"	"The dug un er back, cat"	,,	—	GO T	,,
The man and the cat	"One dag, man, cat, cat"	"Uzz man oo er cat"	"The man er ther cat"	,,	M	MENT	,,
The dog and the man	"Gag, gags, gug an man"	"Gad un er man"	"The gag us er more. The bag uz er man"	,,	GO	GOT MEN	,,
The cat and the dog	"One cat avedee, gag, gag"	"Cat un er gadge"	"The cat un ther dug"	,,	T	T GON	Finally correct
The cat and the man	"Cat ave man"	"Cat un er man"	"The cat uz er man er"	,,	TO	CAT MEN	Correct
The man and the dog	"One man er er gag, gug, gag"	"Ur man ur er gadge"	"Er man er zur bag"	,,	M	MEN GO	,,
The dog and the cat	"One gag er er cat"	"Gad gadge ur er cat"	"Gags er er cat"	,,	GO	GO CAT	Finally correct
The man and the cat	"One man er er cat"	"Urs man urs er cat"	"Ther man er er cat"	,,	MON CAT	MEN C	,,
The dog and the man	"Wul gag, gags un er man"	"Ur gadge un er man"	"Thog er the man"	,,	T	G MEN	Correct
The cat and the dog	"One cat er gags"	"Ur cat un er gadge"	"Er cat un er dug, dag, dug"	,,	COT GO	CAT G	Finally correct
The cat and the man	"One cat er er man"	"Er cat un er man"	"Er cat uz er man"	,,	TH	CAT MEN	Correct

He had extreme difficulty in producing these simple words in response to print or pictures. In fact, there was no material or characteristic difference between these two serial records.

He could copy the words in capital letters with his left hand, but was unable to transcribe them into cursive script. Writing to dictation was impossible. He wrote somewhat better to pictures, although no single instance was exactly correct. Throughout all his writing there was a tendency to spell dog, "go," "got" or "gon." Cat was more often correctly spelt than any other word of the series.

Given a set of block letters, he succeeded in putting together the two nouns in each phrase accurately in response to pictures. But he was slow and tried many combinations before he was satisfied. For instance at the fifth test, when shown the cat and dog, he began by selecting T; this he removed and chose C O. He then put together C A T. D A G, replaced the last three letters by G A, and then finally by D O G.

(4) *The clock tests.*

He showed no hesitation in setting the clock in direct imitation, or to oral and printed commands. But he had extreme difficulty in telling the time aloud and frequently gave up altogether, saying, "No, sir." At other times he named the position of the minute hand according to the number on the clock face to which it pointed, as for instance "six seven" for twenty-five minutes to six and "one eight" for five minutes past eight. Moreover, the words, even when recognisable, were badly articulated.

Table 4.

	Direct imitation	Oral commands	Printed commands	Telling the time	Writing down the time shown on a clock
25 minutes to 3	Correct	Correct	Correct	"No, sir"	53
20 minutes to 6	,,	,,	,,	"Tanty to"	20-6
Half-past 2	,,	,,	,,	"Harves do do"	30-2
20 minutes past 9	,,	,,	,,	"No"	9-40
A quarter to 12	,,	,,	,,	"No"	"No, sir"
25 minutes to 3	,,	,,	,,	"No"	55-3
5 minutes to 2	,,	,,	,,	"Two, one, two"	5-2
Half-past 1	,,	,,	,,	"No, sir"	1-30
5 minutes past 8	,,	,,	,,	"Eight, to, one, eight"	8-5
20 minutes to 4	,,	,,	,,	"Three four, eight to four"	40-4
10 minutes past 7	,,	,,	,,	"Tence to seven"	10-7
10 minutes to 1	,,	,,	,,	"Ten to one"	50-1
A quarter to 9	,,	,,	,,	"Eight, nine, nine half nine"	45-9
20 minutes past 11	,,	,,	,,	"Leven, twelve, leven; no"	54-11; "No, sir"
25 minutes to 6	,,	,,	,,	"Six, seven, six, seven"	53-6

To indicate the time in writing he used figures only, but combined the usual nomenclature with railway time. As a rule he placed the minutes first if they were "to" the hour (e.g. 20-6, for twenty to six) and in the usual position of railway time if they were "past" (e.g. 8-5, and 1-30). But, even with the broadest interpretation, the time was frequently given incorrectly and the words were badly formed.

(5) *The coin-bowl tests.* He could carry out both oral and printed commands, showing his complete understanding of the significance of the lower numbers.

(6) *The hand, eye and ear tests.*

Table 5.

	Imitation of movements made by the observer	Imitation of movements reflected in a mirror	Pictorial commands	Pictorial commands reflected in a mirror	Oral commands	Printed commands
R. hand to R. eye	Correct	Correct	Reversed	Correct	R. hand to L. eye	Traced letters with his fingers; no movement
L. hand to R. ear	L. hand to L. ear	,,	,,	,,	Correct	L. hand to L. *eye*
R. hand to L. eye	R. hand to R. eye	,,	,,	,,	,,	L. hand to L. eye
R. hand to L. ear	Correct	,,	,,	,,	,,	L. hand to L. ear
L. hand to L. eye	,,	,,	Correct	,,	,,	Correct
R. hand to R. ear	,,	,,	Reversed	,,	R. hand to R. *eye*	R. hand to R. *eye*; then correct
L. hand to R. eye	L. hand to L. eye	,,	L. hand to R. *ear*	,,	Correct	Correct
L. hand to L. ear	Correct	,,	Reversed	,,	L. hand to L. *eye*; then correct	,,
L. hand to R. ear	,,	,,	,,	,,	Correct	L. hand to L. ear; then R. hand to R. ear
R. hand to L. ear	L. hand to L. ear; then R. hand to R. ear	,,	,,	,,	,,	R. hand to R. ear
R. hand to R. ear	Correct	,,	Correct	,,	,,	Correct
L. hand to L. ear	,,	,,	,,	,,	,,	,,
R. hand to R. eye	,,	,,	Reversed	,,	,,	R. hand to R. *ear*; then correct
R. hand to L. eye	R. hand to R. eye	,,	,,	,,	,,	R. hand to R. eye; then L. hand to L. eye
L. hand to L. eye	Correct	,,	,,	,,	,,	Correct
L. hand to R. eye	Correct; then L. hand to L. eye	,,	,,	,,	,,	L. hand to L. *ear*; then R. hand to R. eye

When he attempted to imitate my movements sitting face to face, or to carry out pictorial commands, he made many mistakes. But he executed both tasks accurately if either my movements or the pictures were reflected in a mirror.

His response to oral and printed commands was slow and imperfect and he showed a tendency to confuse eye and ear.

Physical Examination.

He was a small, well-built, strongly right-handed man.

He had not suffered from convulsions or seizures of any kind and, throughout his stay in hospital, was free from headache.

There was complete right hemianopsia, which included central vision to this half of the middle line (Fig. 22). Over the blind area form and movement were equally abolished and the reaction of the pupil was absent, or greatly diminished. Vision was perfect over the left half of the field.

Hearing, smell and taste were not affected.

The pupils responded well, except from the hemianopic area, and there was no nystagmus or ocular paralysis. Movements of the right angle of the mouth were less perfect than those of the left and the tongue was protruded distinctly to the right.

All the deep reflexes on the right half of the body were exaggerated and stimulation of the sole of the foot gave a characteristically upward response. The reflexes obtained from the right half of the abdomen were distinctly abnormal; dragging a pin across the surface evoked a slow, undulating contraction, in which the rectus did not participate, confined to the neighbourhood of the part scratched. On the left side such stimulation was followed by a general movement of withdrawal, which included contraction of all the muscles of this half of the abdomen.

On the motor side he showed all the signs of a severe hemiplegia. The grasp of the right hand was greatly diminished (R. 20 kg., L. 60 kg.) and individual movements of the fingers were impossible. When he held out his arms in front of him, the digits of the right hand were out of alignment; this increased and they dropped away still further, on shutting his eyes. Incoordination was present on attempting to touch his nose with the right forefinger, but it was greatly exaggerated, when his eyes were closed. There was no spastic rigidity or hypotonia. Movements of the right elbow and shoulder were carried out well against resistance, though less powerful than those of the left arm.

He now walked easily, although the gait was still characteristically hemiplegic. He could support his weight with difficulty on the right foot, falling immediately his eyes were closed. Dorsiflexion and plantar extension of this foot could be carried out to command, but were weaker than on the normal side. There was distinct incoordination of the right leg and, when his eyes were closed, he found

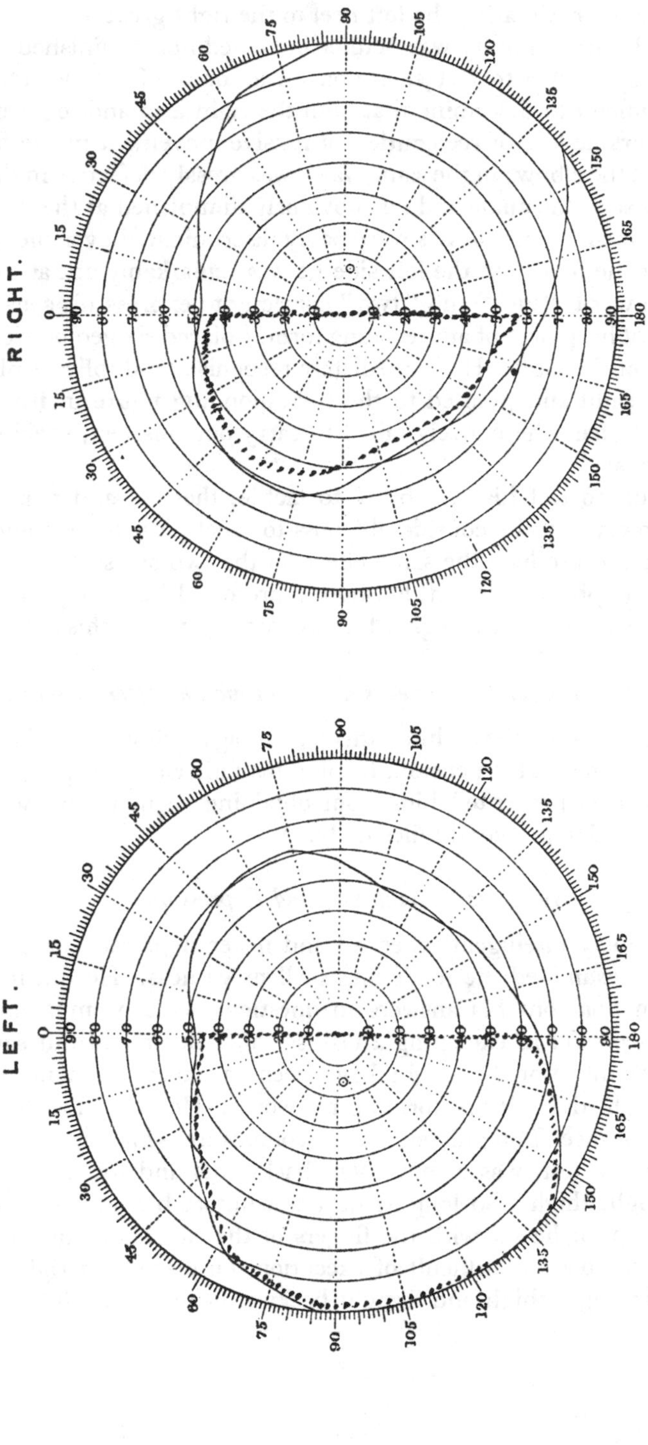

Fig. 22. To show the limitation of the fields of vision in No. 9.

more difficulty in approximating the left heel to the right great toe than vice versa. The tone of the lower extremity was neither increased nor diminished.

It was no easy matter to test sensation on account of his defective speech; but it was not difficult to determine that both the right arm and leg were affected. There was measurable loss of recognition of passive movement in the fingers and, to a less degree, at the elbow; in the same way it was grossly defective in the great toe, considerably less so at the ankle and not obviously diminished at the knee and hip.

The two points of the compasses were badly discriminated over the right index, palm and sole of the foot. On the left side he was remarkably apt at this test and he could use the words "one" and "two" correctly to express his sensations.

In order to test his power of appreciating form, I placed six geometrically shaped blocks in a row on the table. He immediately recognised a duplicate placed in his left hand out of sight and pointed to the corresponding figure in front of him. But with the right hand he entirely failed to carry out this test, shaking his head and saying, "No, sir."

It was difficult to test his sensibility to tactile, thermal and painful stimuli; there seemed, however, to be considerable loss to touch, less to heat and cold, and pricking appeared to produce the same effect on the two sides.

Thus, from the physical aspect, he showed profound hemianopsia and obvious right hemiplegia, with loss of the higher forms of sensation over this half of the body.

CONDITION IN APRIL 1922 (*three years and eight months after he was wounded*).

I had the opportunity of examining this patient again thoroughly in April 1922. He was living at home on his pension, helping his father and keeping a few fowls. The right hemiplegia prevented him from obtaining regular paid work, but he led an active life, walking several miles daily.

Symbolic Formulation and Expression.

He was extremely intelligent, cheerful and never depressed or bored. Quiet and willing to be examined, he made an excellent witness. He did not as a rule volunteer information, but his answers to questions were prompt and accurate. When he was successful in executing a task set him, he smiled but said nothing. On superficial examination he might have been mistaken for a normal person, except for the slight difficulty in forming his words. He never lost his temper or flushed with annoyance. The only sign of discomposure which appeared, when he had difficulty over a test, was a movement backwards and forwards of the right hand over the right thigh. So long as he was comfortable and at ease the right hand lay in his lap, or he sat with the fingers of the two hands interlocked; but, as soon as any task became difficult of execution, he placed his right hand palm downwards on his right thigh and drew it backwards and forwards.

Articulated speech. He talked very little spontaneously and the following conversation gives a fair example of his defects of speech.

Q. When did you enlist?

A. Fomb...I can't tell you.

Q. October? *A*. No.

Q. November? *A*. Yes.

Q. The year? *A*. Nineteen four, sir. (1914.)

Q. You became a sergeant? *A*. Nineteen seventeen.

Q. How do you occupy yourself?

A. I've some fowls...I give 'em corn in mornings...At night I give 'em what you call mash...marley...barley meal.

Q. What is your father?

A. A hare-taker (care-taker). He's blind, sir.

Q. What does he look after?

A. Parish room.

Thus, although there was a great economy of words, syntax and rhythm were not otherwise materially affected. Moreover, when he made a mistake he retraced his steps and attempted to correct it frequently with success.

Familiar objects could be named correctly and the pronunciation of the words was on the whole good; but he had greater difficulty with colours. The sounds he uttered obviously corresponded to their usual designation, but the verbal form was defective; thus black became "ber-lack," white "wide" and green "gree."

He could repeat words said to him somewhat better than when they were employed for naming objects; but his pronunciation showed similar faults to those audible during spontaneous speech, though to a less degree.

Understanding of spoken words. His comprehension of single words and simple phrases was good and in general conversation he seemed to understand everything said to him. He carried out oral commands perfectly, provided they did not necessitate elaborate choice; thus he chose familiar objects or colours correctly and even set the hands of the clock to orders given by word of mouth. But he made several mistakes with the more complex hand, eye and ear tests. If, however, he was asked to perform a single movement only, such as "Shut your eyes," "Give me your hand," the command was perfectly executed. The combination of two such actions, as for instance "Put out your tongue and touch your nose," made him uncertain and led to several erroneous responses.

Reading. He obviously understood the greater part of what he read to himself and carried out most printed commands successfully. But he failed with the more complex hand, eye and ear tests. When the act required was reduced to a single movement, such as "Put out your tongue," a printed order was correctly executed; but he made several mistakes and responded very slowly, if the command was double, i.e. "Put out your tongue and touch your nose." He seemed to have difficulty in formulating even to himself these more complex orders.

But to show how accurately he could read, he selected without material mistakes and in silence the printed card which bore a description of movements carried out by me. Here he had no need to remember a complex order; he recognised my actions and chose the appropriate card accordingly.

Asked, however, to say what he gathered from his reading, he not only had difficulty in finding the words to express himself aloud, but also in evoking them for internal speech. He did not omit any significant point, although the phrases were defective and suitable words were discovered with considerable difficulty.

When he read aloud, his enunciation showed the same kind of faults as voluntary speech; many words were badly pronounced and were separated by pauses of undue length and frequency. The harder the task the worse the results and he succeeded far better, when I set him to read an account of his daily life, than with a paragraph chosen from the newspaper.

Writing was profoundly affected. He wrote his Christian name and surname, but was unable to append his address. He could not even write the alphabet spontaneously and failed altogether with the months of the year.

He was unable to put down on paper the name of a colour shown to him or of any of the familiar objects except "key." Some of the simple phrases of the man, cat and dog tests were written correctly in response to pictures, but in many instances even these monosyllabic words were badly formed. He could not write down in words the time shown on a clock, although he did so accurately in figures.

He wrote somewhat better to dictation. Thus he not only wrote his full name, but was able to append part of the address, though in an insufficient form for the post. When the alphabet was dictated to him, he printed each letter as a capital and so succeeded in writing all but P. The months were written extremely badly, although he was slightly more successful than when he tried to put them on paper unaided. With the man, cat and dog tests every combination was given correctly, but the words were malformed.

Given his full name and address in printed characters, he was unable to copy it completely in cursive script, although he was somewhat more successful than when he wrote to dictation. He copied the alphabet and the names of the months in printed capitals exactly, but failed grossly to translate them into cursive script.

Throughout all these tests he wrote with the left hand; for, though always strongly right handed, he had long given up all attempts to use the hemiplegic limb and had learnt to write with the left hand.

The alphabet. He said the alphabet unprompted as follows: "A B C D E... G H I K L M O P Q R S T..." He then tried again without success, "A B C G ...E G H I J K L M N O P Q R S T...Double X Y Z."

He repeated the letters after me and also read them aloud correctly, except that on both occasions W was again called "Double."

Asked to write the alphabet spontaneously, he produced the printed capitals A B C D E and saying, "No, sir," gave up all further attempts. To dictation he was able to print the letters very slowly in capitals, except P which baffled him altogether. He copied printed capitals exactly, but when he attempted to translate them into cursive script he failed grossly. He wrote, A — C — — *b* — — *i 𝒥 ℋ l ℳ 𝒩* O *p* — R — — *𝒰 𝒱* — — —. I then gave him the twenty-six block letters and asked him to construct an alphabet with the following result: he rapidly produced the series A B C D E F G; then after much manipulation and many changes he placed the letters in the order:

A B C D E F G H I J M N L O P U R S T Q... W V Y X Z.

The last five were put together independently and K was omitted altogether.

The months. He said the months of the year spontaneously as follows: "Jar-u-ary," "Fob-dry," "March," "April," "June," "May," "July," "August," "Sump-tem-ber," "Org-ut," "Can't say any more, sir."

He failed even to repeat them correctly after me, saying, "Jar-ury," "Feb-le-ry," "March," "April," "May," "Jew," "July," "August," "Sump-tembr," "Og-tobr," "Nover...Nover-er," "Dēc-ĕr."

On reading aloud from print, he produced the following sounds: "Jar-ury," "Feb-ry," "March," "April," "May," "Jew," "July," "August," "Semp-temb-er," "Og-tob-er," "No-veb-er," "Dez...Dē...Dē-zembr."

He failed entirely to write the months spontaneously. After writing "March, Aril, m, Jus, N," he said, "No, sir" and gave up all further attempts.

He was almost equally bad to dictation and, taking the months in order, he wrote "J" for January, nothing for February, "Marol" for March, "A" for April, "May," nothing for June and July, "A" for August, nothing for September, October, November and December.

Yet he copied each one of them correctly in printed capitals, an act of purely imitative drawing. When he attempted to translate the printed names of the months into cursive script, he again failed badly, writing, "January," "Feo," "March," "April," "May," nothing for June and July, "August," "Sepb," "Octebr," "Nov," and nothing for December. Thus it is obvious that the disability lay not in the act of writing but in the power to evoke words and to translate them into written symbols.

A printed paragraph. He chose the following paragraph from the daily paper to test his power of understanding what he read.

"Shipbuilding Stoppage. Suspension of Lock-out Notices.

Steps towards the settlement of two big Labour disputes were taken yesterday. Lock-out notices to the forty-seven engineering unions which have broken away, have been suspended pending negotiations, which will open on Monday afternoon. The notices which would have expired to-day affected 600,000 men."

This he read to himself silently and, asked what he had gathered from it, said "In the lock out...forty-seven unions have broke away...Start work Monday afternoon...six...six hundred...six und thousand..."

He then read the passage aloud as follows: "Ship...buildin...stoppages... See...pep...I don't know the word...of lock-out notice...Steps to-fore...toward...settle...of two big...Labour...de-speds...are taken yesterday...Lock-out notice to the...forty-seven...inde...inder...unions which have broke away ...have been...sus-pes-ed...I don't know that...which will...open on Monday afternoon...The notice which will have...expied...to-day...affect...six unded thousand men."

I then asked him to tell me again what he had learnt from this paragraph and he replied, "Lock-out, sir...Forty-seven unions broke away...They start work on Monday afternoon...Six hundred thousand, sir." Thus, it is obvious that he understood the main points of what he read; his difficulty lay in defective verbal formation both for external and internal use.

I then prepared a simpler paragraph embodying information he gave me about his daily life. This was presented to him in typed form:

"I spend much time with my fowls. I have twelve Leghorns and thirteen Anconas. Last Friday they laid twenty-two eggs. I feed them in the morning with corn and in the afternoon with barley meal mash. The eggs now fetch twopence a-piece."

After reading this silently, he said, "I've twelve white Leg-hors...and thirteen Anconas...Last Friday I got twenty-two eggs. I fed on 'em corn in the morning and night barley meal...I had twenty-two eggs last Friday. Eggs fetch twopence each."

He read these sentences aloud as follows: "I spent much time with my fowls. I have twelve...Leghorns and thirteen Anconas. Last Friday...they laid... twenty-two eggs...I've...I've feed...from in the morning...with corn...and in...the after-noon...with barley meal. The eggs was fetching...fetched... twopence each."

I then asked him to repeat the phrases after me and, even under these conditions, he occasionally hesitated in finding the words. He said, "I spend...much...time with my fowls. I have twelve Leghorns and thirteen Anconas. Last Friday they laid twenty-two eggs. I feed 'em in the morning with corn and after-noon I feed with barley meal mash. The eggs na fetch tupce (twopence) each."

Numbers. He counted slowly but correctly up to a hundred, which he called "ondre" or "ondred." All the other decades were so well pronounced that I could not record any definite deviation from the normal.

Arithmetic. He was still somewhat puzzled by the simple problems in addition and subtraction, although his power of bringing out a correct answer had greatly increased.

Addition.

325	458	567
432	122	359
757	580	1016 (wrong)

Subtraction.

586	653	422
242	215	148
344	437 (corrected to 438)	274

Coins and their relative value. Every coin was named correctly though some of the words were badly pronounced; thus shilling was called "shill-un" or "shill-ful." Asked to state the relative value of any two coins placed before him, he was rather slow in evoking the number he wanted, but in every case his answer was finally correct. He had no difficulty with change in ordinary life.

Drawing. Using his left hand entirely, he made a remarkably accurate drawing of a spirit-lamp from a model, showing the relation of the various parts correctly. This he reproduced from memory somewhat less accurately. On the other hand, his drawing of an elephant was poor and he became confused between the tusks and the trunk; finally he called the appendage he drew below the mouth the "trump" or the "truck."

Plan drawing and orientation. Taken into another part of my house, he drew an excellent ground-plan of the room in which we habitually worked, naming each salient feature in turn. He repeatedly answered "I see the room."

He could find his way about perfectly and even travelled alone from the hospital, of which he was temporarily an inmate, to my house.

Images. He evidently visualised strongly for the purposes of memory. As he said he could recall the ward at the London Hospital and "see it" clearly, I asked him about the colours of the curtains to the beds. He gave white and blue correctly and added that a "red thing" was lying on the bed (the red shawl). He also said that the dress of the Sister was "be-loo" (blue), thus accurately differentiating her uniform from that of the Nurses.

Games. He played a splendid game of draughts, beating me by a clever combination of kings. He also amused himself with cribbage and whist, which, as his sister informed me, he played excellently.

Serial Tests.

(1) *Naming and recognition of common objects.* (See Table 6.)

He could carry out oral and printed commands and named all the familiar objects correctly; he had, however, slight difficulty in pronouncing scissors, which he called "ziz-ors" or "ziz-urs." Some of the other words were a little slurred, as if he was talking with a sticky sweet in his mouth. When he read the names aloud, these faults were also evident.

He copied the printed characters exactly, but could not translate them into cursive script. He failed equally badly, when he attempted to write the names of objects shown to him; but, asked to choose a card bearing the name of any one of them he had just seen, he carried out the task perfectly. Thus it was obvious that he knew the names and could decipher print accurately; it was verbal formation that was at fault.

This was evident when he was shown a familiar object and was asked to put together its name out of a set of block letters. He tried the most unlikely combinations and occasionally succeeded, at other times failing completely; yet the combination of letters usually corresponded in some way, even if remotely, with the name he was seeking.

Throughout he remembered the order in which the objects lay on the table. When making his choice to oral or printed commands, he frequently thrust out his hand to the place where the one he was seeking lay, before I had removed the screen. The fact that he knew their names ensured recognition of their position in space.

(2) *Naming and recognition of colours.* (See Table 7.)

Here again oral and printed commands were well executed and he had no difficulty in choosing a card bearing the name of a colour shown to him.

Asked to name the colours, the words were badly pronounced though each bore a distinct relation to the one he was seeking. Told to read the names aloud from print, his pronunciation was imperfect, but he chose the colour without fail.

He was entirely unable to write down the name of a single colour.

(3) *The man, cat and dog tests.* (See Table 8.)

He read aloud both from print and pictures and repeated these simple phrases after me correctly. There was a slight tendency to stumble over the words, but he always corrected any inaccuracies of pronunciation by repeating the phrase.

When he wrote in response to pictures, the content was accurate, but even these simple words were in many instances badly formed. Thus cat was written "cot," dog became "gog." To dictation the results were equally defective. Even copying was carried out slowly and imperfectly. But it is noticeable that in all these tests he wrote in cursive script.

Table 6.

	Pointing to object shown	Naming object indicated	Oral commands	Printed commands	Duplicate placed in left hand out of sight	Reading aloud and choosing object from printed commands		Writing name of object indicated	Copying from print in printed characters	Copying from print in cursive characters	Expressing in block letters name of object indicated	Choosing printed card bearing name of object indicated
						He said	He chose					
Knife	Perfect	Correct	Perfect	Perfect	Perfect	"Naive"	Correctly	Kig	Correct	Knife	Correct	Correct
Key	,,	,,	,,	,,	,,	"Kay, key"	,,	Key	,,	K	,,	,,
Penny	,,	,,	,,	,,	,,	Correctly	,,	P	,,	"No, sir"	Corrected	,,
Matches	,,	,,	,,	,,	,,	,,	,,	"No, sir"	,,	Ma	M C H E; "No, sir"	,,
Scissors	,,	,,	,,	,,	,,	,,	,,	"No, sir"	,,	"No, sir"	K E S S . . . K E I S S . . . K E I S S E Y; "No, sir"	,,
Pencil	,,	,,	,,	,,	,,	,,	,,	"No"	,,	"Can't"	P N E E I Y . . . P N E I N Y; "No, sir"	,,
Key	,,	,,	,,	,,	,,	,,	,,	Key	,,	K	Corrected	,,
Scissors	,,	,,	,,	,,	,,	,,	,,	8	SCISSOR	No response	C S E E	,,
Matches	,,	,,	,,	,,	,,	,,	,,	N	Correct	Ma	M C A C . . . "No, sir"	,,
Knife	,,	,,	,,	,,	,,	,,	,,	H	,,	K	K N E F E . . . "No, sir"	,,
Penny	,,	,,	,,	,,	,,	"Pencil"	Pencil	LE	,,	P; "no"	Correct	,,
Matches	,,	,,	,,	,,	,,	Correctly	Correctly	"No, sir"	,,	Ma	M C H E S; "That's wrong"	,,
Scissors	,,	,,	,,	,,	,,	,,	,,	Z	,,	S	C I H	,,
Pencil	,,	,,	,,	,,	,,	,,	,,	PI	,,	"No, sir"	P E N I N Y; gave up	,,
Penny	,,	,,	,,	,,	,,	,,	,,	PEEY	,,	"No, sir"	P E E N Y	,,
Knife	,,	,,	,,	,,	,,	"Naive"	,,	KE	,,	Knif	K N E I F E; "No"	,,
Key	,,	,,	,,	,,	,,	Correctly	,,	KEY	,,	K	Correct; quick	,,
Pencil	,,	,,	,,	,,	,,	,,	,,	PIL	,,	No response	P E N S I Y	,,

He was then asked to put together the block letters to correspond with each combination of pictures shown to him. In every instance the content was correct, although the words were badly formed. It is therefore obvious that it was not the act of writing as such which was at fault, but the power to form words correctly even out of a set of given letters.

Table 7.

	Pointing to colour shown	Naming colour shown	Oral commands	Printed commands	Printed name read aloud and colour chosen		Choosing card bearing name of colour shown	Writing down name of colour shown
					He said	He chose		
Black	Correct	"Ber-lack"	Correct	Correct	Correctly	Correctly	Correct	B
Red	,,	Correct	,,	,,	,,	,,	,,	"No, sir"
Blue	,,	"Ber-loo"	,,	,,	,,	,,	,,	"No, sir"
Green	,,	Correct	,,	,,	,,	,,	,,	GEED
Orange	,,	,,	Yellow	,,	,,	,,	,,	"No, sir"
White	,,	"Whide"	Correct	,,	,,	,,	,,	THI
Violet	,,	"Don't know"	,,	,,	"Viol"	,,	,,	VO
Yellow	,,	"Red"	,,	,,	Correctly	,,	,,	"No, sir"
Red	,,	Correct	,,	,,	,,	,,	,,	R
White	,,	,,	,,	,,	,,	,,	,,	THI
Yellow	,,	"Yell-er"	,,	,,	"Well, yell, rell"	,,	,,	"No, sir"
Blue	,,	"Be-loo"	,,	,,	Correctly	,,	,,	B
Green	,,	"Gree"	,,	,,	,,	,,	,,	GEEN
Black	,,	Correct	,,	,,	,,	,,	,,	B
Orange	,,	"Red"	,,	,,	,,	,,	,,	"No, sir"
Violet	,,	"Slate"	,,	,,	"Viol"	,,	,,	VI

Table 8.

	Reading aloud	Reading from pictures	Repetition	Copying	Writing from dictation	Writing from pictures	Words composed of block letters to correspond with pictures
The dog and the cat	Correct	Correct	Correct	Correct	Correct	The dog and the cot	Correct
The man and the dog	,,	,,	,,	The man and the gog	,,	Correct	,,
The cat and the man	,,	,,	,,	Correct	The cot and the man	The cot and the man	CO...CAT MAN
The cat and the dog	,,	,,	,,	The cat and the gog	The cot and the dog	The cot and the dog	COT DAN
The dog and the man	,,	,,	,,	The gog (corrected) and the man	Correct	Correct	Correct
The man and the cat	,,	,,	,,	Correct	The man and the cot	The man and the cot	MAN COT
The dog and the man	,,	,,	,,	,,	Correct	Correct	Correct
The cat and the man	,,	,,	,,	,,	The cot and the man	The cot and the man	TO COT MAN
The dog and the cat	,,	,,	,,	,,	Correct	The gog (corrected) and the cat	Correct
The man and the dog	,,	,,	,,	The man and the god	Correct	Correct	,,
The cat and the dog	,,	,,	,,	Correct	The cot and the dog	The cot and the dog	COT DAG
The man and the cat	,,	,,	,,	,,	The man and the cot	The man and the cot	MAN TOC

(4) *The clock tests.*

Table 9.

	Direct imitation	Telling the time	Oral commands	Printed commands: In words	Printed commands: Railway time	Writing down the time shown on a clock: In railway time	Writing down the time shown on a clock: In words
5 minutes to 2	Perfect	Correct	Correct	Correct	Correct	Correct	Impossible
Half-past 1	,,	,,	,,	,,	,,	,,	,,
5 minutes past 8	,,	,,	,,	,,	,,	,,	,,
20 minutes to 4	,,	,,	,,	,,	,,	,,	,,
10 minutes past 7	,,	,,	,,	,,	,,	,,	,,
20 minutes to 6	,,	,,	,,	,,	,,	,,	,,
10 minutes to 1	,,	,,	,,	,,	,,	,,	,,
A quarter to 9	,,	,,	,,	,,	,,	,,	,,
20 minutes past 11	,,	,,	,,	,,	,,	,,	,,
25 minutes to 3	,,	,,	,,	,,	,,	,,	,,

This is a remarkably instructive set of observations. For he was able to tell the time accurately with perhaps a little slurring of some words; he carried out perfectly oral or printed commands whether they were given in words or figures. Moreover, he cleverly shifted the hands round the face of the clock so as to reach the goal with the least expenditure of effort; sometimes he set the hour first, at others the minutes, skilfully converting the previous setting into the next answer.

Asked to write down the time, he at once adopted railway time unprompted and every response was accurate. But, asked to employ words, he was entirely unable to write a single letter. This is further evidence that the defect lay mainly in verbal formation.

(5) *The coin-bowl tests.* He was extremely quick and certain in executing the movements required to oral or printed commands, whether the orders were given in numbers or were expressed fully in words.

(6) *The hand, eye and ear tests.*

Table 10.

	Imitation of movements made by the observer	Imitation of movements reflected in a mirror	Pictorial commands	Pictorial commands reflected in a mirror	Oral commands	Printed commands
L. hand to L. eye	Correct	Correct	Reversed	Correct	R. hand to L. eye	L. hand to R. eye
R. hand to R. ear	,,	,,	,,	,,	R. hand to L. ear	R. hand to R. *eye*
R. hand to L. eye	R. hand to R. eye	,,	,,	,,	Correct	Correct
L. hand to R. eye	Correct	,,	,,	,,	,,	,,
L. hand to L. ear	,,	,,	,,	,,	L. hand to R. ear	L. hand to R. *eye*
R. hand to R. eye	,,	,,	,,	,,	R. hand to L. eye	Correct
L. hand to R. ear	,,	,,	,,	,,	Correct	L. hand to R. *eye*
R. hand to L. ear	L. hand to L. ear	,,	,,	,,	,,	R. hand to L. *eye*
L. hand to L. eye	L. hand to R. eye	,,	,,	,,	L. hand to R. eye	L. hand to L. *ear*
R. hand to R. ear	Correct	,,	,,	,,	R. hand to L. ear	Correct
R. hand to L. eye	,,	,,	,,	,,	Correct	,,
L. hand to R. eye	L. hand to L. eye	,,	R. hand to R. eye	,,	,,	,,
L. hand to L. ear	L. hand to R. ear	,,	Reversed	,,	L. hand to R. ear	,,
R. hand to R. eye	Correct	,,	L. hand to L. *ear*	,,	Correct	,,
L. hand to R. ear	Reversed	,,	R. hand to R. ear	,,	,,	,,
R. hand to L. ear	,,	,,	Reversed	,,	,,	,,

He had great difficulty in imitating movements made by me sitting face to face and in carrying out pictorial commands. But, when my movements on the diagrams were reflected in a mirror, he was quick and accurate.

For the first time in all these serial tests he failed to execute oral and printed commands; evidently the task required was too difficult. I therefore arranged the following tests of graduated severity.

Single command. He was asked to imitate the following movements and to carry them out to oral and to printed commands. "Put out your tongue," "Touch your nose," "Shut your eyes," "Give me your hand," "Touch your nose," "Put out your tongue," "Give me your hand," "Shut your eyes." All these were performed correctly.

Table 11.

	Imitation of movements made by the observer	Oral commands	Printed commands	Printed commands read aloud and acted upon		Choosing a printed card corresponding to movements made by the observer
				He said	Movement performed	
Put out your tongue and give me your hand	Correct	Correct	Correct	Correctly	Correct	Correct
Touch your nose and give me your hand	,,	Touched nose, closed eyes and gave hand	Correct; very slow	,,	Put out tongue and gave hand	,,
Shut your eyes and put out your tongue	,,	Correct	Correct	,,	Correct	,,
Touch your nose and shut your eyes	,,	,,	,,	,,	Shut eyes, put out tongue and touched nose	,,
Put out your tongue and touch your nose	,,	Put out tongue, touched nose and closed eyes	Put out tongue, closed eyes and gave hand	"Put out your hand, tongue and close your eyes"	Shut his eyes, put out tongue and gave hand	Chose reversed order—"Touch your nose and put out your tongue"
Shut your eyes and give me your hand	,,	Correct	Correct	Correctly	Correct	Correct
Touch your nose and put out your tongue	,,	Closed eyes, put out tongue and gave hand	Closed eyes, touched nose and put out tongue	"Touch your nose and give me your . . . and put out your tongue"	Closed eyes, put out tongue and touched nose	,,
Shut your eyes and touch your nose	,,	Correct	Correct	Correctly	Correct	Chose reversed order—"Touch your nose and shut your eyes"
Put out your tongue and shut your eyes	,,	,,	,,	"Put out your tongue and close your eyes"	Closed eyes, put out tongue and gave hand	Correct

Double command. Every test consisted of a combination of two of these commands. Asked to imitate my movements, he carried out the whole series correctly, for little or no internal verbalisation is necessary since there is no question of right or left. But oral and printed commands were not accurately executed, even when the latter were read aloud. He was, however, able to choose correctly a printed card which bore a description of the double movements made by me; twice he reversed the order in which they stood upon the card, but this can scarcely be reckoned a serious mistake.

Physical Examination.

He was happy and cheerful and his general health was extremely good.

The wound was represented by a tough deeply depressed scar, which did not pulsate even when he stooped. The area from which bone had been removed could now be measured accurately; it was roughly oval in shape, about 5 cm. vertically and 3 cm. in breadth. It lay somewhat obliquely distant from the middle line, 1 cm. above and 3 cm. below. The superior limit was opposite a point 21·5 cm. and the lowest portion 26·5 cm. along the nasion-inion line.

He rarely suffered from headache, which if present lay over the forehead and was never situated in the neighbourhood of the scar or in the occipital region. It was not induced by stooping, riding in a motor or train; nor was it caused by fatigue or intellectual effort, such as reading. It was never accompanied by nausea or vomiting.

He had suffered from no epileptiform attacks of any kind except in April, 1921. He had been sawing with his right hand all the afternoon in the hot sun and the same evening became unconscious; the right arm, leg and face "twitched," but he did not bite his tongue or pass water. Since that time he has shown no symptoms of "dizziness" or any form of seizure.

There was complete right hemianopsia, which included half of central vision, and was associated with loss of the pupillary reaction from the blind portion of the field. The discs were in every way normal.

Movements of the eyes and face were unaffected, but the tongue deviated on protrusion a little to the right and was withdrawn somewhat to the left of the middle line.

All the deep reflexes on the right half of the body were greatly exaggerated; the plantar gave a characteristic upward response and the abdominal reflexes were absent on the right side.

He never used the right hand for writing or other fine movements and the grasp was definitely weaker than that of the left. Individual movements were badly executed and, when he attempted to approximate one finger to the thumb, all the digits moved together. If he held out the hands in front of him, the fingers of the right were out of alignment and fell away from the horizontal, when he closed his eyes. There was distinct incoordination to all the tests. Tone was not greatly increased or diminished. Movements at the elbow and shoulder were much less affected and showed little incoordination compared with those of the hand and wrist.

Power had greatly improved in the right lower extremity, but there was still considerable incoordination. He could dorsiflex and plantar-extend the foot and tone was not obviously affected. He walked, however, with a typical ataxic hemiplegic gait and could not stand on the right leg with the eyes closed.

Obviously the loss of power both in arm and leg was mainly afferent in origin; this was borne out by the sensory examination. He failed to appreciate passive movements in the fingers of the right hand and at the wrist; but he recognised an excursion of 5° at the elbow and of 2° at the shoulder. In the same way there was total loss of recognition of passive movement in the right great toe, although he responded to 5° at the ankle and 2° at the knee.

This examination was not easy owing to his inability to find the requisite words sufficiently quickly; this difficulty I overcame in the following manner: I moved the normal fingers or wrist through 3° and then desisted, asking "what is it?" He invariably answered "front," "back," "bent," or "straight" correctly. But no excursion of the right index or great toe, however wide in range, enabled him to state in which direction it had been moved; he invariably replied "Don't know" to my questions.

He discriminated the compass points at 1 cm. on the left palm and palmar surface of the left index; on the sole of the normal foot he gave a good record at 3 cm. On the affected palm and sole he invariably answered "one," even at the maximum possible distance.

Localisation of the spot touched was extremely defective both on the right hand and foot and he usually said "I feel it, I don't know"; on the normal side he was remarkably good in pointing out on the assistant's hand or foot the spot I had stimulated in him.

All power of recognising differences of shape was lost in the right hand. The test was carried out as follows, owing to his difficulty in finding words. The six wooden geometrical figures were ranged on the table before him in a row; a duplicate was then placed in his hand out of sight and he was asked to indicate the corresponding one. On the left side he did not hesitate and made no mistakes; but, when the object was placed in the right hand, he never gave the slightest indication that he recognised its shape or attempted to make a choice from the set in front of him. In the same way appreciation of differences in weight was grossly affected in the right hand.

Tactile sensibility was extremely difficult to test; but it was without doubt disturbed over the right hand, though not over the right foot. There was no gross loss to heat and cold and he denied that there was any difference in this respect between the two hands. The threshold to prick was about the same on the fingers of either hand and on the two palms.

No. 10

A case of Semantic Aphasia, due to a wound with a hand-grenade in the region of the left supra-marginal gyrus. Observations extending over seven years showed considerable variations in the degree but not in the character of the disturbance of function.

There were no abnormal physical signs of any kind. But on two occasions, during periods of worry and mental distress, he suffered from a true epileptiform attack; the first of these occurred five months after he was wounded, the second six years later.

He could name objects and colours shown to him and had no difficulty in finding or articulating words to express his ordinary needs; all his phrases were perfectly formed and spaced. But, in general conversation, he paused like a man confused, who had lost the thread of what he wanted to say. Words and sentences were repeated correctly, provided they did not contain a number of possible alternatives. He chose an object or colour named by me, but had obvious difficulty in setting the clock or carrying out complex oral commands. He was easily puzzled and became confused with regard to the aim of the task set him. He understood the significance of printed words and short sentences, provided they did not contain a command. But he gave a poor account of a paragraph read silently to himself; his narration tailed away aimlessly, as if he had forgotten the goal for which he was making. He read aloud simple sentences without mistakes, but tended to doubt the accuracy of the words he had uttered correctly. He wrote with extreme rapidity, as if afraid of forgetting what he wanted to transfer to paper; at first he tended to employ the same symbol for several different letters. He showed similar defects to dictation and not infrequently forgot what he had been told to write. Apart from the defects in handwriting, he could copy correctly. Although he counted excellently, he was unable to carry out the simplest arithmetical operation; this was the more remarkable as he had been an accountant, accustomed to handle complex masses of figures. He was confused by the relative value of coins and had much difficulty with change in ordinary life. Although he appreciated the various details of a picture, he was liable to miss its general meaning. He could not draw from the model or from memory nor delineate an elephant to command. He failed entirely to draw the ground-plan of a familiar room and was unable to express the relative position of its salient features. Orientation was gravely affected; he was liable to lose his way in the street and had difficulty in finding his own room in the hospital. He could play no games and puzzles worried him greatly.

In this case the sole disturbance produced by the lesion was want of capacity to comprehend and to retain in consciousness the general significance of some symbolic representation, or the intention of an act he was about to perform, either to command or on his own initiative. He could deal with the details of a situation, but not with its general aspects.

Lieutenant Robert M., who was an accountant before the war, enlisted in September, 1914, obtaining his commission in June, 1915. At the time of his wound he was 32 years of age and a most intelligent Scotchman.

He was bombing officer to his regiment, and on March 17, 1916, during a course of instruction to his men on the use of hand-grenades, he was wounded accidentally. He remembers nothing of the occurrence, or of anything that happened on that day.

He was admitted to hospital at Le Tréport on March 18, with two small wounds over the left parietal area, which affected the brain, together with scattered injuries of little import over the chest, abdomen and arms. He was semi-conscious and rambled in his speech. The pupils were equal and reacted to light. There was no paralysis.

On March 18 he was trephined; on enlarging the openings the dura mater was found to have been perforated in two places and two small fragments of depressed bone were removed. A small drainage tube was inserted through each opening into the brain. These were removed on March 22, and his progress was reported to be satisfactory.

When admitted under my care to the Empire Hospital for Officers on April 20, 1916, there was a healed wound in the left parietal region. Bone had been removed over an oval area 2·5 cm. by 1·25 cm., extending from 15·5 cm. to 18 cm. along the nasion-inion and 8 cm. to the left of the middle line. The total distance from nasion to inion was 34 cm. The wound was firmly healed and did not pulsate (cf. Figs. 12 and 13, Vol. 1, pp. 460 and 461).

On physical examination, I could find no abnormal signs of any kind except the disorders of speech. His vision was R. $\frac{6}{6}$, L. $\frac{6}{9}$, with slight myopia. The visual fields were not restricted and the discs showed no changes. Motion, sensation and the reflexes were unaffected.

He was a strongly right-handed man, who could neither throw, nor cut left-handed with the loose-jointed scissors (Gordon's test). He could tie a reef-knot and had no difficulty in using knife, fork, spoon or other tools. He made the movements of brushing his hair without a brush in his hand and could pretend to take a cigarette from his case, to light it and to blow out the imaginary match.

He had not suffered from fits or any other attacks. His headache varied greatly; it was never acute or associated with nausea and vomiting, but was "dull" and diffused mainly on the left half of the head. It was greatly increased by fatigue and concentrated mental effort. He was conscious of an abnormal sensation when he stooped to do up his boots, but not with less extreme changes of posture. Once induced, the headache required some days before it passed away.

CONDITION BETWEEN MAY AND JUNE 1916 (*ten weeks after he was wounded*).

He was a remarkably intelligent man and a most willing subject for examination. His temper was unusually equable, even when he found difficulty in expressing himself, and he was bright and happy throughout his stay in the hospital.

Symbolic Formulation and Expression.

Articulated speech. He had no difficulty in finding or articulating words to express his ordinary needs and all his phrases were perfectly formed and spaced. Syntax was entirely unaffected. But in general conversation he paused like a man confused, who had lost the thread of what he wanted to say.

He could say the days of the week and months correctly and counted without hesitation or error.

He had no difficulty in repeating anything said to him, provided the sentence did not contain a number of possible alternatives; any mistake he might make depended on faulty comprehension or memory, and not on want of power to repeat what was said.

Understanding of spoken words. At first sight he appeared to understand all that was said to him, choosing both geometrical shapes and colours correctly, though with some hesitation, to oral commands. But with the more complex clock tests he failed lamentably, evidently unable to comprehend the full significance of the order. His responses to the hand, eye and ear tests were even worse; eye and ear were confused and he tended to fail in executing an order which required him to bring his hand across to the opposite half of the face. Moreover, in general conversation he was liable to become confused, because he did not understand the full meaning of what was said. This he explained as follows: "I don't seem to understand all you say and then I forget what I've got to do."

Reading. He could understand the significance of printed words and short sentences without fail, provided they did not contain a command. But, when asked to read silently to himself a series of paragraphs in the newspaper, he gave a poor account of their full meaning; he lost the thread of what he wanted to say and his narration tailed away aimlessly

He chose the following message from the King on the Battle of Jutland: "I am deeply touched by the message you sent me on behalf of the Grand Fleet. It reaches me on the morrow of a battle, which has once more displayed the splendid gallantry of the officers and men under your command. I mourn the loss of brave men, many of them personal friends of my own, who have fallen in their country's cause; yet even more do I regret that the German High Seas Fleet, in spite of its heavy losses, was enabled by the misty weather to evade the full consequences of an encounter they have always professed to desire, but for which, when the opportunity arrived, they showed no inclination. Though the retirement of the enemy immediately after the opening of the general engagement robbed us of the opportunity of gaining a decisive victory, the events of last Wednesday amply justify my confidence in the valour and efficiency of the fleets under your command."

After he had read it through to himself, he said, "The King refers to the loss of the many brave men under his command, many of them personal friends of his own. He refers to the loss of the many brave men. He lays great stress on the fact that the Germans were evidently unable...to come to grips...with our men."

He could read aloud simple sentences perfectly without mispronunciation; but in the course of a long or difficult passage he tended to become confused, even though he was reproducing the words correctly. Given the King's message, he read it aloud correctly until he reached "yet even more"; thence he continued in jerky sentences of a few words apiece until he came to "for which...they have always professed a desire...for which they have...they have the opportunity... arrive they show no inclination," when he stopped and said, "That's funny, I seem to be getting the wrong sense somehow. Shall I go on?" Encouraged to do so, he read to the end correctly.

He was then asked what he understood from the paragraphs he had read aloud, to which he answered, "You see, Doctor, it's like this; I've got a general epitome of what I've been reading in the paper. When I tell you, I may get it mixed up. About the King's message...The fleet was at the...If they hadn't had the opportunity to fully engage the German fleet...the, ah yes, misty weather spoilt things ...notwithstanding our men's keenness to force a general action, the misty weather and the enemy's disinclination to fight robbed us of victory."

He had no difficulty in reading and understanding a letter written by himself or by others, provided it did not deal with matters which would have confused him however they had been presented.

Writing. His handwriting was profoundly altered; he wrote his name and address with extreme rapidity, twice employing the peculiar letter like a 𝒬, which formed so prominent a feature of his script at this stage.

Asked to compose a letter to me, he wrote as follows, saying the words aloud: "Dear Dr Head, I have a vase containing some beautiful flowers. My wife brought me some lillies of the valley." At the same time he wrote with considerable difficulty a scrawl which was comprehensible only if his intention was known. This he read aloud exactly as if it had been perfectly written. Throughout he showed a peculiar tendency to use a figure resembling 𝒬 for D F O R T and V.

I dictated to him, "The lilies of the valley, which are standing on my table, were sent to me by my wife from Cork." This he wrote with difficulty; he dashed off the first few words, paused, and suddenly wrote "which are standing on my table," and then stopped. I repeated several times, "which were sent me by my wife" before he could put the next phrase on to paper, and even then he omitted "wife"; and yet he read what he had written exactly as if it were a perfect reproduction of the sentences I had dictated.

He could copy the names of the colours from print, but wrote extremely rapidly and tended to employ the curious sign *Q* in place of several of the initial letters. Asked to copy the simple man, cat and dog phrases, he tended to reproduce a common fault, which ran throughout these tests, substituting in this case "man" for "cat."

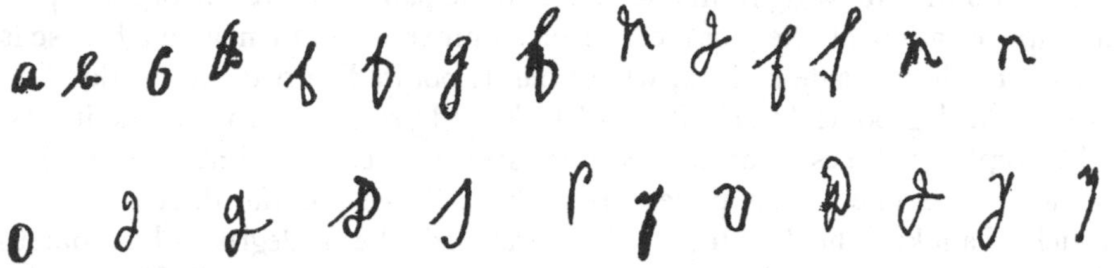

Fig. 23. The alphabet, written spontaneously by No. 10.

The alphabet. He could say the alphabet perfectly and repeat it without fail. But, when asked to write the letters, he said each one aloud once or more and wrote the above script (fig. 23). He added, when he had finished, "I seem to get mixed between capitals and other letters." To my dictation he produced an almost identical sequence.

General significance of pictures and print. Shown a picture and asked to describe what he saw, he went over it in detail, usually beginning at one side and working across to the other: but, as a rule, he failed to appreciate its general significance. For instance, he was shown a photographic reproduction of the tower with the leaning Virgin at Albert; at the top of the picture was printed, "When the end of the war will be; a prophecy." After examining it with care and reading the superscription, he said that it reminded him of something he had seen before; "In the other picture I saw, there was a piece of statuary. I don't know if that is a confusion in my mind or not. It was a piece of old building tumbling down; like the leaning tower of Pisa. That building has fallen over much more than this; the local French people believe that the statue of the Virgin Mary... they believe that the statue has fallen and that then the war will end...just in that place the war will end." During the narration he looked away from the picture, evidently recalling some previous memory, and I therefore said: "What bearing has this picture on the story you have just told me?" He then looked at the picture again, passing his finger over the various details as he mentioned them. "This is simply a building, that has been bombarded, in ruins; one tower, as often happens, seems standing unmolested. I can now see the statue quite plainly; I can see the arms quite plainly. I think I might have been confused about the statue if I hadn't known the story." It was not until after he had recounted to me the familiar legend and recalled previous illustrations he had seen of the church at Albert, that he suddenly noticed the most salient feature in the picture before him.

In consequence of this difficulty in recognising the full significance either of pictures or of printed matter, most jokes were incomprehensible. Suppose, however, that the humour consisted solely in the detail of the drawing, it might be appreciated; but any demand for co-ordination between its various parts, or with the text beneath it, met with little response.

I showed him a drawing from one of the comic papers where the point depended on the appreciation of the significance of summer-time, then a much discussed novelty. Standing beside a clock, whose hands pointed to two, the bride of a day says to her bridegroom: "Look, it's 2 o'clock, and yesterday at this time it was 1," and he replied: "Yes, darling; and yesterday at this time we were two, and now we are one." The patient remarked: "I've got the drift of that. It's not much of a joke. They've stupidly been married; the bridegroom has something stupid to say about yesterday we were two and now we are one." Then, pointing to the clock, he said: "I could have told the time there better than when you were trying me...two o'clock." I asked: "What happened at two o'clock, just a fortnight ago?" He replied: "Oh! I see, Daylight Saving Act." To my question, "What happened to the clocks?" he answered: "They were put back an hour. That's a thing I'm rather hazy about. I have to think of that...forward...back, no, I have to give that up; I've been trying to think that out, and haven't got to a conclusion yet, somehow."

Then I told him "The clock was put forward; at twelve o'clock it was put forward to ——?" and he replied: "Put forward...well at twelve o'clock it was put forward to half-past eleven. I shouldn't think it was half an hour, anyhow; half-past eleven, no, eleven o'clock. I can't get it; I seem to have got the idea, but I can't get hold of it."

General intention of an act to be performed. This inability to grasp the general significance or intention of an act he is asked to perform was well illustrated during the tests for the spacial aspects of sensation. When the index finger of either hand was moved passively, even with the eyes open, he did not give consistently appropriate replies. Sometimes he said correctly "the same," "two together" (for two movements in the same direction), "different," "not the same"; or if I asked: "Which way is it moving?" he would answer "forwards," "backwards," "bending," or "straightening." But, if I remained silent, he usually simply replied "yes," or wagged the finger of the other hand aimlessly backwards and forwards without indicating the direction.

If, during the compass tests, he was touched with a single point more than once successively, he tended to count "one," "two," "three"; then he would exclaim: "Oh! bother I've muddled it again." Although sensation was unaltered, he could not hold fast in his mind that the intention of the test was to determine his power of discriminating contact with one or two points.

Asked to point to the spot on either hand touched by me, he did so without difficulty; but, unless the command was repeated every time, he would forget what he had to do and held the indicating finger poised in the air. If I repeated the order he would exclaim "Oh! yes, of course," and carry it out correctly.

His power of appreciating the addition or removal of weights placed on the palm of either hand was certainly unaffected. But he frequently failed to give a consecutive reply, saying, "I don't know what you mean by on and off; I get confused"; and yet on more than one occasion he volunteered the statement "You touched the weight, you did not take one off," which was quite correct. I laid two weights on the table in front of him and requested him to place one on to the other, or to take it off silently, in order to indicate whether I had added or removed a weight from his hand. This confused him profoundly and he made no attempt to carry out the command, although he had been previously answering correctly by word of mouth.

Arithmetic. Although he counted excellently and with ease he was entirely unable to carry out the simplest arithmetical operation. He could not even add 231 and 356 or subtract 432 from 865. He said "I seem to get tangled up in the process." This is the more remarkable as he was an accountant in civilian life, accustomed to handle complex masses of figures.

Coins and their relative value. He named every coin with perfect ease. But, as soon as two of them were presented to him and he was asked, "How many of this one (of lower value) go into this one (of higher value)?" he became confused. The following are some of his answers:

A penny and sixpence—"Twelve."
Sixpence and a shilling—"Twelve...yes, twelve, sixpence."
Sixpence and half-a-crown—"Let me see, twenty-two...I thought of twenty-four, but it's not."
A halfpenny and a penny—"Penny and halfpenny, penny and two pence...no, penny and halfpenny."
A halfpenny and sixpence—"Six and twelve is it?...No."
One penny and a shilling—"Twelve."
Sixpence and half-a-crown—"Six...twenty-four."
Sixpence and one shilling—"Six...twelve."
One penny and sixpence—"Twelve."

Drawing. He was unable to delineate a vase of simple form either from the model or from memory. Asked to draw an elephant, he failed entirely to produce a figure of any kind, but scrawled idly on the paper.

Plan drawing and relation of objects in space. Told to draw a plan of his room in the hospital, he failed entirely; he made no attempt even to put the pencil to paper, saying: "I've all sorts of ideas, but I can't carry them out."

But, with his eyes closed, he had no difficulty in pointing to the position of the window, fireplace, wash-hand stand, chest of drawers and other pieces of furniture. When asked to say how the wash-hand stand stood in relation to the fireplace, or the latter to the door, he entirely failed to do so; allowed, however, to say: "The fire is there and the door there," he pointed to their position with complete accuracy. He knew exactly where they were and was certain that he could "see them in his mind," but was unable to express their relative position to one another.

Orientation. He was extremely liable to lose his way in the hospital and had difficulty even in finding his room. This feature of his affection was more fully investigated when he was up and about, and is considered more in detail later.

Games. He could play no games such as chess, draughts or cards; nor could he put together jigsaw puzzles, so popular an employment amongst wounded soldiers.

Serial Tests.

(1) *Naming and recognition of common objects.*

Table 1.

	Pointing to object shown	Oral commands	Printed commands	Duplicate placed in hand out of sight	Naming an object indicated	Writing name of object indicated
Cylinder	Correct	Correct	Correct	Correct	"The cube"	C
Cone	,,	"A cone and a pyramid; but I can't." Correct	,,	,,	Correct	Wrote nothing
Cube	,,	Correct	,,	,,	,,	C
Sphere	,,	,,	,,	,,	,,	Sp
Ovoid	,,	,,	,,	,,	,,	O
Pyramid	,,	,,	,,	,,	,,	𝒬
Sphere	,,	,,	,,	,,	,,	Sp
Cone	,,	"Pyramid; no"; chose correctly	,,	,,	,,	Clo
Ovoid	,,	Correct	,,	,,	,,	𝒬ov
Cube	,,	,,	,,	,,	,,	Scrawl
Cylinder	,,	,,	,,	,,	,,	Wrote nothing
Pyramid	,,	,,	Chose cone; then correctly	,,	,,	Sype

During the observations on sensibility I found he was unusually accurate in his nomenclature of geometrical figures, and I therefore selected them as the objects to be named or indicated in this test. With the general run of patients the names applied to these solid figures are so inconstant and uncertain, that it is not advisable to use them in this manner; but in this case they distinctly added to the value of the results obtained.

He showed little difficulty in pointing to an object named orally or in print and made one mistake only in nomenclature. But he failed entirely to write their names; he not infrequently hit upon the correct initial letter, although he showed a tendency to use the same symbol for different capitals.

When he was told to say each name aloud before putting it into writing, he did so correctly; but he produced an illegible scrawl which, however, contained the same number of signs as the word he had uttered. For instance, he said "Cylinder yes, C Y L I N D E R," and as he spelt each letter he made a mark upon the paper, which might or might not correspond to its normal shape. "Pyramid" was correctly articulated; but he then said "P Y R I M D" and wrote a word consisting of six more or less incomprehensible letters.

(2) *Naming and recognition of colours.*

Table 2.

	Pointing to colour shown	Oral commands	Printed commands	Naming	Writing name of colour indicated	Copying names from print	Printed name read aloud and colour chosen	
							He chose	He said
Blue	Correct	Correct	Correct	Correct	𝒬lue	𝒬lue	Correctly	Correctly
Yellow	,,	,,	,,	,,	Orange	𝒬ellow	,,	No reply
Red	,,	,,	,,	,,	𝒬ed	𝒬ed	,,	Correctly
Black	,,	,,	,,	,,	𝒬lack	Black	,,	,,
Orange	,,	,,	Yellow	"Red"	Orange	𝒬range	,,	"Yellow"
White	,,	,,	Correct	Correct	Whide	White	,,	Correctly
Violet	,,	,, (slow)	,,	,,	𝒬iolet	𝒬iolet	,,	,,
Green	,,	Correct	,,	,,	𝒬reen	𝒬reen	,,	,,
Blue	,,	,,	,,	,,	𝒬lue	𝒬lue	,,	,,
Yellow	,,	,,	,,	,,	𝒬range	𝒬ellow	,,	"Green"
Red	,,	,,	,,	,,	𝒬ed	𝒬ed	,,	Correctly
Black	,,	,,	,,	,,	Black	Black	,,	,,
Orange	,,	Yellow	Yellow	"Red"	𝒬range	𝒬range	,,	"Yellow"
White	,,	Correct	Correct	Correct	White	White	,,	Correctly
Violet	,,	,,	,,	,,	𝒬iolet	𝒬iolet	,,	,,
Green	,,	,,	,,	,,	Green	Green	,,	,,

Asked to point to a colour corresponding to one he had been shown, he answered correctly, but tended to forget the order in which they lay on the table before him. He swept his finger backwards and forwards along the row until he found the one he wanted; then he answered without doubt or hesitation.

Printed commands were carried out somewhat more easily than those given orally, though both were on the whole correctly executed; the choice of yellow for orange can scarcely be reckoned as a mistake. When he attempted to name the various colours, he responded quickly and with assurance, but made two errors, twice calling orange "red."

Told to write these names, he produced in each case something which distinctly represented the colour shown to him, although the letters were badly formed and there was a peculiar tendency to use a common sign for B G R V and Y.

When he was asked to copy these names from print, he almost exactly repeated his previous performance; to write words evoked on seeing a colour and to copy them from a card seemed in this case to be an almost identical task.

(3) *The man, cat and dog tests.*

Table 3.

	Reading aloud	Reading from pictures	Writing from pictures	Writing from dictation	Repetition	Copying print into handwriting
The dog and the cat	Correct	Correct	Dog and Cat	(Illegible word) the Cat	Correct	The Dog and the Cap asp
The man and the dog	,,	,,	Man and "No, I'm done"	The man and the Dog	,,	The man and the Dog
The cat and the man	,,	,,	Cap and man	The cat and the man	,,	The cat and the man
The cat and the dog	,,	,,	D Cap and "No, I can't"	The cat and the man	,,	The man and the Dog
The dog and the man	,,	,,	Dog and man	The Ɋog and the man	,,	The Dog and the man
The man and the cat	,,	,,	Man and cat	The man and the cat	,,	The man and the cat

He had no difficulty in reading from print and from pictures or in repeating after me the series of short sentences of which this test is composed.

But his writing showed the same peculiar changes noticed with previous methods of examination. He wrote with extreme rapidity, as if afraid of forgetting what he intended to do. Thus, when the pictures of the dog and the cat were placed before him, he gazed at them for a time; suddenly he exclaimed, "I've got it," dashed off "dog and," paused and then added a scrawl to represent "cat." Shown the man and the dog, he wrote "man and," adding "now I'm done." Writing from dictation seemed to be equally uncertain and was carried out at extreme speed. Even copying showed the same peculiarities; thus, when a card bearing "the dog and the cat" was laid before him he wrote rapidly "the dog and the," paused, added "cap," said "No, that's not it...cat," wrote "asp" and finally gave up, saying "No, I can't do it."

(4) *The clock tests.*

Although he was able to reproduce exactly by direct imitation the position of the hands on a clock set by me, his method of action was clumsy. Thus, in order to place the minute hand at 45, he would move it all round the clock from 50, its previous position; to set 7.10 after 3.40, he moved both hands round to 7 and then swung the long hand to ten minutes past the hour. He did not appreciate quickly the relation of a task he had solved successfully to one he was about to perform.

Both oral and printed commands were carried out with extreme difficulty and uncertainty. He failed to differentiate the symbolic value of the two hands and confused "to" and "past" the hour. Similar mistakes were apparent when he attempted to tell the time, and still more when he wrote it down silently. If he was permitted to say it aloud before writing it, what he wrote depended entirely upon the words he uttered. Even copying from a printed card was imperfectly carried out.

Table 4.

	Direct imitation	Oral commands	Printed commands	Telling the time	Writing down the time	Telling the time and writing it down at once		Copying print in handwriting
						He said	He wrote	
5 minutes to 2	Correct	Set 2.10	Both hands at 2	Correct	Wrote nothing	"Two o'clock ... about two o'clock"	Qwo o'clock	Correct
Half-past 1	,,	Set 1.10	Both hands at 1; "I seem to think there is something wrong"	,,	Correct	Correctly	Correctly	,,
5 minutes past 8	,,	Both hands at 8	Both hands at 8	,,	Ten minutes past eight	,,	,,	Ten past eight
20 minutes to 4	,,	Both hands at 4; then 4.25	Long hand at 4; short hand at 7	"Twenty-five minutes to four"	Gave up	"Twenty minutes past seven"	Twenty minutes past seven	Correct
10 minutes past 7	,,	Long hand at 7; short hand at 5	Correct	"Ten minutes past eight... seven"	Correct	Correctly	Correctly	,,
20 minutes to 6	,,	Set 6.20	Set 6.15	"Twenty-five to six"	Ten minutes past seven	,,	Twenty minutes to sis	Twenty minutes to sis
10 minutes to 1	,,	Set 1.10	Both hands at 2	"Five to eight... no, that's ten"	Correct	,,	Correctly	Correct
A quarter to 9	,,	Correct	Correct	Correct	Quarter to eight	,,	,,	,,
20 minutes past 11	,,	Long hand at 11; short hand at 10	Long hand at 11; "I've no certain opinion"	"Ten minutes past eleven; I get confused between hour hand and long hand"	Ten minutes past four	"Twenty past twelve"	twenty minutes past twelve	twenty past ilfion
25 minutes to 3	,,	Long hand at 3; then gave up	Set 3.35	"A quarter past seven"	Half past seven	"Quarter past seven"	Quarter past siven	Correct

(5) *The hand, eye and ear tests.*

Table 5.

	Imitation of movements made by the observer	Imitation of movements reflected in a mirror	Pictorial commands	Pictorial commands reflected in a mirror	Oral commands	Printed commands	Reading aloud printed com-mands
L. hand to R. ear	Touched chin with L. hand	Correct	L. hand to L. ear	L. hand to L. ear	R. hand to R. ear	Held up L. hand	Correct
R. hand to L. eye	R. hand to R. eye	R. hand to R. *ear*	L. hand to L. eye	Correct	Correct	R. hand..."I couldn't follow so much"	,,
R. hand to L. ear	L. hand to L. *eye*	R. hand to R. ear	R. hand to R. ear	R. hand to R. ear	R. hand to R. ear	R. hand to R. ear	,,
L. hand to L. eye	R. hand to R. eye	Correct	R. hand to R. *ear*	Correct	Correct	Correct	,,
R. hand to R. ear	Correct	,,	Reversed	,,	,,	,,	,,
L. hand to R. eye	R. hand to R. eye	,,	R. hand to R. eye	L. hand to L. *ear*	L. hand to L. *ear*	R. hand to R. eye	,,
L. hand to L. ear	Reversed	,,	Reversed	Correct	L. hand to L. *eye*	L. hand to L. *eye*	,,
R. hand to R. eye	,,	,,	,,	R. hand to R. *ear*	Correct	No answer	,,
L. hand to R. ear	R. hand to R. ear	,,	R. hand to R. ear	L. hand to L. ear	L. hand to L. *eye*	L. hand to L. ear	,,
R. hand to L. eye	R. hand to R. *ear*	R. hand to R. eye	Reversed	R. hand to R. *ear*	R. hand to R. eye	R. hand to R. eye	,,
R. hand to L. ear	R. hand to R. ear	R. hand to R. ear	R. hand to R. ear	L. hand to L. ear	L. hand to L. ear	L. hand to L. ear	,,
L. hand to L. eye	Correct	L. hand to L. *ear*	Correct	R. hand to R. *ear*	Reversed	Reversed	,,
R. hand to R. ear	,,	Correct	Reversed	Correct	Correct	R. hand to R. *eye*	,,
L. hand to R. eye	R. hand to R. *ear*	L. hand to R. *ear*	R. hand to R. eye	L. hand to L. eye	L. hand to L. eye	L. hand to L. eye	,,
L. hand to L. ear	Correct	Correct	Reversed	Reversed	Reversed	Reversed	,,
R. hand to R. eye	,,	,,	,,	R. hand to R. *ear*	,,	Correct	,,

This series of tests puzzled him greatly and reading aloud the orders in print was alone executed correctly. Throughout all these other tasks, he tended to make the same kind of mistakes, confusing eye and ear, or right and left, failing in most instances to recognise that an order required him to bring his hand across his face to touch the eye or ear of the opposite side. Throughout all these observations, he moved his lips and occasionally could be heard to repeat the command, usually incorrectly. He complained, "My initial difficulty seems to be right and left; it confuses me and I forget the rest of what I've got to do."

No wonder that, under such conditions, he failed to imitate my movements sitting face to face, or to carry out pictorial commands; for both require accurate appreciation and reproduction of a somewhat complex formula. But his uncertainty of general intention led him even to confuse these orders when reflected in a mirror; he failed to recognise that he had simply to imitate exactly what he saw in the glass without reasoning about right and left. Oral and printed commands were also badly executed and he could frequently be heard to repeat the order wrongly under his breath. This was not so much due to want of power to understand the actual words as to an inability to formulate and retain in his memory the general intention of what he was told to do.

Subsequent Progress.

So long as he remained in the Empire Hospital, where he occupied a room to himself, he progressed favourably. But, at the end of July, 1916, he was sent to our Convalescent Hospital at Roehampton. Here many of the patients were up and about, occupied in games and other more or less active amusements. There was a large camp close by in Richmond Park; bands played, men marched and the sound of explosions from the bombing school were distinctly audible. He wandered about unhappily and complained that there was "too much going on, it puzzles me. They are always going by with a band and I want to think what they are. It bothers me." He suffered from headache, mostly over the left side, but nausea and vomiting were absent. The discs were normal.

On *August* 23, 1916, he had a definite epileptiform convulsion, which was seen by Dr Riddoch, who was talking to him at the time. He ceased speaking, turned towards the right side; his eyelids closed. The right arm became flexed and rigid, but there were no clonic contractions and the leg was not obviously affected. The conjunctival reflex was absent. He did not bite his tongue or evacuate urine or fæces. After the attack was over the right plantar reflex gave an upward response.

In *September*, 1916, he was moved back to the Empire Hospital for closer observation, and his general condition improved greatly under the influence of quiet and restricted surroundings. His headache almost disappeared and nausea and vomiting were absent. The discs were unaffected and visual fields normal. There was neither paralysis nor paresis, and all the reflexes, including the abdominal and plantar, were unaffected.

On *October* 16, 1916, Mr Walton explored the wound. A small flap was turned down and an irregular trephine hole was discovered, filled with tough fibrous tissue. This was dissected away carefully and a small piece of bone (0·8 by 0·5 by 0·2 cm.) was taken away from the superficial part of the cortex. When the scar tissue was removed, this fragment was visible without further dissection. The wound healed by first intention.

He was sent to the country and his general condition greatly improved. All headache disappeared; he remained free from attacks and showed no physical signs of a lesion to the nervous system, beyond the condition of his speech.

In *June*, 1917, he was again put through a complete examination. The tests with common objects were now carried out perfectly and those of the man, cat and dog series were noticeable only for the extreme rapidity with which he wrote. He asked to be permitted to leave out the "thes" in writing, for "I keep track of it better" if allowed to shorten the sentence in this way. The clock tests still showed all the previous faults in executing oral and printed commands, and the results of the hand, eye and ear tests were almost identical with those set out on Table 5. He made the definite statement that, when attempting to carry out oral and printed commands, "I seem to act more spontaneously, but I still say it over to myself. Though I don't say it aloud, I say it to myself." If he was permitted to say it aloud his actions were almost perfectly in accord with the order given by word of mouth or in print.

He could write an excellent letter, but had extreme difficulty in reducing the alphabet to writing. In the course of what he wrote spontaneously in my presence, occurred the following passage: "Shall I now try to tell you a very Diffcul tast you set me, that is trying to write the Letters of the alphabet. This test is one which I always felt would be Difficut. he trouble is mostly in beginning the Letters i.e. actual Letters of the alphabet wihle I can write straight on beginnin a new letter or sentence troubles me. This may not be very intellegible to you, but if I may, I shall try to explain my somewhat rambling..." He then ceased and appended his signature. He had no difficulty in reading this whole letter, when written; he appreciated where he had gone wrong and corrected some of the mistakes.

Arithmetical operations were impossible, except the first or simplest addition and subtraction sums. He had no difficulty in naming coins, but was still slow in recognising their relative value, though his answers were on the whole correct.

He was given a brightly coloured picture of a jetty with a small lighthouse projecting into the sea; moored close to shore was a fishing boat that filled up at least one-third of the picture. Holding it in his hand he began to describe what he saw: "It's a picture of the sea...and it shows the harbour and...the...this might be a light house...and there's a steamer out at sea...Life boat, on rollers ready for launching...there's a small boat here [pointing to the shore]. There's a ship here possibly for pulling up any sort of boat." He entirely missed, in this detailed description, the large fishing boat, which filled up a considerable portion of the picture. After it was removed he again enumerated from memory the various objects he had seen, entering into even closer detail. The picture was then replaced in his hands and he suddenly exclaimed, "Oh! I left out the very large boat, fishing boat, sailing boat. I think I missed it from the beginning."

After an attack of influenza in *July*, 1918, he regressed and did not recover his powers of speech, up to the point he had previously reached, until the beginning of 1919. In March of that year his condition was much the same as that I have just described, but by June he showed distinct improvement.

I pass over all my observations during the next two years, which simply confirmed and amplified those already recorded.

CONDITION BETWEEN APRIL 28TH AND MAY 4TH, 1921 (*five years after the injury*).

He was in splendid physical health and did not suffer in any way from his head. But he complained that he easily became tired especially if he had to think much and then lost "the grip of things." "If I've got to hurry it puts me out directly."

He had been through a course of training in apiculture under the ægis of the Pensions Ministry. His wife, an extremely able young woman, took part in this instruction, and it was she who managed all the business and administration, whilst he carried out the physical work required for the industry.

Articulated speech. He could find all the words and names he required for daily use; his sentences were perfectly formed and spaced and syntax was unaffected; but he still showed a tendency to become confused in the give and take of conversation. He was able to say the days of the week or the months correctly and counted without mistake or hesitation. Repetition was perfect, provided the phrases were not long and complicated in their significance.

Understanding of spoken words. On superficial examination he seemed to understand all that was said to him. He had no difficulty in choosing familiar objects or colours to oral commands, but he failed grossly to set the hands of the clock, or to carry out the hand, eye and ear tests, to orders given by word of mouth.

In ordinary intercourse he was frequently unable to comprehend with uniform exactitude what he had heard and so became easily confused. Of this several characteristic instances are given below.

Reading. He still had profound difficulty in grasping the full significance of what he read silently, although he could read aloud without mistakes and with perfect enunciation (vide infra, p. 166).

Writing. He wrote with undue rapidity and formed his letters carelessly, as if in fear that he might forget what he intended to express. But his script was now legible and he had ceased to employ a common sign for several different capital letters.

The following excellent letter was composed and written spontaneously in my presence: "Dear Dr Head, London seems very beautiful at present. The trees look so fresh and green that one might almost imagine oneself in the country. Nearly two years ago I was in London and was very much impressed by the beauty of the trees. London must, I think, look at its best in early May. My mother visited London at Easter and was full of enthusiasm for the natural beauty of the surroundings, the blossoms on the fruit trees particularly taking her attention. I do not mean to say that London is more beautiful than the country—it is very beautiful in some respects wonderfully so—but what seizes the imagination is that so much beauty should exist around a great city. The cause may, I should say, be given in one word—trees."

Here the only faults were poor handwriting and careless spelling, corresponding to the hurried manner in which he carried out his task. He read this letter over aloud to me perfectly and did not notice any of the mistakes.

He could write to dictation and copy correctly, but his handwriting tended to show the same faults as when he wrote spontaneously.

The alphabet. He could say, repeat and read aloud the alphabet in perfect order, quickly and without mistakes.

But, when he came to write the letters, he lost the thread in the middle; he paused after J, started again with I, and then, except for two illegible scrawls before L, wrote the remainder correctly. To dictation he made the same sort of mistakes, writing mainly in capitals: *A B* C D *E F G* H *J I J K L m n* O *P Q* R *S T* *u v w x y z*. When I said G he wrote *J*, and followed it rapidly by *G* in response to a second command; but for I, he again substituted *J*, correcting it on repetition of the order. He was then asked to copy the printed alphabet:

this he carried out in cursive handwriting, slowly and with evident difficulty. For k he first wrote *h* and added *k*; r was preceded by two illegible attempts, and for t he first wrote *d*, and he made the following explanatory remarks: "I found some difficulty. I always have difficulty with a k; I always write h; then I know it is different; I can't get started somehow with the r, the same with the t. I thought it was simple; I took the risk it would come right, and it came right. I wasn't sure until I came to put the stroke and then I found I was right. I had to risk it."

A printed paragraph. I gave him the following passage from Landor's letters, asking him first of all to read it to himself and then to tell me what he had gathered from it.

"On Wednesday last, I was present at a wedding; the only one I was ever at, except one other. There was bride-cake and there were verses in profusion, two heavy commodities! But what an emblematic thing the bride-cake is! All sugar above, all lumpiness below. But may Heaven grant another, and far different destiny, to my sweet-tempered, innocent, sensible young friend."

Four minutes later he handed the paper back, saying, "On Wednesday last I was present at a wedding. The...the only one except one other at which I was present. There were...presents...and verses...and bride-cake in profusion... The...the bride-cake all sugared above...lumpiness below...The one, the cake ...yes, the cake suggested to be emblematic of the future state of the married couple...I wasn't able to quite follow what was really meant by the emblematic state. There seemed to be in the writer's mind some meaning, but I couldn't find what it really was."

He then re-read the contents silently and wrote as follows:

"On Wednesday last I was present at a wedding, the only one except one other at which I was present. There were verses in profusion and a brides cake, both heavy commodities. The one all sugar above, all lumpiness below, simmingly an emblem of the future state. May the future state of my innocent young friend be..." He ceased to write and said, "I've rather lost the trend of things."

He was asked to read the passage aloud, which he did correctly; then he copied it in cursive handwriting clearly and without mistakes.

Finally I asked him, "What was it that bothered you?" and he replied, "Well at first it was an ordinary conventional wedding with cake and I suppose in those old days verses; they are not so prevalent nowadays. He seemed to regard the wedding cake as an emblem of the future state of his young friend, who was about to be married...and the writer's mind...he seemed to...regard the wedding cake as...as...as..." Then he gave up all further attempts to explain his meaning.

I demanded, what is an emblem? He answered at once, "Oh! an emblem is a...well...the Cenotaph might be taken as an emblem of sacrifice and adhesion to a great principle."

Significance of pictures. He was given a coloured picture of a motor car standing before a large country house; the driver, a young man, was talking to two girls, one of whom held a greyhound by the collar. Asked the meaning of this picture he went over it in detail from left to right and then back again without the least evidence of constructive appreciation. He said: "There are two trees on the left-hand side and a house, perpendicular columns. There's a doorway on the right and a window just above it. There are chimneys. Then there are the side windows. Then there are some small buildings at the back, out-buildings or a lodge, something like that. Behind that there are trees. Then there's a small hill; at the bottom of it there's a lake. In the foreground there's a motor car; it's standing. The driver's a man, looks like the owner of the car, not a chauffeur. He is speaking to two ladies. He appears to be addressing more directly a lady with a red hat and another lady standing by is holding a hound." Every detail was recognised correctly; but he did not weld them into a coherent whole and express the meaning of the picture in a set of general propositions.

He was then shown a series of humorous sketches representing a spectator who, arriving late at a play, strips off inadvertently both his coats, and is taking his seat in shirt sleeves to the horrified amusement of the audience. When I asked the patient what he saw in these pictures, he entirely missed the point. "There's an audience, possibly a concert audience. The audience is seated, waiting and...a man comes along wearing his coat. He has some difficulty evidently in taking it off, whether real or assumed. The audience seems greatly interested. I'm not sure about it...I was trying to think it might have been part of the performance...or he might have got there and seem to be rather prominent. It often happens in a theatre that somebody comes late."

But, on the other hand, he was sometimes surprisingly quick in seeing the point of a picture, if it depended on details, especially if each bore its explanatory label. Thus, I showed him a cartoon of Winston Churchill trying on a hat which was too small for his head; behind on a shelf lay the head-gear appropriate to the Home Office, Board of Trade, Admiralty, War Office, Air Minister and Ministry of Munitions, each bearing a label. Above stood an unopened band-box marked "The Premier." He said at once, "That, of course, is Mr Winston Churchill. Shortly, the point is the statesman is suffering from what is commonly called swelled head; his head is too big for his hat. There are many different shapes and the caricaturist has it in his mind that he has worn them all at one time or another. There's the civilian bowler hat, the admiral's peaked hat, the War Office; forage cap it's called in the Air Ministry, the Flying Corps; then the Ministry of Munitions cap, indicated by something connected with the workman, the labourer." Then he returned to the left of the picture and pointing to the first on the shelf said, "This must be a policeman's helmet" (correct); but he entirely missed the hat-box marked "The Premier" and all that it implied.

Comprehension of general significance. He still showed the same lack of power to grasp the general aim or significance of a question, order, or series of propositions. For instance, on a sunny spring morning I said, before we began work, "I hope you don't find it cold; shall I put the window up?" He answered "Yes," but as soon as I began to raise it he called out "No, no." Then he explained, "When you said 'have the window up,' I thought you meant open...more air. You went to put the window like that" (waving his hand upwards) "and I thought no, no, more air, that's what I want." This is a good example of the confusion which is liable to arise in his dealings with others.

Starting from errors of this kind, he was perpetually liable to arrive at mistaken conclusions. One day he was waiting on the station platform of his native town, when he saw a young lady who was an old acquaintance. His brother told him her name, said she had gone away some time ago and added that she was now married. This the patient strenuously denied, asserting she wore no wedding ring. He had looked for it on what seemed to him to be her left hand, but was in reality her right.

He still had serious difficulty in appreciating the significance of summer-time. He gave a perfect definition of summer as "the season at which the sun approaches nearest to the earth and the days are longer and the heat more intense." Asked what he understood by time, he answered, "Time is the length of a day reckoned as twenty-four hours subdivided into day and night." He now recognised that summer-time consisted in arranging the hands of the clocks on a certain date "so that there may be more day-light during ordinary working hours." But he could not be certain what happened to the clocks. "This bothers me," he said, "very much all through, more especially when we come back again to winter-time at the end of the season; I seem to want to tell you in one clear sentence what happened, when the clocks were altered to normal time; I seemed to get muddled between two things."

Arithmetic. He was extremely slow in carrying out the simplest arithmetical exercises and took twenty minutes over the following examples without being able to complete the last one:

Addition.			Subtraction.		
231	648	856	865	782	912
356	326	275	432	258	386
587	974	1131	433	524	26

He brought out the answer to the first sum fairly quickly, but the second caused him extreme difficulty; he gave it up, but insisted on returning to it later, and finally completed it correctly. The answer to the first subtraction came with moderate ease, but the second was enormously prolonged, and the third of the series was not completed.

He complained, "I found difficulty in them all. I found the subtraction more difficult than the addition. When there was a carry, it seemed to be more difficult.

What I feel about it is...if I were to begin my education, like a boy at school, I shouldn't know where to begin. In those sums you gave me I did the addition almost involuntarily, I think the results of former practice. The subtraction...the simplest one, I did it in the more or less involuntary way...but with the more difficult I had to think what subtraction really meant."

Coins and their relative value. Money in all its forms was named accurately and with great rapidity; even notes were distinguished without fail. But, when he was asked to state the relative value of any two coins, he answered slowly and with hesitation, although he made one actual mistake only in a series of eighteen observations, saying that twelve sixpences went to a shilling.

He still had extreme difficulty in calculating the change he should receive after making a purchase. His tobacco now cost him a shilling an ounce. He would ask for two ounces, placing a two-shilling piece on the counter; if he wanted a box of matches in addition, he waited until the first transaction was over and then took a penny from his pocket, so as to avoid the difficulties of change. Should he happen to have nothing less than a ten-shilling note, with which to pay for his tobacco, he asked the tobacconist to give him florins only (two-shilling pieces); these he counted, "one, two, three, four," and he knew that four was the right number. But, if he was given the change in shillings, he was lost. "I don't like getting a half-crown (two and sixpence) in change; it puzzles me. I know the tobacconist, if he liked, could cheat me[1]."

Drawing. A glass jug of simple form was placed on the table in front of him and he made a feeble representation of its outlines. Ten minutes later, on attempting to reproduce the jug from memory, he exactly repeated his previous drawing; he was evidently recalling his motor acts and did not rely on his visual images to help him in this task.

Asked to draw an elephant, he produced a scrawl which bore no relation to any known animal; he omitted the trunk and, when I enquired if he had left out anything, he said, "Elephant's nose; I'm not sure where the nose ought to be." I then told him to draw the head only and he became completely confused.

He then said, "I'll draw you a bee-skep" and proceeded to do so accurately, giving the exact form of the Dutch hive they were using, together with the stand and the metal cover to keep off the rain.

Plan drawing and relative position of objects in space. When removed into another room, he was unable to draw a plan of the one in which we had so often worked; the windows were placed on the wrong side and the relation of the main door to the fire-place was reversed. So far this examination confirmed, but added

[1] On a previous occasion (June 1919), when tobacco was somewhat cheaper, I asked him how much it cost an ounce. He replied, "If I buy two ounces of tobacco at a time...if I put down a florin I get...I ought to get change amounting to...well at any rate, I get threepence." He knew exactly the change he should receive from a two-shilling piece, when he purchased two ounces of tobacco, but could not tell me the price per ounce.

nothing to, my previous observations. But from this point onwards I modified my procedure as follows. I made him shut his eyes and point to the position of the various objects as I named them, which he did perfectly. His eyes were then opened and I put before him an outline plan, on which he indicated with his finger the place of the various pieces of furniture; this he carried out correctly in every instance. Finally, I asked him again to draw a plan of the room in which we worked and he was now able to do so, at any rate as far as its main features were concerned. He said, "When you asked me to do this first I couldn't do it. I couldn't get the starting point. I knew where all the things were in the room, but I had difficulty in getting a starting point, when it came to setting them down on a plan. You made me point out on the plan and it was quite easy, because you had done it. After things were pointed out, I retained them in my memory and got them down on paper quite easily."

Visual images. A few days after I had tested his power of drawing, he volunteered the following introspective remarks: "I thought of what you asked me to do, drawing the glass. In bed I was trying to think about it. I was trying to see the glass bottle; the picture seemed to evade me. I knew it was a bottle and I could describe the shape of it, and I remember making a drawing of it, and I could describe the drawing. But then, when it came to seeing it as a picture, I was more or less nonplussed. I often seemed to have got the picture, but it seemed to evade me."

"There is a photograph of my wife, which is hanging in the bedroom. I can see that; the expression in that photograph is very good, I can see that."

"I can see the bee alighting on the alighting board. I see it quite clearly. Now, for instance, our hives are painted in two colours, one green, one white. I can see a bee alighting on the alighting board, say, for instance, yellow-coloured pollen. Yes, I can see that quite clearly."

"The more I try to...to make them come the more difficult it is to get in touch with them, as one might say."

Orientation. He was completely unable to find his way alone. He never took his bearings and, if he was going to a place for a second time, did not recognise landmarks or appreciate that he was passing over the same ground again. He did not know which way to turn, and if he chanced to take the opposite side of the road, became confused and was ignorant in which direction to walk.

Given the number of a turning to the right or left, he could never find it correctly; but, told to take the "next on this side," he was able to do so. Left and right puzzled him greatly; he tried to work them out by thinking which was the left half of his body and frequently brought out an incorrect answer.

Relation of objects to one another. His inability to remember the relation of external objects to one another came out when he was given a mechanical task. He made the four portions of a bee-hive under supervision of the instructor, but was unable to put them together. He was incapable of wiring his bee-frames except by passing the wire backwards and forwards in direct sequence from side to side.

I placed before him all the breakfast utensils requisite for one person, and asked him to set the table. He quickly placed the cup, the saucer and the plate correctly. Then he became confused, laid the knife across the plate and removed it, set the spoon to the right of the plate and took it away again; finally, after much hesitation, he placed the fork to the left, the knife to the right and the spoon above the plate. Subsequently he set the remaining objects such as the sugar basin, salt-cellar and pepper-pot in their appropriate positions.

He explained his difficulty in carrying out the task as follows: "There was something missing, something unusual. I got the knife and fork, I couldn't find...let us say the bacon and eggs. Then the spoon puzzled me; I wasn't quite sure why it was there. If I was laying my own breakfast table I should know, because I always take porridge. If I saw the spoon, I should look for the bowl for the milk and so on; but there seemed nothing like that, and so I thought the best way out of the difficulty was to place the spoon in a position in which it might be convenient for any purpose."

"I always try to have the things in my bedroom in exactly the same position. If I've got to think where they are and look for them, I get muddled; I lose time. I have them all in the same order; then I don't have to think. If I have to look for them I am bothered. If I go to a strange room, it's a more difficult job to dress and takes an appreciably longer time than if I am at home."

Games and puzzles. He could not play any games or amuse himself with puzzles. I played draughts with him, simplifying the game by removing one of the three rows of men on either side. He complained, on being beaten with the greatest ease, "The chief bother was trying to follow the consequences of the next move. I couldn't foresee what would happen."

He had never been good at billiards and now could not play at all. "Somehow the three balls put me out of it. Even with two balls my stroke was indifferent, but if I wished to cannon I seemed to think of the three actions necessary to be made. As a consequence I became muddled, I couldn't make a cannon. A straight shot with two balls was not so bad, but the third ball confused me. I seemed to think of the three functions at the same time and got muddled."

I therefore tried the following experiment. A basket was placed at the end of the room and he threw balls of paper into it, even more accurately than I could; but, when I placed a screen in front of it, his shots became extremely bad, and he said, "When I could see the basket, I could follow the line of vision; when it was covered, I didn't seem to feel so confident it was in the same place, I don't know why. I'd seen the basket before you'd put the screen there; I knew you hadn't changed the position, but in some odd way I didn't feel perfectly confident in my own mind that it was in that position."

Serial Tests.

(1) *Recognition and naming of common objects.* All these tests, except that of writing the name of an object shown to him, were now carried out perfectly. His handwriting had greatly improved, he spelt the words correctly, but still tended to hurry as if he were afraid of forgetting what he had to do. During these observations he said, "I feel quite confident. But there was an odd thing the other day. I was down at carpentry; the man had different bits of wood, he was going to number them. I couldn't make the A and the C; I made the B, I couldn't make the D."

Thus in spite of his perfect writing he is still uncertain about the formation of individual letters to command; this corresponds with the results obtained when he was made to write the alphabet.

(2) *Recognition and naming of colours.* He carried out all these tasks without any material mistake, but evidently found some difficulty in writing the names of the colours, although he spelt them correctly. This he explained as follows: "The only difficulty had nothing to do with the colours. You called it violet; I named it mauve. The same with orange; the colour was quite familiar, but the term orange did not seem to come to me. I compromised by calling it light brown, which was not quite the correct colour. But, when you said orange, I was quite certain that it was orange." Whenever he was in doubt, his handwriting deteriorated and he formed the word hurriedly.

(3) *The man, cat and dog tests.* He was already able to carry out these tests perfectly in June, 1919, and the records obtained in May, 1921, were equally good.

At the close of these observations he volunteered the following statement: "I can see a man with his trousers cleanly cut. He is tall and straight; he has a hat on, and is clean-shaven." I said, "Tell me about the dog." He answered, "The dog has short legs, like a terrier, roughish coated; maybe a Scotch terrier." *Q.* "Now about the cat?" *A.* "It's an ordinary cat; the whiskers are rather evident. I think she is sitting, not lying down; but a cat rests on her hind legs, the position a cat has when she's...Her weight is on that part of her...it corresponds to our...let me see...the femur isn't it? She's just sitting up, on her haunches, that's the word I wanted."

(4) *The clock tests.*

Direct imitation was carried out exactly, and he set the hour hand in a position proportionate to the minutes. Oral and printed commands were badly executed, he made many mistakes, mistook the hands, and was slow, hesitating, and uncertain of the correctness of his final choice. Commands given in railway time yielded better results, especially if they were printed; he held the card before him until he had finished setting the clock, looking back repeatedly for correction and reassurance. He said, "It was much easier; I could get a starting point. You see the main thing that really mattered was the unit, two o'clock; the other matters were subsidiary." Thus, when the order was given in railway time, he set the hour and then the minutes; whereas if these preceded the number of the hour, as with the ordinary nomenclature, he became confused. He could now both tell the time and write it correctly.

Table 6.

	Direct imitation	Oral commands		Printed commands		Telling the time	Writing down the time	
		Ordinary nomenclature	Railway time	Full words	Railway time		In words	In railway time
5 minutes to 2	Correct	Reversed hands; long hand at 2	Correct	Set 2.5	Correct	Correct	Correct	Correct
Half-past 1	,,	Slowly, correct	,,	Correct	,,	,,	,,	,,
5 minutes past 8	,,	Reversed hands; long hand at 8	,,	Hour hand between 7 and 8; long hand at 5 minutes past	,,	,,	,,	,,
20 minutes to 4	,,	Set 4.20	Set 4.20	Set 4.20	,,	,,	,,	,,
10 minutes past 7	,,	Both hands at 7	Correct	Correct	,,	,,	,,	,,
20 minutes to 6	,,	Hour hand at 6; otherwise correct	,,	Correct (very slow)	,,	,,	,,	,,
10 minutes to 1	,,	Correct	Reversed hands; long hand at 12	Correct	,,	,,	,,	,,
A quarter to 9	,,	,,	Correct	,,	Hour hand at 8; long hand correct	,,	,,	,,
20 minutes past 11	,,	,,	,,	,,	Correct	,,	,,	,,
25 minutes to 3	,,	Set 3.25	Set 2.25	Hour hand at 3; long hand correct	,,	,,	,,	,,

(5) *The coin-bowl tests.* In June, 1919, his answers to verbal commands were slow and somewhat uncertain, but finally correct. He made no mistakes and was quicker and more certain to printed commands; but he held the card in his hand and repeatedly referred to it for confirmation.

By May, 1921, all hesitation had disappeared and these tests were carried out perfectly. "I have practically no difficulty. I take the penny and I say 'first into third' (no word is uttered). I just consider for a moment and then I get it."

(6) *The hand, eye and ear tests.*

He still had difficulty in imitating movements made by me, or represented pictorially. Reflection in the glass did not materially improve his answers. Oral and printed commands, carried out silently, gave better results and, when he was allowed to read the order aloud, he executed it without fail. Writing down the movements made by me gave him considerable trouble; he was slow and hesitating and made several mistakes.

Table 7.

	Imitation of movements made by the observer	Imitation of movements reflected in a mirror	Pictorial commands	Pictorial commands reflected in a mirror	Oral commands	Printed commands	Reading aloud and executing printed commands: He read	Reading aloud and executing printed commands: Movements made	Writing down movements made by the observer
L. hand to L. eye	Correct	Correct	Correct	Correct	Correct	Correct	Correctly	Correct	Right hand to left eye
R. hand to R. ear	,,	,,	,,	,,	,,	,,	,,	,,	Reversed
R. hand to L. eye	,,	,,	L. hand to L. eye	,,	,,	Reversed	,,	,,	,,
L. hand to R. eye	L. hand to R. *ear*	R. hand to R. eye	Correct	R. hand to R. eye	,,	Correct	,,	,,	,,
L. hand to L. ear	Correct	Correct	,,	Correct	,,	,,	,,	,,	,,
R. hand to R. eye	,,	,,	Correct (slow)	R. hand to R. *ear*; corrected	,,	,,	,,	,,	Correct
L. hand to R. ear	,,	L. hand to L. ear	Correct	R. hand to R. ear	,,	,,	,,	,,	Reversed
R. hand to L. ear	L. hand to L. ear	Correct	,,	R. hand to R. ear	,,	,,	,,	,,	Correct
L. hand to L. eye	L. hand to R. eye	,,	L. hand to L. *ear*	Correct	L. hand to R. eye	,,	,,	,,	Reversed
R. hand to R. ear	Correct	,,	Correct	,,	Correct	,,	,,	,,	Correct
R. hand to L. eye	,,	L. hand to L. eye	Reversed	,,	L. hand to L. eye	,,	,,	,,	,,
L. hand to R. eye	L. hand to L. eye	Correct	,,	R. hand to R. *ear*	Correct	,,	,,	,,	,,
L. hand to L. ear	Correct	,,	Correct	Correct	,,	,,	,,	,,	,,
R. hand to R. eye	,,	,,	R. hand to L. eye	,,	,,	,,	,,	,,	,,
L. hand to R. ear	,,	R. hand to R. ear	Reversed	R. hand to R. ear	,,	Correct (slow)	,,	,,	,,
R. hand to L. ear	R. hand to R. ear	Correct	R. hand to R. ear	L. hand to L. ear	,,	Correct	,,	,,	,,

CONDITION BETWEEN FEBRUARY 27TH AND MARCH 5TH, 1923 (*seven years after the injury*).

He took a cottage in the West of England in order to carry on his business of bee-keeping. At first all went well and he was happy; but gradually the strain and worry of the hard work began to tell upon him. The little house was badly constructed and the winter storms beat upon its corrugated iron roof like hail, preventing him from obtaining a sufficient amount of sleep. The new hives, ordered from the makers to an exact measure, deviated from scale and could not be readjusted; this troubled him greatly. Finally, the bees turned out to be infected with disease; they had to be destroyed and all the capital and labour expended by the two young people were lost.

Throughout this year he steadily deteriorated and on August 25, 1922, was seized with an epileptiform attack whilst in bed; he lost consciousness, became rigid, but there was little "jerking." He did not bite his tongue or pass urine. This fit was followed by greatly increased "nervousness" and tendency to confusion. The weather was extremely bad and he went out of doors very little; sleep deserted him and he ceased to take sufficient food. Finally, with the close of the year, he and his wife were forced to give up the experiment.

When I saw him in February, 1923, the wound was in perfect condition, firmly covered with tough scar tissue, painless and not tender to the touch; it did not pulsate. The discs were unaffected and there were no abnormal physical signs of any kind, apart from his disorders of speech.

Articulated speech was not affected except that he tended to become confused and to pause in narration like a man who has lost the thread of what he wanted to say. Verbal formation and syntax were perfect. He could name common objects, geometrical shapes or colours without difficulty and repeated everything said to him with ease.

Understanding of spoken words. He was still in exactly the condition described on p. 165. He chose any object shown to him with certainty and even carried out the hand, eye and ear tests to oral commands. But he made many mistakes in setting the hands of a clock, provided the order was given in words; if however it was in the form of numbers, the so-called railway time, he executed it correctly.

This tendency to confusion was even more apparent in general intercourse; but, in spite of these misunderstandings, he gave repeated evidence of considerable powers of appreciation.

Reading. He still had considerable difficulty in grasping the full significance of what he read to himself, although he could choose common objects, geometrical shapes and colours accurately to printed commands. The hand, eye and ear tests were executed slowly but correctly, and yet he made many errors in setting the hands of a clock, when the order was given in the usual nomenclature. On the other hand commands in railway time were carried out with no mistakes though sometimes slowly.

He read aloud perfectly; enunciation and rhythm were normal, and he was able to understand the meaning of printed sentences better if he was permitted to articulate the words.

Writing. He still wrote with great rapidity, as if he were afraid of forgetting what he intended to place upon paper, and his handwriting suffered in consequence. Name and address were written correctly and he composed a letter of considerable length, which was on the whole remarkably coherent.

He wrote well to dictation and copied accurately from print, but his handwriting was hurried and poorly formed.

The alphabet. He could say the letters in correct sequence, repeat them after me and read them aloud perfectly. But, when he attempted to write the alphabet, he was liable to become confused. Thus he wrote: *a b b c d e f g h s 𝒥 i 𝒥 j k*. The remainder were written correctly. At the end he said, "I made a mistake there" (pointing to the letter preceding *c*), "I was conscious of it; I had c in my mind's eye; I went to make it, but it seemed to act of its own accord and I went wrong. With i, just the same sort of thing occurred; I couldn't get on with the j properly and I put a capital, which seemed to come easier." It is noticeable that he wrote each letter very quickly, as if afraid of forgetting what he wanted to write. To dictation he made exactly the same mistakes, writing *a b b c d e f g H i h j i j k*, etc. Even when copying from printed capitals he wrote *j i* for I, and *s j* for J, although the other letters were correctly written in cursive script. Given the twenty-six block letters, he put them together in the right sequence, saying: "That's quite easy because I do one thing at a time; I know what ought to come next and seeing the letter confirms it."

A printed paragraph. I selected the following description from Dickens, to serve as a test: "The gentleman spoken of had a very ugly squint and a prominent chin. He was wearing a tall white hat with a narrow flat brim and riding breeches with yellow leather gaiters. He carried in his hand a switch, with which he tapped his boots, as he talked in a hoarse voice."

Asked what he had understood, after reading these sentences silently, he replied: "The passage tells of a peculiar looking man. He had a prominent chin and an ugly squint. He wore riding breeches and yellow gaiters. He carried in his hand a switch, with which he tapped his riding breeches...his gaiters..."

He read this paragraph through once more to himself and wrote down the following account: "The gentleman spoken of had a prominent chin and an ugly squint. He wore riding breeches and yellow gaiters. He carried in his hand a switch with from time to time he tapped his riding." The spelling was correct but the writing was bad and became worse towards the end; two words were omitted in the last sentence.

These sentences were read aloud from print perfectly and he both copied and wrote them to dictation without error or omission; but the writing was hurried and poor. During the act of copying he said, "Sometimes when I'm writing, I don't form a letter properly, and when I go back over it again, I get puzzled... from the fullstop the continuity is lost and the writing doesn't flow easily."

I then asked him to narrate to me what he remembered of the paragraph he had so often read and transcribed. He replied, "The gentleman spoken of had a prominent chin and an ugly squint. He wore...he wore riding breeches and yellow gaiters...He...carried in his hand a switch...with which...from time to time... he rapped...his riding boots. There's another point I have left out; he wore a tall hat with a narrow flat brim...There is still another piece...It's all chopping and changing...I have forgotten pieces of it and things occur to me as I go over it again."

I then handed him a list of the various details mentioned in this description, arranged in a vertical column (ugly squint; prominent chin; tall white hat; narrow flat brim; riding breeches; yellow gaiters; carried a switch; tapped his boots; talked in a hoarse voice). The whole set were reproduced correctly from memory, although in changed order. In fact, his memory tested in this way was remarkable, and he explained, "If I get them in any order, just as recollection comes to me... as soon as a word comes to me, I must grasp it in case it escapes me."

Numbers and arithmetic. He counted accurately and without hesitation, each number following its predecessor in rapid sequence.

He still found great difficulty in carrying out simple exercises in arithmetic, and his answers, even when correct, were given slowly and with hesitation:

Addition.			Subtraction.		
231	648	856	865	782	912
356	326	375	432	258	386
587	974	1131 (wrong)	433	544 (wrong)	524 (wrong)

Coins and their relative value. Coins and notes were named accurately and he was now able to state their relative value without mistakes, although he was somewhat slow and uncertain. But he still found much difficulty with change in the transactions of daily life.

I gave him a ten-shilling note and asked him to pile up its equivalent from amongst the coins on the table; this he carried out with some effort correctly. I then handed him the same note, and telling him I had bought something for two-and-six, asked for change. This puzzled him greatly; for although he said "seven-and-six," he had great difficulty in collecting the coins to make up this sum. I gave him the same note once more and said I had purchased something for "three-and-three"; this he was entirely unable to work out. He complained, "It is parts of a shilling that bother me and a halfpenny makes it worse; I get confused and lose the significance of the figures."

Drawing. When a painted jug was placed before him he made a recognisable outline drawing, poorly executed and omitting the pattern. The lines were feeble and uncertain, and a child could have done better.

A quarter of an hour later he reproduced it from memory with the same faults and omissions, saying, "I can see the jug in front of me as I draw it. I can see the general shape, the colours; there's blue and green and an eastern colour. I didn't take notice of the pattern. Then there was the shape of the jug, a sloping shape, wider at the base than farther up. The lip was slightly broken. Then there was the handle, an ordinary old-fashioned handle, except that there were one or two excrescences or rather knobs." All these details were absolutely correct, but they were not represented on his drawing; in fact, this is another example of his remarkable power of remembering isolated aspects of some object or event without the ability to combine them into a general whole.

Asked to draw an elephant, he produced a childishly inadequate body and legs, and was hopelessly puzzled over the head. He said, "It's awfully difficult; it's hard to work in the details, to find where the details ought to go." But when I drew an outline of the animal, leaving blank the eye, ear, trunk and mouth, he inserted all but the ear correctly, naming them as he did so.

Told to draw anything he liked, he made an excellent outline picture of a Dutch beehive, pointing out the high entrance which distinguished it from the English form, and indicated the bees on guard before the opening.

Memory and images. There can be little doubt that he still retained considerable powers of visual imagery, although he could not always employ it at will for the purposes of language. He not only described to me the colour and form of the jug given him as a model, but when I asked him, "Do you remember the man, the cat and the dog I showed you yesterday?" he replied as follows: "Yes, a tall thin man; I think he had a tall hat; I see him, but I'm not clear of other details. He must be clean shaven...he had ordinary trousers...I can't remember any detail about his coat. The dog...the dog was a short thick-set type of dog, something like an Aberdeen terrier...There was shading on the picture to show his rough coat... I think he was looking to the left. The cat was sitting on her haunches...she had the usual...the usual prominence was given to her whiskers." I asked if he could see them clearly, and he answered, "Yes, I can see the cat sitting, and the shaggy dog, and the man...yes."

He frequently gave evidence of a startling memory for detail; for instance, set to write me a letter, he remembered what he had written some years before and amplified it on the second occasion. He visited a friend who had been a fellow officer in the same regiment, and astonished him by an extensive memory of the men's names and peculiarities. Even when he did not know the name, he could describe the man sufficiently accurately to be recognisable. His mind contained a mass of detail which he had difficulty in utilising for the logical sequence of a general statement.

Significance of pictures. These tests revealed the same difficulties as before, and he entirely failed to appreciate the meaning of the humorous picture of the man who inadvertently removed his two coats on entering a theatre. He added, "Apparently there's a joke somewhere, but I haven't been able to see what it really is."

Orientation and plan drawing. He still had extreme difficulty in finding his way, and, although he had passed down a street many times, he never recognised which turning to take. When travelling by the Underground Railway, his wife was obliged to push him off the moving staircase; for he was always completely puzzled how to step from it at the end.

Another set of observations to test his power of drawing a plan, carried out in the same order, brought out exactly similar results to those described on p. 169.

Serial Tests.

(1) *Recognition and naming of common objects* and

(2) *of colours* were carried out perfectly and the names were written down without mistakes.

(3) *The man, cat and dog tests* gave him no difficulty.

(4) *The clock tests.*

Table 8.

	Direct imitation	Oral commands: Ordinary nomenclature	Oral commands: Railway time	Printed commands: Ordinary nomenclature	Printed commands: Railway time	Telling the time	Writing down the time: In words	Writing down the time: In railway time
5 minutes to 2	Correct	Correct	Correct	Set 5 minutes to 10	Hour hand at 1; long hand at 55 min.	Correct	Correct	Correct
Half-past 1	,,	,,	,,	Correct	Correct	,,	,,	,,
5 minutes past 8	,,	Gave up puzzled	Correct (slow)	Long hand correct; hour hand between 7 and 8	,,	,,	,,	,,
20 minutes to 4	,,	Set 4.20	Correct	Correct	,,	,,	,,	,,
10 minutes past 7	,,	Very slow; finally correct	Correct (slow)	,,	,,	,,	,,	,,
20 minutes to 6	,,	Set 6.35	Correct	Correct (very slow)	,,	,,	,,	,,
10 minutes to 1	,,	Correct	,,	Correct	,,	,,	,,	,,
A quarter to 9	,,	,,	,,	,,	,,	,,	,,	,,
20 minutes past 11	,,	Long hand at 20 to; hour hand at 11	,,	,,	,,	,,	,,	,,
25 minutes to 3	,,	Correct	,,	Long hand correct; hour hand between 3 and 4	,,	,,	,,	,,

This table shows a remarkable resemblance to that obtained two years before (p. 173), ample testimony to the trustworthiness of the tests. He could tell the time and write it down correctly. Oral and printed commands still gave him considerable difficulty if presented in ordinary nomenclature, but could be executed, though slowly, if the order was in railway time.

(5) *The coin-bowl tests* were performed without mistakes.

(6) *The hand, eye and ear tests.*

Table 9.

	Imitation of movements made by the observer	Imitation of movements reflected in a mirror	Pictorial commands	Pictorial commands reflected in a mirror	Oral commands	Printed commands	Reading aloud and executing printed commands: He read	Reading aloud and executing printed commands: Movement made	Writing down movements made by the observer
L. hand to L. eye	Correct	Correct	Reversed	Reversed	Correct (slow)	Correct (slow)	Correctly	Correct	Correct
R. hand to R. ear	,,	,,	Correct	,,	Correct	Correct	,,	,,	,,
R. hand to L. eye	Reversed	,,	,,	,,	,,	,,	,,	,,	,,
L. hand to R. eye	Correct	R. hand to R. eye	,,	,,	,,	Correct (slow)	,,	,,	,,
L. hand to L. ear	,,	Correct	,,	Correct	,,	Correct	,,	,,	,,
R. hand to R. eye	,,	,,	,,	R. hand to R. *ear*; corrected	,,	R. hand to R. *ear*; corrected	,,	,,	,,
L. hand to R. ear	R. hand to R. ear	R. hand to R. ear	,,	Correct	,,	Correct	,,	,,	,,
R. hand to L. ear	Correct	Correct	,,	,,	,,	,,	,,	,,	,,
L. hand to L. eye	Reversed	,,	,,	,,	,,	,,	,,	,,	,,
R. hand to R. ear	Correct	,,	,,	,,	,,	,,	,,	,,	,,
R. hand to L. eye	L. hand to R. *ear*	,,	Reversed	,,	,,	,,	,,	,,	,,
L. hand to R. eye	Reversed	,,	Correct	,,	Correct (slow)	,,	,,	,,	,,
L. hand to L. ear	,,	,,	,,	,,	Correct	Correct (slow)	,,	,,	,,
R. hand to R. eye	,,	,,	,,	,,	,,	Correct	,,	,,	,,
L. hand to R. ear	,,	,,	,,	,,	,,	,,	,,	,,	,,
R. hand to L. ear	,,	,,	,,	,,	,,	,,	,,	,,	,,

Although the actual results were somewhat better, these records corresponded closely to those obtained two years before. He had regained some further power to imitate my movements and to perform pictorial commands; but he was still puzzled when they were reflected in the glass, and, although the actual errors were not numerous, his actions were slow and uncertain. He could, however, write down my movements without fail.

He continued to be worried and depressed, and in May, 1923, began to develop the idea that he ought not to take food. This reached such proportions that he was admitted to a hospital under the Pensions Ministry devoted to patients with mental disorders, where he still remains (1925). Throughout he was quiet, easily managed, and after the first few weeks took food on persuasion. He had no initiative and could not be employed successfully in the workshops. He still showed the same semantic defects even on superficial examination. Articulated speech was not affected and he understood what was said to him in conversation. He could carry out simple orders correctly, but was easily confused. He read the newspaper daily and could give a brief account both orally and in writing of any paragraphs that had interested him. He showed no signs of progressive dementia.

No. 11

A case of bullet wound in the left occipital region, which produced a gutter fracture 4 cm. in length running upwards and inwards, together with a smaller opening in the skull situated in and just to the right of the middle line of the scalp.

Central vision alone was preserved in the right eye, whereas the left showed right hemianopsia with maintenance of central vision for 10° to the right of the fixation point.

There were no other abnormal physical signs. But the patient occasionally suffered from attacks in which, though consciousness was fully preserved, he either "felt numb" down the right side or seemed to go suddenly blind.

He talked slowly, but articulation and syntax were not essentially affected and he could repeat all that was said to him, if the sentences were not long and complex. He showed considerable hesitation in naming common objects and, at the first examination, failed several times with colours. He read to himself with difficulty and made many mistakes when reading aloud. In neither case could he obtain a clear notion of the meaning of the passage he had read. He wrote with great effort and employed capitals and small letters indiscriminately. When writing the monosyllabic words of the man, cat and dog tests, he tended to reverse the order and to substitute one name for another. Writing to dictation and even copying print into cursive script were very defective. He could count slowly up to a hundred, but hesitated over the higher decades. Numbers stated categorically seemed to convey little to him and he failed to place a certain coin into a definite bowl to orders given by word of mouth or in print. Moreover, his answers were equally defective, whether the command was printed in figures or in words, showing it was the idea of number that was at fault. He failed to solve simple problems in arithmetic and had difficulty in stating the relative value of two coins, although he could build up the equivalent of any one of them from various pieces of money lying on the table before him. He was able to draw spontaneously, or from a model and from memory. But asked to draw an elephant, he produced a figure without its most characteristic features; these he named and added one by one in response to my question as to what he had omitted. He could not construct a ground-plan, tending to represent all the salient objects of my room in elevation. In spite of the gross lesion of the visual centres, he undoubtedly still possessed visual imagery and he showed no evidence of this form of agnosia. There was no general loss of orientation in space; he was liable to make mistakes, because he could not formulate to himself or to others the exact details of the route he should take. But he did not lose himself, for he recognised familiar landmarks, when they came into sight, and so guided himself to his ultimate destination correctly. He played draughts, but not card games and was easily confused by puzzles.

My first set of observations was made five months after he was wounded and I carried out a more complete examination eight and a half years later. On both occasions the records showed defects of essentially the same nature, consisting mainly of loss of capacity readily to select the symbol, which exactly fitted a situation, or to appreciate its full meaning when presented orally or in print.

Private William L., aged 38, a reservist of the Middlesex Regiment, was recalled to the Colours on the outbreak of war from his occupation as a merchant seaman.

He went to France in January 1915, and, on some unascertainable date in February, was struck by a rifle bullet in the occipital region. He could not remember being wounded, but had a clear recollection that he was in the trenches and that his officer gave him a cup of tea before he was removed to the field ambulance. Here he seems to have undergone some operation.

He arrived in England without notes of any kind and was admitted to the surgical side of the London Hospital on March 1st and was discharged on March 18th, 1915, with the wound healed. He returned from a convalescent home on May 20th and remained in the hospital until June 14th. During these early days of the war, a wound of the head was considered as an injury to the skull and little or no attention was paid to its neurological aspects. Thus, there are no records of any value with regard to the condition of this patient, when he was admitted for the first time. But owing to the unbounded energy and perspicacity of the late Dr E. G. Fearnsides, then acting as Medical Registrar, we possess a complete account of the physical state of this patient during his second sojourn in the surgical wards of the hospital. Anxious to give me the opportunity of investigating the speech defects of this patient, Dr Fearnsides admitted him for a further period from June 24th to July 10th.

Physical Condition between May 20th and 25th, 1915 (*about three months after the injury*).

The wound, which was now completely healed, consisted of a gutter fracture of the skull, 4 cm. in length, situated obliquely in the left occipital region. The track of the bullet was continued for a short distance superficial to the bone and then produced another smaller fracture extending from the middle line for about 1 cm. to the right.

The lower end of the left-sided fracture lay 4·5 cm. distant from the middle line, opposite a point about 29 cm. along the nasion-inion; the upper extremity of this opening in the bone was 1·5 cm. from the middle line and 25 cm. back from the nasion. The fracture in the middle line and to the right lay at about 24·5 cm. along the nasion-inion, which measured in all 35 cm. (Fig. 24).

He had suffered from no convulsions, giddiness, headache or vomiting.

He could count fingers with the right eye, but sight was reduced to central vision only. With the left eye vision was $\frac{6}{6}$ in spite of right hemianopsia. These fields were worked out on many occasions perimetrically and as the records differed little I prefer to give those obtained in June 1915 (vide p. 184).

The optic discs were normal.

The pupils responded to light, even over the blind area, and there was no hemianopic reaction, although it was somewhat more sluggish from the right than the left half of the field.

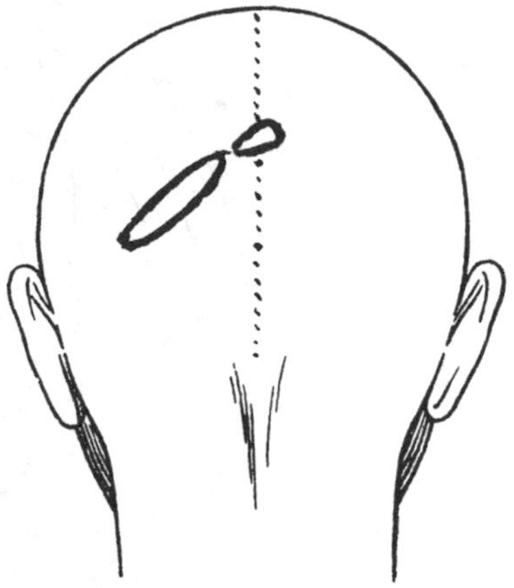

Fig. 24. To show the situation of the bullet wound in No. 11.

Hearing, smell and taste were unaffected.

Movements of eyes, face and tongue were perfect.

All the reflexes, superficial and deep, were normal.

There was no paralysis, paresis, incoordination or change in tone anywhere.

The patient complained that the right half of his body did not "feel the same" as the left, but no alteration could be discovered in sensibility. Vibration was recognised equally well on the two sides and localisation was not affected. The compass points were accurately discriminated at 0·75 cm. over the finger tips, and size, shape and weights were equally well appreciated on the two hands.

Condition in June and July, 1915 (*about five months after the injury*).

All the results obtained in conjunction with Dr Fearnsides were exactly confirmed and the condition of sight was again examined with especial care. With the right eye he could count fingers at about 30 cm.; with the left his vision was $\frac{6}{6}$ and Jäger 1.

Plotted with a 5 mm. white square, the field in the right eye was confined to an area 10° from the fixation point (Fig. 25). In the left eye there was definite right hemianopsia, which did not occupy central vision to the right of the middle line. Colour vision was maintained even over the restricted central field of the right eye.

The pupils certainly reacted to light from the blind areas of the retina.

Symbolic Formulation and Expression.

Mentally he was somewhat dull and, although fairly intelligent and attentive, he rarely volunteered any information. He complained mainly of lack of memory and the salient feature of his condition was inability to recall events which had happened even during his last stay in hospital. He could not remember dates or the names of people and places.

Articulated speech and understanding of spoken words. There was no gross abnormality in articulated speech; words were well pronounced on the whole and

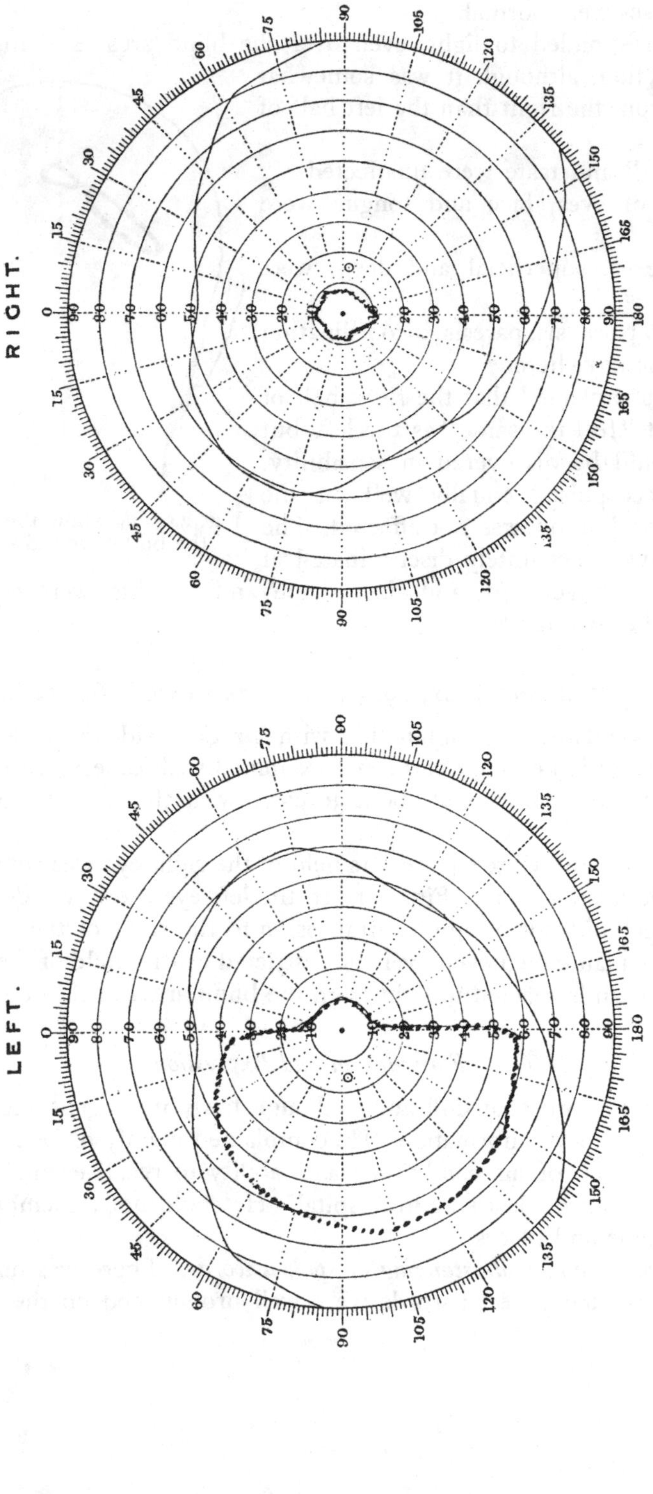

Fig. 25. To show the limitation of the fields of vision in No. 11 (June 1915).

syntax was not affected. He had considerable difficulty in naming colours and on two occasions failed to give any reply. He could repeat what was said to him correctly.

He was slow at understanding ordinary conversation and oral commands were executed hesitatingly and with occasional errors.

Reading. He failed to understand the meaning of a printed passage read silently and printed commands were badly performed. When he read aloud, the more difficult words were so badly deformed as to make nonsense, and there is little doubt that a similar want of appreciation confused him when he read to himself.

These defects were obvious, when the following passage, chosen by the patient from the daily paper, was employed to test his power of reading.

"Several kinds of bombs are dropped from Zeppelins. Some of them are explosive, causing a violent but local detonation. Another type, which is here illustrated, is known as an incendiary bomb. It readily fires buildings and their contents owing to the fierce nature of the flames and the molten metal generated by the chemicals used."

After reading this to himself he said, "Many kinds of Zeppelins...flying about, sir," and then ceased.

He read the passage aloud as follows: "Several kind of bombs are dropped from Zeppelins. Some of them are explosive causing a violent but lotical donation. Another type which is her illustrated is known as an indencery bomb. It readily fires buildings and their contents owing to fierce nature of flames by the molten... metal."

I then asked him to tell me what he had understood from the words he had just read. He replied simply, "Zeppelins flying over head dropping...bombs...on various places."

Q. "Tell me about Zeppelin bombs, what do they do?"

A. "They drop and explose...the force of them come to the ground...they go off, sir."

Q. "What do they do when they explode?"

A. "They spread out...kill people...make a hole in the ground."

Writing. He wrote his name and address correctly and produced the following short letter to me slowly and with much effort: "I write these few lines to you in hoping to find you in the Best of Health as I am the same at present. as I enjoy myself at the London Hospital as I am looking after some men who are ill as we Have good nurse to Look after us." To dictation this was almost exactly reproduced with its faults in punctuation and the use of capital letters.

When writing the simple phrases of the man, cat and dog tests from pictures or to dictation, he showed a tendency to reverse the order or to substitute one name for another.

He could not say the letters of the *alphabet* in order and, after four attempts, he finally reached T and then stopped puzzled. He wrote them spontaneously as follows, slowly and with considerable difficulty: *A B C D E F G H I J K L M N o p q R S T W X y Z.*

Arithmetic and the relative value of coins. He could count, but was unable to use numbers with ease; thus, he knew that three times eight was twenty-four, although he could give no answer when he was asked the question in the reversed form, "How many is eight times three?" He was very slow in solving simple problems in arithmetic and failed altogether with the last subtraction.

Addition.

215	258	258
323	433	963
538	691	12.21
Quick and accurate	Very slow	Very slow; he was greatly puzzled by the third column and hesitated long before writing 12

Subtraction.

234	652	631
122	438	456
112	214	7
Quick	Slow	Gave up, saying, "No, I can't"

All the coins were named correctly; he gave the following answers, when two of them were laid on the table and he was asked to state their relative value:

A halfpenny and sixpence—"Sixpence halfpenny."
A penny and half-a-crown—"Twenty-four."
A two-shilling piece and a pound—"Ten" (correct).
A half-crown and a pound—"Four, eight" (correct).
A sixpence and a pound—"Don't know."
A shilling and a pound—"Twenty" (correct).
A sixpence and a pound—"Forty" (correct).

Visual images. When in my room at the hospital, he could describe the various objects around his bed in the ward, indicating their position and colour with accuracy. He knew the difference between the uniform of a Sister and a Nurse. He said he could see the former clearly; "I see her...sitting down...a white thing...a white hood on her head...white things going down her back...blue dress."

He drew a good representation of a horse and of a cup and saucer spontaneously, but unfortunately his power of drawing to command was not fully recorded.

Orientation. He had no difficulty in finding his way about the wards or garden of the hospital, but was liable to be puzzled in the street "until I get the main roads."

Serial Tests.

At this time these tests were still in an experimental form and I should not have reported this case had not the records been elucidated and explained by the results obtained more than eight years and a half later.

(1) *Naming and recognition of colours.*

Table 1.

	Pointing to colour shown	Naming colour shown	Oral commands	Printed commands
Violet	Correct	"Don't know"	Red	Red
Yellow	,,	Correct	Correct	Correct
Black	,,	"Bl...black"	,,	,,
Red	,,	Correct	,,	,,
Blue	Violet	,,	Correct; very slow	,,
White	Correct	,,	Correct	,,
Orange	,,	"Red"	Yellow	Yellow
Green	,,	Correct	Correct	Correct
Violet	,,	"Don't know"	Red	Orange
Yellow	,,	Correct	Correct	Correct
Black	,,	,,	,,	,,
Red	Orange	,,	Orange; then correct	Orange
Blue	Correct	,,	Correct	Correct
White	,,	,,	,,	,,
Orange	,,	"Red"	Yellow	Yellow
Green	,,	Correct	Correct	Correct

He was in no sense colour-blind; but he had considerable difficulty in naming a colour shown to him and made a choice very slowly to oral or printed commands.

(2) *The man, cat and dog tests.*

Table 2.

	Reading aloud	Reading from pictures	Copying from print	Writing from dictation	Writing from pictures
The man and the dog	Correct	"The man and the cat"	Correct	Correct	Correct
The dog and the cat	,,	Correct	,,	The cat and the dog	The cat and the dog
The cat and the man	"The cat and the dog"	,,	The cat and the dog	Correct	Correct
The dog and the man	Correct	,,	Correct	The man and the dog	,,
The cat and the dog	,,	,,	,,	Correct	The cat and the man
The man and the cat	,,	"The man and the... dog"	,,	The man and the	Correct
The man and the dog	,,	Correct	,,	The dog and the man	,,
The dog and the cat	,,	,,	,,	The cat and d	The dog and the man
The cat and the man	,,	"The cat and the dog"	,,	The cat and the dog	The man and the cat
The dog and the man	"The dog and the cat and the man"	Correct	,,	Correct	Correct
The cat and the dog	Correct	,,	,,	The dog and the cat	,,
The man and the cat	"The man and the dog"	,,	,,	The dog and the cat	,,
The man and the dog	Correct	,,	,,		
The dog and the cat	,,	,,	,,		
The cat and the man	,,	"The...cat and the dog"	,,		
The dog and the man	,,	Correct	,,		
The cat and the dog	,,	,,	,,		
The man and the cat	,,	,,	,,		

He read these simple phrases aloud from print or from pictures, but showed a tendency to substitute one name for another. From pictures or to dictation, he wrote them poorly, although he copied them from print on the whole correctly in cursive script.

(3) *The hand, eye and ear tests.*

Table 3.

	Imitation of movements made by the observer	Imitation of movements reflected in a mirror	Pictorial commands	Pictorial commands reflected in a mirror	Oral commands	Printed commands	Pictorial commands translated into words
R. hand to L. ear	Correct	Correct	Reversed	Reversed	Correct	Reversed	Correct
L. hand to R. eye	Reversed	,,	Correct	Correct	,,	R. hand to L. *ear*	,,
R. hand to R. ear	Correct	Reversed	,,	,,	,,	R. hand to L. ear	,,
R. hand to L. eye	,,	,,	R. hand, then L. hand to R. eye	Reversed	R. hand to R. eye	Correct; doubtful	,,
L. hand to R. ear	Reversed	Correct	Reversed	Correct	Correct	Reversed	,,
R. hand to R. eye	Correct	,,	Correct	,,	,,	R. hand to L. eye	,,
L. hand to L. ear	,,	Reversed	,,	,,	L. hand to R. ear; corrected	L. hand to R. ear	,,
L. hand to L. eye	Reversed	,,	,,	Reversed	Correct	L. hand to R. eye	,,
R. hand to L. ear	Correct	Correct	Reversed	Correct	Correct; slow	Reversed	,,
L. hand to R. eye	Reversed	,,	Correct	Reversed	Correct	Correct	,,
R. hand to R. ear	Correct	,,	,,	,,	,,	R. hand to L. ear	,,
R. hand to L. eye	,,	,,	Reversed	,,	,,	Reversed	,,
L. hand to R. ear	Reversed	,,	Correct	Correct	L. hand to R. *eye*	,,	,,
R. hand to R. eye	Correct	,,	,,	,,	Correct	R. hand to L. eye	,,
L. hand to L. ear	Reversed	,,	,,	,,	,,	L. hand to R. ear	,,
L. hand to L. eye	,,	R. hand to L. eye	L. hand to L. *ear*; then correct	,,	L. hand to L. *ear*	L. hand to R. eye	,,
R. hand to L. ear	Correct	Correct	Reversed	Reversed	Correct	Reversed	,,
L. hand to R. eye	Reversed	,,	Correct	Correct	,,	,,	,,
R. hand to R. ear	Correct	,,	,,	Reversed	,,	R. hand to L. ear	,,
R. hand to L. eye	,,	Reversed	Reversed	,,	,,	Reversed	,,

When imitating my movements sitting face to face or executing pictorial commands, he showed a tendency to perform the reversed action. This fault was also present, to a less degree, if either my movements or the diagrams were reflected in a mirror; he was evidently puzzled by this simple form of the tests.

Both oral and printed commands were badly executed, but he was able to translate the pictorial cards into words without a single mistake.

Condition between January 18th and March 9th, 1924 (*nine years after the injury*).

I lost sight of this patient until the end of 1923, when he again came under my care and I was able to make a complete series of observations, which threw an interesting light on his previous condition.

The firmly healed wound in the occipital region was covered by tough tissues which did not pulsate; it was not tender. He complained of occasional sharp pains in the head which, starting in the left occipital region, passed over the vertex to the right half of the forehead. This throbbing and aching headache might come on two or three times in the day or even at night when he was in bed. It was not increased by stooping or jolting, as for instance on an omnibus. Reading or even mental and bodily fatigue did not induce the pain, although they increased it if it was present. It was not accompanied by nausea or vomiting.

He had suffered from no fits or epileptiform seizures of any kind. But he complained that he sometimes became weak down the right side; the hand seemed to drop and became "numb," whilst the power of the leg was diminished. Consciousness was in no way disturbed. These attacks usually lasted a few moments only, during which he ceased working and stood still; they might occur as often as three or four times a day.

Occasionally, but much more rarely, he suffered from another form of attack in which it seemed as if he lost his eyesight. "Everything went blank" before his eyes, but he did not lose consciousness. On one occasion he was in his own kitchen and could not see the objects on the wall.

He asserted that he could see "quite well," although he confessed that he frequently ran into obstacles as he walked; "I run into people in the street and if I stoop I hit my head." When the left eye was covered, he said his sight became "misty" and seemed "dazed," he was, however, ignorant of the extreme restriction of his visual field in the right eye.

Vision with the right eye was $\frac{6}{24}$, with the left $\frac{6}{9}$. The field in the right eye was reduced to central vision only and extended for 10° at most around the fixation point. With the left eye only there was right hemianopsia with retention of vision for a short distance around the fixation point to the right of the middle line (Fig. 26).

The discs and fundus were absolutely normal in both eyes.

The pupils reacted to light, even over the blind areas of the retina; there was no hemianopic reaction.

Hearing, smell and taste were unaffected.

All the movements of eyes, face and tongue were normal.

The reflexes, including the plantars and abdominals, were brisk and equal on the two sides.

There was no paralysis, paresis, tremor, alteration in tone or incoordination.

Sensibility was unaltered. He could recognise passive movements of 1° in all the fingers and in both great toes. The compass points were discriminated at 1 cm. on the palmar aspect of the digits and at 3 cm. over the soles of the feet. Localisation was not affected. He could appreciate the various tests for shape correctly, provided he was not asked to name them, and could select from the various geometrical objects on the table before him the one which corresponded to that he held in his hand out of sight.

Symbolic Formulation and Expression.

He was very quiet and unresponsive, neither volunteering an explanation of his mistakes nor garrulously attempting to correct them. Introspectively he was a poor subject of examination and, although willing and anxious to do well, he never asked

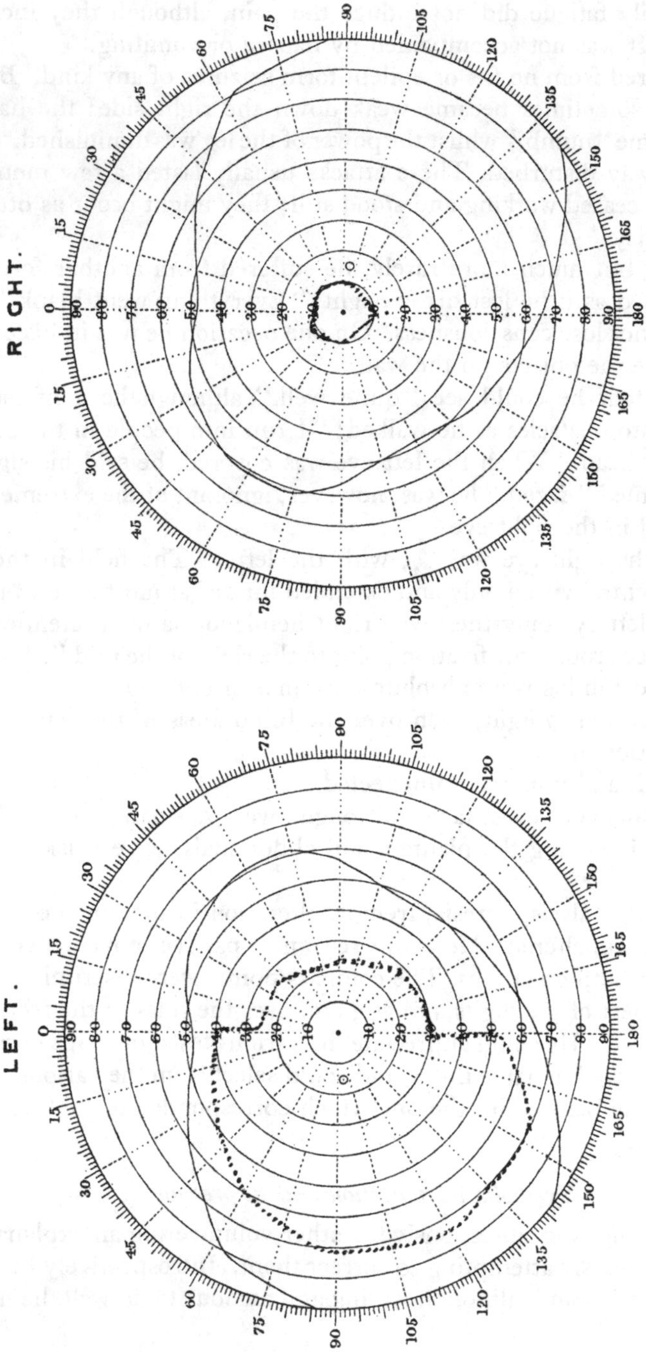

Fig. 26. To show the limitation of the fields of vision in No. 11 (March 1924).

if he was right or wrong. He was employed as a street sweeper under the Borough Council, and his chief disabilities were revealed by the following conversation:

Q. What difficulty do you find in your work?
A. Getting the question or answering.
Q. Give me an example?
A. When we are told to go anywhere or to get things.
Q. What happens?
A. I have to think; I get the wrong things.
Q. Have you difficulty in understanding orders?
A. Yes, I do wrong things.

Articulated speech. Words were correctly formed and intonation was not grossly affected. He complained, "I can't hardly get my words out...it's fetching them out...I can't hardly find the names." This difficulty in discovering exactly the word he required spoilt the freedom of his phrases, but syntax was not otherwise disturbed. He named common objects and colours accurately, though with some hesitation. He could repeat without fail any simple group of words said by me and articulation was perfect.

Understanding of spoken words. He chose familiar objects or colours and set the clock correctly to oral commands; but he failed grossly with the coin-bowl tests and made several mistakes in carrying out the movements of hand to eye or ear.

He was evidently puzzled by general conversation and particularly by any phrase that was either complex in meaning or full of details. When a short passage was read aloud to him, he was unable to retail its significance and complained that he "forgot" what it was about.

Reading. He selected common objects or colours and set the clock to printed commands without mistakes, though somewhat more slowly than when the same orders were given by word of mouth. He made many errors with the movements of hand to eye or ear and failed entirely to execute the coin-bowl tests, whether the command was printed in words or figures.

Handed a passage selected by himself and asked to read it silently, he was unable to give an account of what he had gathered from it. He had evident difficulty in recalling the details and complained, "It's difficult, I can't remember."

Although he could read aloud a series of consecutive sentences without mistakes, his power of reproducing their meaning was extremely poor. Moreover, reading a command aloud did not materially aid its correct execution. This was particularly evident with the coin-bowl tests; he read aloud every order correctly, whether in figures or words, but executed them wrongly.

Writing. He could write his name and address, but even the short letters he wrote to me contained gross errors and corrections. Writing was evidently difficult, his spelling defective and he interjected capitals irrelevantly. Thus he wrote: "Dear

Sir, I am sorry to say that I keen on (erased) Loseing myself and menory and weakness Down Right side and my Right Leg it seems to Drag

Im yours Truly

William L. . . ."

[Dear Sir, I am sorry to say that I keep on losing myself and memory and (have) weakness down (my) right side and my right leg seems to drag. I am, yours truly.]

On another occasion he wrote with great slowness in my presence, "as I wont to go ary where I am alway Behind and does not (illegible erasure) Relize I am late. or be in time." Asked to read this aloud he said, "When I want to go anywhere, I am always behind and does not realise I am late or be in time."

When writing the phrases of the man, cat and dog tests from pictures, he showed a tendency to forget the names or to reverse the order. He succeeded in executing this task to dictation without mistakes, provided I repeated the words more than once, and the short phrases were copied from print on the whole correctly.

As soon, however, as he was asked to communicate in writing what he had gathered from a printed paragraph, not only was the content gravely defective, but his writing and spelling deteriorated. The results were equally bad when the passage was dictated by me. If he was allowed to copy it, he succeeded somewhat better, although the words were badly formed and capitals and small letters were used indiscriminately. This was evidently due to want of ease in translating print into cursive script, for even when he copied the printed alphabet he committed the same fault; and yet, when given the alphabet in small cursive script, he reproduced it without any such lapses. His difficulty throughout lay in finding the form of symbol which exactly fitted the situation.

The alphabet. He said the letters spontaneously, repeated them after me and read them aloud without mistakes. Asked to write the alphabet, the order was correct, but he used capitals and small letters indiscriminately as follows: *𝒜 ℬ c d ℰ f g ℋ ℐ 𝒥 𝒦 l m n o 𝒫 q ℛ s t u v w x y z*. To dictation he wrote, *𝒜 ℬ c d e f g h ℐ 𝒥 𝒦 l m n o 𝒫 q ℛ s t u v w x y z*. I then gave him the alphabet in printed capitals, urging him to copy them in small cursive script; but he produced the following mixture, A B C D E *f g* H *ℐ 𝒥 𝒦 ℒ m n o* P *q* R *s t v u w x y z*. When, however, I gave him the letters in handwriting, he copied them exactly with great ease and rapidity; for this task demanded no translation of any kind. The twenty-six block letters were put together very slowly as follows: A B C D E F G H I J F (reversed); then he continued J K L M N O P Q R T U V W X Y Z. The S which had been omitted was finally inserted in its right position after much hesitation and uncertainty.

A printed paragraph. He selected as a test the following passage from Dickens:

"The gentleman spoken of had a very ugly squint and a prominent chin. He was wearing a tall white hat with a narrow flat brim and riding breeches with yellow leather gaiters. He carried in his hand a switch with which he tapped his boots, as he talked in a hoarse voice."

This he read silently and, when asked what he had understood, replied, "The gentleman spoken of... Can't remember any more... I read it, I can't remember it."

Again he read it through to himself and wrote as follows: "There was a gentleman was walking along had a Proimt chin and a Pair of Gatters Brim hat and a swish."

The whole passage was read aloud correctly, except for a slight error in the last sentence; he said, "a switch, with which he tapped his boots, as he walked along...as he walked in a hoarse voice."

To dictation he made many errors and I was compelled to repeat the words in short groups many times in succession, before he could place them on paper as follows: "the genleman spoken of. hand Very ugley and Proment Chin He was wearing a hat Brod Brim Rindig Brechis with yellow Gatters He carried in his hand a swich which He taf his Boots as he tack in a Horse Voice."

Asked to copy the passage in cursive script, he wrote "the genleman spoken of had a very ugly squint and a prominent chin he was wearing a tall white Had with a narrow flat Brim and Riging Breeches with yellow leather gatters He carried in His hand a swich witt whch he taf his Boots as He walk in a horse Voice."

Finally I requested him to tell me what he had gathered from the sentences he had read, written and copied. He replied, "There was a prominent gentleman... walking...which he had...squint...chin...and he wore...broad brim...hat... which...wore a pair of yellow gaiters...and...as he walked...he has a hoarse voice"; he added, "It's difficult, I can't remember."

Numbers and arithmetic. He counted up to a hundred without mistakes, but paused in doubt at the beginning of the decades 70, 80 and 90. He wrote down all these numbers correctly, except that he omitted 77 and 90 from the series and was compelled to rectify several errors in sequence.

The first two addition sums were worked out from left to right; this made no difference to the first answer, but profoundly affected the second. He therefore reversed the method with the third problem, although this answer was also given incorrectly. I could obtain no clue to the cause of the confusion over the third addition and third subtraction sums.

Addition.			Subtraction.		
432	564	486	854	562	624
343	328	245	412	238	256
775	8812 (wrong)	2621 (wrong)	442	234 (wrong)	2458 (wrong)

Coins and their relative value. All the coins were named correctly. He had, however, considerable difficulty in stating the relative value of any two of them placed before him.

	1st series	2nd series
A penny and a shilling	"thirteen times"	Correct
A sixpence and half-a-crown (2s. 6d.)	"twenty-eight"	,,
A sixpence and ten shillings	"thirteen"	,,
A penny and sixpence	"seven"	,,
A two-shilling piece and a pound note	"twenty-two"	,,
A shilling and a ten-shilling note	Correct	,,
A sixpence and a pound note	Correct (very slow)	"forty-six"
A penny and a two-shilling piece	Correct	"forty-eight"
A sixpence and a shilling	,,	Correct
A penny and half-a-crown (2s. 6d.)	"thirty-four"	"sixty-four"
A shilling and a pound note	Correct	Correct
A halfpenny and a sixpence	,,	,,
A sixpence and a two-shilling piece	,,	,,

The first mistake was obviously due to the common fault of adding the two coins together, instead of stating their relative value.

If a coin, or even a Treasury note of the value of ten shillings or a pound, was placed on the table, he could build up from a heap of loose money its exact equivalent. He knew its value, but was unable to formulate a relation with ease and certainty.

He complained of much difficulty with change in the monetary transactions of daily life. "When I'm sent for anything, I find afterwards I'm short; I can't get, at the moment, how much it is. I sent the girl last night to get some milk and sugar; I gave her two and six, she brought back a penny. I didn't realise that she was sixpence short until several hours afterwards."

Drawing. He made an excellent drawing of a spirit-lamp from a model and reproduced it correctly from memory, not only ten minutes, but even a week later.

On his own initiative he drew a horse and a rough representation of the house in which he lived.

But he made an incomplete drawing of an elephant to order. Asked if he had left out anything, he replied, "His ear," and made a mark on the side of the head. When I enquired, "Has an elephant got anything else?" he answered, "Trunk," "Eye," "Tail," "Toes," marking in each object in turn as he named it; but he forgot the tusks.

Plan. Asked to make a ground-plan of the room in which we habitually worked, he drew a series of objects, bookcase, table, couch and filing cabinet in elevation. When, however, I asked him to point to the position of these salient features on a plan sketched by me, he did so readily and without mistakes. I then handed him an identical outline sketch and, on this occasion, he was more successful in marking the situation of the prominent pieces of furniture; but he again tended to represent them in elevation, the door had a handle, the couch had four legs and the bookcase a projecting flap.

Images. There can be no doubt that he still possessed the power of visual imagery. A week after he had drawn the spirit-lamp from a model, I asked him what I had given him to draw; he replied, "A testing glass," and to my question, "Can you see it?" answered, "Yes, I see it in my mind." He then took the pencil in his hand and made a good representation of the lamp, showing the wick, neck and general shape correctly.

He insisted that, when attempting to draw a ground-plan, he saw my room and the objects he was trying to indicate. He added that he could see a picture of his wife and of the barrow he used when at work.

Orientation. He found his way about London alone and habitually came to my house unattended. He knew that he caught a No. 13 omnibus at London Bridge and alighted at the Marble Arch. But he could not state what turnings he would have to take to traverse the short distance to my house. He complained, "I often go wrong; difficult finding the turnings; I don't seem to remember where I am and which way to go; I know, when I see them; I know your house, when I see it." Thus he had no difficulty in recognising familiar landmarks, although he could not formulate them either to me or to himself with ease.

Games. He could play draughts, but not cards, and he failed with jigsaw puzzles; "I've tried, but I don't seem to get on with puzzles."

Serial Tests.

(1) *Naming and recognition of common objects*. He could name familiar objects slowly and make an accurate selection to oral or printed commands. When writing down the name, he made one mistake only, substituting "pencel" for penny, but there were several errors in spelling which may have been due to his somewhat defective education; thus pencil became "pencal," "pencel," and scissors, "sicers," "serries" and "securs." To dictation he wrote the whole series in an almost identical manner. His handwriting greatly improved when he copied from print, although he still found difficulty in spelling scissors and wrote "pinny" and "pencal" for penny and pencil.

(2) *Naming and recognition of colours*. All these tests were carried out correctly; but he was noticeably slower in naming or in selecting colours to printed commands than when the order was given by word of mouth. He wrote down their names somewhat laboriously though without gross errors in spelling.

(3) *The man, cat and dog tests*. He could read these simple phrases from print or in response to pictures and repeated the words after me without fail. If he wrote them from pictures, however, he made several mistakes, reversing the order of the two nouns or failing to complete the phrase. Even when copying the words from print, he showed some uncertainty and once wrote "the man and the cat" in place of the dog and the cat. To dictation every phrase was written correctly; for, after he had put down the first half, I reinforced his memory by saying the whole to him again.

(4) *The coin-bowl tests.*

Table 4.

	Oral commands	Printed commands (not read aloud)		Printed commands read aloud and executed			
				In figures		In full words	
		In figures (e.g. 2nd into 3rd)	In full words (e.g. Second penny into third bowl)	He said	Movements executed	He said	Movements executed
2nd into 3rd	Correct	3rd into 2nd	3rd into 2nd	Correctly	3rd into 2nd	Correctly	2nd, then 3rd into 1st
1st into 3rd	4th into 2nd	4th into 2nd	4th into 2nd	,,	4th into 2nd	,,	2nd into 1st
2nd into 1st	3rd into 4th	3rd into 4th	3rd into 4th	,,	3rd into 4th	,,	3rd into 4th
3rd into 2nd	2nd into 3rd	2nd into 3rd	2nd into 3rd	,,	2nd into 3rd	,,	2nd into 3rd
1st into 4th	4th into 1st	4th into 1st	4th into 1st	,,	4th into 1st	,,	4th into 1st
4th into 3rd	1st into 3rd	1st into 3rd	1st into 2nd	,,	1st into 3rd	,,	1st into 3rd
2nd into 4th	3rd into 1st	2nd, then 3rd into 1st	3rd into 1st	,,	3rd into 1st	,,	3rd into 1st
4th into 1st	1st into 4th	1st into 4th	1st into 4th	,,	1st into 4th	,,	1st into 4th
3rd into 1st	2nd into 4th	2nd into 4th	2nd into 4th	,,	2nd into 3rd	,,	2nd into 4th
1st into 2nd	4th into 3rd	4th into 3rd	4th into 2nd	,,	4th into 3rd	,,	4th into 3rd
3rd into 4th	2nd into 1st	2nd into 1st	2nd into 1st	,,	2nd into 1st	,,	2nd into 1st
4th into 2nd	1st into 4th	1st into 3rd	1st into 3rd	,,	1st into 3rd	,,	1st into 3rd

This was a remarkable series of observations, for he seemed to experience greater difficulty than with any other set of tests. He was completely unable to execute oral or printed commands and it seemed to make little or no difference whether the order was expressed in figures or in words. Although he read the printed commands aloud correctly, this did not increase the number of times he made an accurate choice of coin or bowl.

The same sort of mistakes recurred time after time and he was particularly liable to be misled by fixing his mind on one number and guessing the other one. Frequently it was impossible to discover why he pitched on either of them. Asked what was his difficulty, he replied, "It seems to be the thinking or the memory," and he added, "I seem to have to think first before doing anything."

(5) *The clock tests.* All these tasks could be performed and he wrote down the time on the whole correctly though slowly. Writing and spelling were, however, somewhat defective and he substituted "20 minutes to 2" for 5 minutes to 2. He complained throughout that when writing he found difficulty in "getting the letters."

(6) *The hand, eye and ear tests.*

Except that there were somewhat fewer mistakes, these records, taken nine years after the injury, were identical in character with those of an earlier period; but he now made no errors when my movements or the pictorial commands were reflected in a mirror. This showed that his powers of reasonable deduction had distinctly improved.

He imitated my movements poorly, when we sat face to face, and failed to execute orders given in the form of pictures. Oral and printed commands were also executed slowly and imperfectly.

Yet he could write down my movements and he translated them correctly into spoken words. But throughout these tests he watched my actions intently and wrote down the first half of the phrase; then he looked at me again and determined the eye or ear to which I had approximated my finger. In this way he simplified the task by dividing it into two separate portions.

Table 5.

	Imitation of movements made by the observer	Imitation of movements reflected in a mirror	Pictorial commands	Pictorial commands reflected in a mirror	Oral commands	Printed commands	Writing down movements made by the observer	Movements of the observer translated into words
L. hand to L. eye	Correct	Correct	Reversed	Correct	Correct	L. hand to L. *ear*	Correct	Correct
R. hand to R. ear	,,	,,	Correct	,,	R. hand to L. ear	Correct	,,	,,
R. hand to L. eye	Reversed	,,	Reversed	,,	Correct	,,	,,	,,
L. hand to R. eye	Correct	,,	Correct	,,	,,	R. hand to R. eye	,,	,,
L. hand to L. ear	,,	,,	Reversed	,,	,,	Correct	,,	,,
R. hand to R. eye	Reversed	,,	Correct	,,	R. hand to L. eye	R. hand to R. *ear*	,,	,,
L. hand to R. ear	Correct	,,	,,	,,	Correct	Correct	,,	,,
R. hand to L. ear	Reversed	,,	,,	,,	,,	,,	,,	,,
L. hand to L. eye	L. hand to R. eye	,,	Reversed	,,	,,	,,	,,	,,
R. hand to R. ear	Reversed	,,	,,	,,	R. hand to L. ear	,,	,,	,,
R. hand to L. eye	,,	,,	Correct	,,	Correct	,,	,,	,,
L. hand to R. eye	Correct	,,	,,	,,	,,	,,	,,	,,
L. hand to L. ear	,,	,,	,,	,,	,,	,,	,,	,,
R. hand to R. eye	,,	,,	,,	,,	,,	,,	R. hand to eye	,,
L. hand to R. ear	,,	,,	,,	,,	,,	,,	Correct	,,
R. hand to L. ear	,,	,,	,,	,,	,,	,,	,,	,,

No. 13

A case of Syntactical Aphasia due to injury of the left temporal lobe by a shell fragment. The skull had been perforated at a spot lying over the upper portion of the first temporal gyrus and the sylvian fissure, on a level vertically with the foot of the post-central fissure. Bone had also been removed by trephining over an area just behind the central fissure.

There was slight loss of power and incoordination in the right hand associated with distinct loss of sensibility; this subsequently passed away entirely. The lower extremity was unaffected and the reflexes were normal.

He talked rapidly; the rhythm of speech was disturbed and syntax was defective whether the words were spoken or read aloud. If hurried he tended to lapse into jargon. He could name objects correctly and repeat all that was said to him. Comprehension of spoken words was unaffected and he could execute oral and printed commands. But he was liable to forget what he had been told or had read silently, if he attempted to say the phrases over to himself in order to remember them. He could write a good letter spontaneously, but made many mistakes if he attempted to put down what he had read or when writing to dictation. Numerals were badly pronounced and arithmetic was defective.

Four and a half years later his condition had improved somewhat, but the form assumed by the loss of speech was identical with that revealed by the earlier observations.

Rifleman William R., aged 19, was wounded on May 20th, 1917, the first day he was in the front-line trenches. A shell burst close to him and blew him into the air; at the same time he was struck by a fragment in the left temporal region. He did not become unconscious, but picked himself up and ran back, unable to speak a word or to understand what was said to him. He told me he suffered from "tremendous pain" in his head, and added, "I went man (mad), kept running, all the time. Did not know where I was going. When I got to dressing station I dropped, was very sick, could not stand any more, fell down."

He arrived in England with no notes of any kind; but he appeared to have been trephined at the casualty clearing station, where he remained for about three weeks, before he was admitted to the London Hospital under my care on June 21st, 1917.

There was a long surgical scar extending from the fronto-temporal to the parietal region on the left side of the head. In the course of this incision were two granulating areas of small size, of which the anterior seemed to be superficial and due to the operation; it healed rapidly. Posterior to this lay a pouting sinus level with a point 16 cm. along the nasion-inion line, and 8 to 9 cm. from the middle of the scalp; this led down to the surface of the brain within the trephined area. Exactly below it, 11 cm. from the middle line, was another small fungating sinus passing down to and apparently penetrating the bone, from which exuded a considerable quantity of pus. It undoubtedly represented one of the original wounds (Fig. 8, Vol. 1, p. 449).

The total nasion-inion measurement was 34 cm., and this was transected by the interaural line at a point 14·5 cm. along its course.

From all these wounds cultures of staphylococcus albus were obtained, pure and in abundance. They healed completely by July 16th under suitable antiseptic treatment.

An X-ray photograph showed that bone had been removed over an irregular area, 6 cm. in length and 4 cm. vertically, which was bisected by the surgical incision. This included the site of the posterior sinus, but not that of the opening above the insertion of the ear, which was certainly one of the original wounds. It looked as if the operation had been performed to expose Broca's area because of the preponderating affection of speech.

On admission to the London Hospital he was in excellent condition mentally; his memory was good and, in spite of his defective speech, I succeeded in obtaining from him a history of his injuries and subsequent treatment.

His speech was a jargon closely resembling that of a child, who is fluent, but has not learnt to form its phrases or articulate clearly. He could find the names for common objects and understood what was said to him.

He suffered from no headache, vomiting or seizures of any kind. The pupils reacted well, eye movements were normal and the optic discs showed no changes. The lower half of the face on the right side was distinctly weak and the tongue tended to deviate somewhat to the right on protrusion. All the reflexes were normal, including those from the sole of the foot and from the abdomen. The right hand showed some loss of sensation, but no motor paralysis, whilst the lower extremity was completely unaffected.

Condition between July 6th and 27th, 1917 (*seven to ten weeks after he was wounded*).

He was an intelligent young man who, at fourteen years of age, had reached the highest standard in an elementary school and had subsequently become a clerk in an insurance office. He was bright, willing and good tempered; but, when his speech was unintelligible and he saw he could not make himself understood, he flushed and became confused.

He had always thrown a ball and played cricket right-handed.

Symbolic Formulation and Expression.

Articulated speech. He talked with considerable rapidity, but slurred the words and tended to omit articles, conjunctions and prepositions. Frequently his pronunciation approximated to that of a baby who is learning to speak.

When giving the history of his injury he said, "He ās (asked) me 'Could I walk down there.' Couldn't speat (speak). Started pitting (picking) 'em up, pitting up. I did like zis (this)", moving his left hand backwards and forwards horizontally to indicate that he did not know where to go or what to do. Asked where they took him from the first aid post he replied, "Nozzer dressin stashn. Took me nozzer hoshl. She, she, ess, they call it. Op-rashn there." (To another dressing station. They took me to another hospital. C.C.S., they call it. Operation there.)

He described the condition of his right hand as "Tiff-rent from uffer 'n. Kā tell ooh, know zis 'un seems strong" (different from the other one; I can't tell you, I know this one seems strong). In the same way he said that contact with the test-hairs "tittles" (tickles).

His attempt to reproduce for my benefit what he had gathered from a picture and its printed legend afforded another excellent example of the character of his spontaneous utterance. The internal structure of the words was deformed, the balance of the phrase disturbed and its syntax defective.

These defects of pronunciation and syntax sometimes became so gross that he seemed to be talking jargon. If, however, he was made to talk slowly and to break up his answers into short phrases, words emerged used correctly and with a definite meaning; and yet, from the inaccurate pronunciation and hurry of his speech, he might seem to be talking incomprehensible nonsense.

The rhythmic beat of his phrases and polysyllabic words was faulty; he could not "touch off" the sounds correctly so as to produce a coherent sequence of properly articulated words or syllables.

He repeated the simple words and phrases of the man, cat and dog tests correctly and his pronunciation was much better than when he said the same words spontaneously in response to pictures. But with longer and more complex sentences he tended to become confused and to lapse into jargon.

The months were given in the correct order and without hesitation; but the words were badly pronounced and the sounds he uttered could be represented somewhat as follows: "Jan-wy," "Feb-wy," "Marse"; April, May and June perfectly articulated; then "Uly," "Augst," "Sep-pembr"; October and November as usual, ending with "Ze-zember."

He was perfectly familiar with the names of common objects and had no difficulty in finding isolated words; but his mispronunciation of the less usual ones, especially if they formed part of a phrase, rendered them unintelligible without a knowledge of the context. I pointed to a white scar on his scalp and he answered "Aevus ah a baby" (Naevus as a baby). Thus he was able to find the name and form the essential part of the word rapidly and with certainty, although it would have conveyed no meaning to anyone unfamiliar with the origin of the scar.

The names he gave to geometrical figures formed an excellent example of how his power of finding the right word was vitiated by difficulties of pronunciation. A sphere was called "Wound" (round), a pyramid "Joy-angle" (triangle), a cylinder "Ope-long" (oblong), a cone "Pyr-mid" (pyramid); cube and ovoid were respectively "square" and "oval." Every name corresponded in some obvious way with the shape of the object, though pronunciation of all but the simplest words was faulty.

Exactly similar defects appeared when he attempted to name the colours; the internal balance of the words was disturbed, especially with those of more than one syllable.

Understanding of spoken words. He understood spoken words and chose a common object or a colour correctly when asked to do so. He set the clock and carried out even the complex hand, eye and ear tests without fail to oral commands.

Reading. There is no doubt that he understood what he read to himself and he could execute printed commands perfectly.

But it is impossible to give an exact reproduction of the sounds he emitted when he attempted to read aloud. The words of any one group or phrase were said with extreme rapidity and were shortened so that they could be hurried into a single breath-pause. Each sentence was said "in one breath"; then after a momentary stoppage, he dashed off again. It was always possible, with the original before you, to recognise the words he was saying; but many of them approached so closely to jargon, that it would have been impossible to do so without the key.

He was asked to read the following printed paragraph aloud, "Blackpool, which was the first town to employ women tramway-car drivers, finds that they are more careful than the men. Thus here we see a woman at the wheel while a man is acting as conductor." This became as nearly as the sounds could be reproduced, "Back-ool which was first noun, town, to employ women frame maine cart drivers fries zat zey are more careful than the men. Sis here we see a woo-mer at the wheel while a man is acting conductor." Told to read the title at the head of the picture, to which this paragraph served as a legend, he said, "Mins bixet oer men" (woman's victory over man).

I then asked him what he had gathered from the sentences he had just read aloud. He replied, "Fane made cars in Bakl. They had boo-men for rīvers and they say more better than the men. The men are actin as conductors."

I enquired what he thought about it and he answered, "They may be bettn barring central nerves. Say for instance they wun over somebody, they would go mad." This was evidently intended for, "They may be better barring their nerves. Say for instance they ran over somebody, they would go mad."

He then indicated the various points in the picture, saying, "Here's lay (lady), here handle, the man condukr (conductor), on the nines (lines), shot steats (it's got seats) on it, zee (three) passengers, two man, lady."

He composed an excellent letter but when he attempted to read aloud what he had written much of his utterance was jargon (vide infra).

Writing. He could write his name and address correctly and composed the following well written letter to his mother. "Dear Mother, just a few lines to let you know I have been wounded in the head but I am glad to say it is going on alright,

I want you to come and see (me) as soon as you can. I am in the London Hospital so it will be quite easy to come. Will close now, From your loving son."

When I asked him to read aloud what he had just written, many of the words were badly articulated and the phrasing was faulty. Owing to the rapidity with which he spoke, his pronunciation was extremely difficult to reproduce with any approach to accuracy. But he read this letter, of his own composition, somewhat as follows: "Bear Mother, Tus a su lines to let you know I have been wounded in the head ber 'm to tay it is dowing on ăl right. I want you to come and see me as soon as er tan. I em in London Topl so it will be quite easy to come. I'll ose now, from your loving son."

He wrote down the names of common objects and of colours accurately. Shown the time on a clock face, he transcribed it correctly, but omitted the word "minutes" as unnecessary to convey his meaning.

In the same way when writing from pictures he left out the conjunction and the articles; thus, the man and the cat became "man cat." Moreover, he reversed the order, reading from right to left instead of in the normal direction; after half this series was completed, I pointed out that we usually read from left to right and he then completed the remaining six tests in the right manner.

He wrote extremely badly to dictation, reproducing the same sort of errors that were so evident in speaking. But he copied even long phrases and paragraphs perfectly.

The Alphabet. Told to say the alphabet he made no mistakes over the first seven letters, but continued: "Ash" (H), "Eh" (I), "Deh" (J), "K L M O M P Q U R S Y Z." The omission of the letters after S seemed to be due to the close approximation of the sound "Esk" he made for S to that of X. Such errors were not fortuitous, for they were repeated exactly on another occasion a week later and also appeared in the written alphabet.

When he read the printed letters aloud, his pronunciation improved; H became "Ash," but the remainder were correctly articulated, and S and X were clearly differentiated.

Asked to write the alphabet silently, he made no mistakes until he came to L; then he continued as follows: *n o m p q r x y z*. Here again he was misled by the similarity of S and X into omitting all the intervening letters.

He copied from print in cursive handwriting perfectly and without omissions.

Interpretation of a picture and its explanatory legend in speech and writing. He selected from the daily paper a picture showing a collecting box for flowers placed on one of the suburban railway platforms. Underneath was the legend, "This box has been placed on the platform at Snaresbrook Station as a receptacle for flowers for the wounded. Many of the passengers contribute nosegays daily from their gardens and these are forwarded without delay to the Bethnal Green Infirmary." As a Londoner in an East End hospital this interested him greatly.

Asked to put down on paper what he had gathered from his reading and from the picture, he wrote, "At Sanbrook Station they have large box which are collicting flowers for the wounded soldiers and they are sending to the Belnah Green Hospital."

I then dictated the printed description with the following result: "This box has been placed on the platform a smatbrook station as sesful for the wounded many of the passengers contic nonsgay from there garndens and these without delay to the Belneth Green infirary." Yet he was able to copy these printed sentences without fault or omission and the words were remarkably well written.

Given the paper and asked to read it aloud he produced the following jargon: "Zis box had been place on the plakform at Senbrook Station as a...for flowers for the wounded...Many ob le pasn-gers contribute nosezays from their gardens and these are for-boarded without delay to Besnal Green Internary."

Shown the picture again, he pointed out all the various significant objects, giving them recognisable names, "Box, flowers for wounded soldiers. On the back plakform, Senfbrook. Ladies, see, putting flowers into box."

He evidently understood the significance both of the printed legend and of the picture, but he could not reproduce his conception in coherent words or in writing, although he copied correctly.

Numbers. He counted freely up to a hundred and showed none of that hesitation in finding the correct word, seen in some other forms of aphasia. The numerical order was accurate and the name he gave to each number corresponded recognisably to its proper designation; but many were badly pronounced.

Three became "free," but otherwise his articulation was fairly correct up to fourteen. Then he counted "hifteen, sick-teen, seventeen, eighteen, ni-teen, twenty." But when he had to combine twenty with some simple numeral, he said, "henty-one, henty-two, henty-free, tenty-four, penty-fi, twenty-six, twenty-seven, twenty-eight, penty-nine." Thirty was sometimes pronounced correctly, at others it became "sirty"; in the same way fifty was "pissy, pifty or pisby." The remaining decades were "sickty, sempy, eighty, ninety, hundred."

One of the most striking features of his counting was the irregularity of his utterances; sometimes the word was accurate, at others it was badly articulated, although invariably recognisable.

Arithmetic. Unfortunately, although he had reached the highest standard at the primary school, he had never cared for arithmetic. He said, "No good, arithmetic at all. I no good at all that at tool" (school).

Addition.			Subtraction.		
243	268	389	876	652	823
325	424	265	243	328	365
568	692	654	4		

He gave no answer to the three subtraction sums.

Coins and their relative value. The names of the various coins were badly pronounced, but were obviously accurate. A two-shilling piece was called "two shins" and two-and-six, or half-a-crown, "two er six, half town."

In the same way he could express the simpler relations, but had difficulty when he was compelled to employ higher numbers.

Sixpence and shilling—"Two."
Penny and sixpence—"Six."
Penny and shilling—"Chelf" (twelve).
Sixpence and half-a-crown—"Wife" or "foif" (five).
Sixpence and two shillings—"Four."
Halfpenny and sixpence—Shook his head, flushed and gave no answer.
Halfpenny and penny—"Two."
Halfpenny and shilling—Shook his head, flushed and gave no answer.

(This series was repeated twice over with the same result.)

He had no difficulty with change, provided he was not compelled to express himself in words.

Drawing. He said that he had never been a good draftsman; but he drew a fairly accurate outline of an object put before him and reproduced it from memory later.

An elephant drawn to command showed all the salient points in this animal. He named them one after the other as follows, "Eye, ear, tusts (tusks), tump (trunk), front les (legs), hine les (hind legs), tail."

Plan. Asked to construct a ground-plan of that part of the ward which contained his bed, he evidently failed to understand what I required. But, when I drew an oblong in the centre of a sheet of paper to represent his bed with his figure on it, he placed around it the various objects in their correct relative position. When he had outlined the next bed with his neighbour lying on it, I asked, "Where is he wounded?" He replied, "In the knee that affek-ed his pook" (in the knee; that affected his foot).

He described from memory the position of his bed, the locker with two doors, the colour of the curtains and all about the other patient. He was evidently a visualiser, but was not ready with his pencil.

Games. He placed the dominoes in order, number to number correctly with the doubles at right angles in the usual way. He found no difficulty with simple card games, so long as they did not demand the calling of numbers.

Serial Tests.

(1) *Naming and recognition of common objects.* He experienced no difficulty in selecting an object he had seen or held in his hand out of sight. He could name the whole series correctly and obeyed oral and written commands. He wrote all the names accurately except scissors, which he spelt "siccios."

(2) *Naming and recognition of colours.*

Table 1.

	Pointing to colour shown	Oral commands	Printed commands	Naming	Writing name of colour	Printed commands read aloud and colour chosen	
						He said	He chose
Black	Correct	Correct	Correct	Correct	Perfect	"Back"	Correctly
Red	"	"	"	"	"	"Rate"	"
Orange	"	"	"	"Ŏn-ache"	"	"Ŏn-age"	"
White	"	"	"	Correcr	"	"White"	"
Green	"	"	"	"Be-leen, ge-leen"	"	"Green"	"
Violet	"	"	"	"Wider"	"	"Viodet"	"
Blue	"	"	"	Correct	"	"Blue"	"
Yellow	"	"	"	"	"	"Yellow"	"
Black	"	"	"	"Back"	"	"Black"	"
Red	"	"	"	Correct	"	"Red"	"
Orange	"	"	"	"Ō-nez"	"	"Ŏn-age"	"
White	"	"	"	Correct	"	"White"	"
Green	"	"	"	"	"	"Green"	"
Violet	"	"	"	"Wi-let"	"	"Viodet"	"
Blue	"	"	"	Correct	"	"Blue"	"
Yellow	"	"	"	"	"	"Yellow"	"

He indicated the colour shown to him and executed with ease oral and printed commands. But, when asked to read the names aloud, his pronunciation was defective, although he chose the right colour without hesitation. The sounds he emitted bore an obvious relation, not only to the correct nomenclature, but also to the true verbal form of the colour-name he was seeking; but the internal balance of the words was defective. The longer ones were on the whole less perfectly pronounced than those of one syllable. When he attempted to name the colours, his speech showed exactly the same defects; orange for instance was called "ŏn-ache" or "ō-nez," and violet "wider" or "wi-let."

(3) ***The man, cat and dog tests.*** As far as the actual content of these tests was concerned, he carried out accurately the task of reading aloud, converting pictures into spoken or written words, writing to dictation, copying print or repeating words said by me. But his answers were very irregular in form and showed two characteristic faults. He tended to omit the article and conjunction, even when reading aloud, repeating words said by me, or writing to dictation; and, if asked to translate pictures into spoken or written words, he reversed the usual order, reading from right to left.

Pictures shown	*He said*	*He wrote*
Man and cat	"Cat and man"	Cat man
Dog and man	"Man and dog"	Man dog
Cat and dog	"Dog and cat"	Dog cat
Cat and man	"Man cat"	Man cat
Man and dog	"Dog and man"	Dog man
Dog and cat	"Cat dog"	Cat dog

Pictures shown	*He said*	*He wrote*
Cat and man	"Man tat"	Cat man
Man and dog	"Dog ă man"	Man dog
Dog and cat	"Cat dog"	Dog cat
Man and cat	"Cat man"	Man cat
Dog and man	"Man god"	Dog man
Cat and dog	"Dog cat"	Cat dog

At the point marked by a line in the second and third columns, I told him that we usually read from left to right and not in the opposite direction; but this led to no result. After he had written the first six tests of the next series again in the reverse order, I repeated the same remark and this time he corrected his manner of reproducing the pictures. None of these faults were evident, when he transcribed print into cursive handwriting; in such circumstances he copied exactly the words before him.

(4) *The clock tests.* He set one clock in imitation of another and carried out oral commands well. Orders given in print were less perfectly executed; he made two mistakes, in both instances setting ten minutes to the hour instead of ten minutes past. When he attempted to tell the time, each phrase was pronounced with great rapidity and some of the words were slurred; thus, he spoke of "Five minutes pass eight," "Spinther pass eleven" (twenty minutes past eleven). But the words always bore a definite resemblance to the correct nomenclature. He wrote down the time directly from the clock face without an error, omitting in every case the word "minutes."

(5) *The hand, eye and ear tests.*

Table 2.

	Imitation of movements made by the observer	Imitation of movements reflected in a mirror	Pictorial commands	Pictorial commands reflected in a mirror	Oral commands	Printed commands	Printed commands read aloud and executed	
							He said	Movements executed
L. hand to R. eye	L. hand to L. eye	Correct	L. hand to L. eye	Correct	Correct	Correct	"Less hand to right eye"	Correct
R. hand to R. ear	Reversed	,,	Reversed	,,	,,	,,	"Right hands and right ear"	,,
R. hand to L. eye	,,	,,	,,	,,	,,	,,	"Right hands and left eye"	,,
L. hand to R. ear	,,	,,	Correct	,,	,,	,,	"Left hand and right ear"	,,
L. hand to L. eye	,,	,,	L. hand to R. *ear*	,,	,,	,,	Correctly	,,
L. hand to L. ear	,,	,,	Reversed	,,	,,	,,	"Left hand and left ear"	,,
R. hand to L. ear	,,	,,	,,	,,	,,	,,	Correctly	,,
R. hand to R. eye	,,	,,	R. hand to L. eye	,,	,,	,,	"Right hands to right eye"	,,

When he attempted to imitate my movements, sitting face to face, he was wrong every time; his mistakes consisted in direct reversal of right and left in all but the first of the series. He was equally incorrect but less constant in the form of his errors to pictorial command. If, however, either my movements or the pictures were reflected in a mirror, the orders were carried out perfectly and without hesitation. He had no difficulty in executing commands given orally or in print, although he read them aloud badly.

Physical Examination.

So long as he remained quietly in bed he suffered from no headache; but, when he walked or stooped, the trephined area began to pulsate and he suffered from pain in the left half of the head. This was not associated with nausea or vomiting and subsided shortly after he lay down. He had not suffered from fits or any other form of seizure.

He had always been a little short-sighted and his vision was $\frac{6}{12}$ in both eyes. The visual fields were normal. A watch was heard at three inches (8 cm.) in both ears and there was nothing to show that his hearing had been materially affected in consequence of his wound.

The pupils reacted normally, all ocular movements were carried out well and there was no nystagmus. The right angle of the mouth was distinctly weaker and moved less perfectly than the left, and the tongue tended to deviate slightly to the right on protrusion.

All the reflexes were normal and equally brisk on the two sides, including those from the abdomen and sole of the foot.

No loss of power was discovered anywhere, except in the right upper extremity. He could carry out isolated movements of the fingers, but the grasp of the right hand was 15 kg., compared with 42 kg. from the left. When he held out both hands in front of him, the digits on the right side were not in complete alinement and tended to fall away on closing his eyes. They were, moreover, somewhat hypotonic. All movements of the elbow and shoulder were executed strongly against resistance and the tone of the muscles, apart from those of the hand, was not materially affected. There was no incoordination or ataxy of the limb as a whole; but on closing the eyes he brought the right forefinger into contact with the nose more clumsily than the left.

That these disorders were of afferent origin was borne out by sensory measurements. The power of appreciating posture and passive movement was definitely affected in the digits of the right hand, for he did not reply to any change of less amplitude than 10°; on the left side, to 2° only, he responded correctly "Ford" or "Back." Elbow and shoulder appeared to be unaffected. Discrimination of two points and localisation of the spot touched did not differ materially on the two hands and weights were correctly appreciated. To measured tactile stimuli there was no considerable difference between the two hands; but he complained that over the palmar aspect of the digits of the right hand "I seems heavier, it goes round and round; on the other (left) it's alright, it tittles" (tickles). The threshold to pricking was equal on the two sides.

CONDITION IN MARCH 1922 (*four years and ten months after he was wounded*).

On his discharge from the Army in November, 1917, he returned to the insurance office where he had been a clerk before the war. But he was no longer capable of carrying out the whole of the work on account of his verbal defects. He said, "Speech at times very bad. I have a job in getting out what I want to say. When I get excited, I can't say a word, when I go to take a message."

The scar of the wound was deeply depressed, firmly healed, and the orifice in the skull was covered with tough tissues; it did not pulsate unless he stooped and then to a slight degree only.

He occasionally suffered from headache, chiefly at the back of the head on both sides, throbbing in character. It might come on at any time of the day or even the night and, if once induced, lasted three or four days. It was associated with tenderness of the scalp in the occipital region. Stooping increased the pain and it was eased by lying down. It did not seem to be induced by jolting, as for instance when riding on a motor omnibus, but came on in the Underground Railway as a kind of "swirling feeling as if my head was going round and round." Reading might bring on the headache, but the most potent cause was the feeling of bored depression he described as "being fed up."

At no time had he suffered from fits or other attacks of an epileptiform nature.

He was slightly myopic and vision was $\frac{6}{18}$ with either eye. The visual fields were unaffected. The discs were absolutely normal.

The pupils reacted well and movements of the eyes, face and tongue were perfect.

The reflexes, even the plantars and abdominals, were unaffected.

There was no paralysis, paresis, incoordination, tremor or defect of tone.

Sensibility was unchanged even to the most elaborate tests. Posture and passive movement were appreciated equally well on the two sides, the compass points were distinguished on the fingers and palm at a distance of 1 cm. from one another, localisation was perfect, and size, shape and weight were equally well recognised on either hand.

Symbolic Formulation and Expression.

Provided the examination was carefully conducted so as not to arouse feelings of anger or disgust, he was a trustworthy and willing witness. But, if he became conscious that he was answering badly, his face would flush and he ceased to attempt to reply to the task set him, saying, "When I keep to the same thing I seem to get fed up" (bored). I had to be careful not to evoke this state of mind, in which it was impossible to continue the examination.

Articulated speech. He talked with great rapidity, rushing his phrases as if he must hurry in order to express what he wanted to say. Single words were well pronounced as a rule, but those of more than one syllable tended to be shortened or slurred. His speech was jerky and the rhythm was defective because of the omission of connecting words. Some phrases were run off glibly as a whole; others were shortened so as to be uttered in one breath, and he explained that if he could not say a sentence "all at once," he was unable to "get it out at all." Conversely, on several occasions, when he had answered correctly and with ease, he said, "simply come automatically; quite simple."

When he had mispronounced a word, he did not go back and try again, but dashed on in the hope that he would be understood. If checked and asked to repeat what he had said, he usually became confused and blushed; he intensely disliked being pulled up. The more he was pinned down to making his meaning clear the more confused he became and the closer his speech approximated to jargon. He explained that it was "Like when I go into one of the man-gers (managers of the insurance company). If I look at 'em, stand there, say nothing, like mesmerised. If I don't look at 'em, I can speak fairly well to 'em." Moreover, he said that, when he was sent on a message, he could deliver it all right if he did not think about it. But if he said it to himself silently as he went along the passage of the office he could not deliver it clearly.

He never had a moment's hesitation over names apart from their verbal structure; nor did he ever use wrong words.

He could repeat everything said to him, even the more difficult polysyllabic words which occurred in the paragraph employed as a test on p. 210.

Understanding of spoken words. Not only was his phrasal utterance defective, but his phrasal memory was transitory. If he did not repeat the words to himself at once, he forgot what he had been told; he complained that he did not hold it long enough. On the whole, however, he understood ordinary conversation, and oral commands were executed perfectly; he even set the hands of the clock and carried out the hand, eye and ear tests without mistakes.

Reading. There is no doubt that he understood most of what he read to himself and printed commands were executed correctly.

When he attempted to read aloud, he experienced the same difficulty and made similar mistakes in pronunciation to those audible when he spoke spontaneously. The longer words were slurred and rhythm was defective, especially if he tried to read quickly.

Writing. He wrote his name and address correctly and gave the time shown on a clock without mistakes, although the words were badly written and "minutes" was either shortened or omitted. Asked to read a paragraph silently and to put on paper what he had gathered, he failed badly and gave up in disgust.

When writing to dictation, his spelling was bad, some words were omitted, others were left incomplete and the mistakes closely resembled those which occurred in articulated speech. Evidently they were the result of defective internal verbalisation.

He could, however, copy print in cursive script perfectly and the character of his handwriting was better than with any other test.

The alphabet. He said the alphabet spontaneously as follows: "A B C D E F G H I J K R S T U V W X Y Z"; but he read aloud and repeated the letters perfectly.

Asked to put down the alphabet unprompted on paper, he wrote, A B C D E F G H I J K L M and then ceased, saying, "It seems diff-ult...when it's like that I'm done."

He copied print in cursive script perfectly and without hesitation.

Given the twenty-six block letters, he arranged them as follows:

A B C D E F G H I J K L M N
O P U R S W T X
Y Q Z, with V left alone on the table.

He then said, "That's wrong somehow," but failed to correct his errors.

Interpretation of a picture and its explanatory legend in speech and writing. I showed him the same picture (see p. 202) showing a collecting box for flowers placed on one of the suburban railway platforms during the war. He looked at it for some time and read the legend to himself silently. Asked to tell me what he had gathered, he replied, "They had a box er-reted (erected) at Snaresbrook Station in aid of contributing flowers for wounded soldiers...Bethnal Green Infirmy (Infirmary)."

He read the legend aloud as follows: "Fresh flowers daily for wounded. This box has been placed on the platform at Snaresbrook Station as a...that gets me now, these words...for flowers for the wounded. Many of the pass-gers cont-bute nosegays daily from the gardens and these are for-ward-ed without delay to the Bethnal Green Infirmary." He then explained, "The more I press myself the worse it gets," and added, "When I'm all right in myself I can ramp off...When I'm not myself, right off, very down."

Yet, when repeating these phrases after me, every word was perfectly articulated and he made no mistakes of any kind.

He was then asked to read the sentences through again silently and to write down what he had gathered. He wrote extremely slowly, "at Snaresbrook Station there has been plased a box on the platform for flowers," and then gave up in disgust.

I dictated the passage to him with the following result: "This box has been placed on the platform at Snaresbrook Staition as a res for flowers for wounded. Many of the passenge cor nosegays da from their garders and these are warded without delay to Bethnal infermy." In conclusion he said, "I seem to have no time for it all."

But he copied the whole of the printed paragraph without a mistake in excellent handwriting, showing that his previous failures were due to defective internal speech.

Numbers. He counted well, but each compound number was ejaculated with great rapidity, although the part indicating the decade was now correctly pronounced.

Arithmetic. He had never been good at arithmetic and disliked "sums" at school. He still made many mistakes with the usual tests in addition and subtraction.

Coins and their relative value. All the coins were named without mistakes and the words were well pronounced. He could now state the relative value of any two of them correctly, although he was a little slow with the higher numbers. He had no difficulty with change in daily life.

Plan. I took him into another room and asked him to draw a plan of the one in which he usually worked. He refused, saying, "I'm no good. It doesn't interest me." Later he added, "I see a picture for a time. It doesn't interest me, so I don't seem to worry about it." But I am certain from the observations made throughout these sittings that he naturally employed visual images, when attempting to recall persons, places or objects.

Orientation. He spent most of his time running errands in the City and never lost his way or had a moment's doubt. "I know where I've got to go and go straight away." But he complained that if he had to tell another person "I shouldn't seem to know."

Serial Tests.

(1) *Naming and recognition of common objects*. All these tasks were carried out correctly, but the words were pronounced with great rapidity. Even when he wrote the names of objects shown to him, the only word wrongly spelt was scissors ("sicurse," "siccsers"); he said, "There's only one word, diff-ty in pronouncing and writing...that's scissors. When find it diff-cult to pronounce a word, it's much harder to write."

(2) *Naming and recognition of colours*. He indicated the colour shown to him and carried out oral and printed commands with ease and certainty.

He named all the colours accurately although his pronunciation of several of the words was defective; thus orange became "orridge," violet "wi-let" or "vi-let." The monosyllables were articulated correctly, but words of several syllables tended to be slurred. He complained, "It seems my tongue gets caught. I'm never the same. Some days I'm right off. Other days just the op-site (opposite). Never two days alike."

All the colour names were written with uniform correctness and he gave the following explanation: "No diff-ulty. Said 'em in my mind. Instantaneous. You've got your eye on the thing. Nach-ly (naturally) you know what it is."

(3) *The man, cat and dog tests*. He read these simple phrases aloud and repeated them after me correctly. When he translated pictures into words, the actual content was accurate, but he showed the same curious tendency to read from right

to left as was the case during the earlier examination. At a point marked by a line in the series I asked if he was not accustomed to read from left to right, and he at once reversed the order.

Pictures shown	*He said*
The dog and the cat	"Cat and the dog"
The man and the dog	"Dog and the man"
The cat and the man	"Man and the cat"
The cat and the dog	"Dog and the cat"
The dog and the man	"Man and the dog"
The man and the cat	"Cat and the man"
The dog and the man	"Dog and the man"
The cat and the man	"Cat and the man"
The dog and the cat	"Dog and the cat"
The man and the dog	"Man and the dog"
The cat and the dog	"The cat and the dog"
The man and the cat	"Man and the cat"

But he wrote the phrases correctly from pictures or to dictation and copied them with complete accuracy.

(4) *The clock tests.*

Table 3.

	Imitation	Oral commands	Printed commands	Telling the time	Writing down the time shown on a clock set by the observer	
					In figures	In words
5 minutes to 2	Correct	Correct	Correct	"Five to two"	2.55	five min two
Half-past 1	,,	,,	,,	"Two thirty"	1.30 (correct)	half past one
5 minutes past 8	,,	,,	,,	"Five minutes pās eight"	8.5 (correct	five past eight
20 minutes to 4	,,	,,	,,	"Twenty to four"	4.40	twenty min four
10 minutes past 7	,,	,,	,,	"Ten minutes pās seven"	7.10 (correct)	ten past seven
20 minutes to 6	,,	,,	,,	"Twenty to six"	8.30	twenty min to six
10 minutes to 1	,,	,,	,,	"Ten to one"	1.50	ten min to one
A quarter to 9	,,	,,	,,	"Quarter to nine"	9.45	quarto to nine
20 minutes past 11	,,	,,	,,	"Twenty past eleven"	11.20 (correct)	twenty min past eleven
25 minutes to 3	,,	,,	,,	"Five and twenty to three"	2.35 (correct)	five twenty to three

He set one clock in imitation of another and carried out oral and printed commands with ease. He told the time accurately, although his pronunciation was somewhat defective.

Asked to write down the time shown on a clock he gave the hour and minutes correctly, but the words were in many instances defective. Thus, he wrote "five min two" for five minutes to two, "twenty min four" for twenty minutes to four, and "quarto to nine" for a quarter to nine. But he made many errors, when he attempted to write down the time in figures, although he adopted this nomenclature on his own initiative. There was a tendency to take the number which lay clockwise of the hour hand instead of the one which was behind it; for instance, he wrote "4.40" instead of 3.40 and "9.45" in place of 8.45.

(5) *The hand, eye and ear tests.*

Table 4.

	Imitation of movements made by the observer	Imitation of movements reflected in a mirror	Pictorial commands	Pictorial commands reflected in a mirror	Oral commands	Printed commands	Printed commands read aloud and executed		Writing down movements made by the observer
							He said	Movements executed	
L. hand to L. eye	Correct	Correct	L. hand to R. eye	Correct	Correct	Correct	"Left hand to right ear, eye"	Correct	Correct
R. hand to R. ear	,,	,,	Correct	,,	,,	,,	"Right hand to right eye, ear"	,,	,,
R. hand to L. eye	,,	,,	,,	,,	,,	,,	Correctly	,,	,,
L. hand to R. eye	Hesitated; correct	,,	Reversed	,,	,,	,,	,,	,,	,,
L. hand to L. ear	L. hand to R. ear	,,	Correct	,,	,,	,,	,,	,,	Left hand to right ear
R. hand to R. eye	Correct	,,	,,	,,	,,	,,	,,	,,	Correct
L. hand to R. ear	L. hand to L. ear	,,	Reversed	,,	,,	,,	,,	,,	Confused; wrote nothing
R. hand to L. ear	R. hand to R. ear	,,	Hesitated, flushed, gave up	,,	,,	,,	,,	,,	Correct
L. hand to L. eye	R. hand to R. eye; corrected	,,	R. hand to L. eye	,,	,,	,,	,,	,,	,,
R. hand to R. ear	Correct	,,	Correct	,,	,,	,,	,,	,,	Right hand to right *eye*
R. hand to L. eye	,,	,,	Reversed	,,	,,	,,	"Right hand to left ear, eye"	,,	Correct
L. hand to R. eye	L. hand to R. *ear*	,,	Correct	,,	,,	,,	Correctly	,,	,,
L. hand to L. ear	Reversed	,,	,,	,,	,,	,,	,,	,,	,,
R. hand to R. eye	,,	,,	R. hand; then L. hand to L. eye	,,	,,	,,	,,	,,	,,
L. hand to R. ear	Correct	,,	Reversed	,,	,,	,,	,,	,,	Left hand to left ear
R. hand to L. ear	,,	,,	L. hand to L. ear	,,	,,	,,	,,	,,	Left hand to right ear

He carried out oral and printed commands with ease and certainty, but made many mistakes when he attempted to imitate my movements sitting face to face. He complained, "It's diff-ult to tell anyone, may be I'm not quick at grasping. Your sitting opposite way to me, that helps make the thing a bit mystery. Say it to myself. Then it's gone again. I lost it. Don't hold it long enough." When, however, my movements were reflected in a mirror, he said, "Simply come automatically. Quite simple."

Pictorial commands puzzled him greatly. "I was trying to picture myself round the way same as picture shows." He became confused, flushed, and at one point in the middle of the series gave up. As soon as the diagram was reflected in the mirror, all hesitation and doubt disappeared and he said, "It seemed to come to me, which is my right and which is my left. Didn't say nothing. Knew what it was."

He had much difficulty in writing down the movements made by me and in the middle of the series became confused, rested his head on his hand and wrote nothing. But he shortly afterwards continued and gave several correct answers.

These tests seemed to arouse in him a consciousness of his daily disabilities and evoked the following remarks: "When I keep to the same thing I seem to get fed up (bored). Same as when I go to pit-chers (pictures, i.e. cinematograph). Sit here ten minutes, then go off to sleep. Pit-chers seem to tie me up. Don't seem to take any interest. Reason why I don't go any more." After he had failed to carry out the series of pictorial commands, he said, "Like when I go into one of man-gers (managers of the insurance company). If I look at 'em, stand there, say nothing, like mesmerised. If I don't look at 'em, I can speak fairly well to 'em."

No. 14

A case of Syntactical Aphasia, due to a wound over the first temporal gyrus and the Sylvian fissure, produced by a fragment of shell casing.

He developed seizures in which he ceased to talk and his right arm fell powerless on the bed; he was never convulsed, did not appear to lose consciousness, but could not speak and was powerless to think. These attacks were preceded by a "tingling feeling" down the right side, accompanied by an hallucination of taste and smell and a peculiar mental state.

At first there was gross loss of power and incoordination of the right arm and leg; movements of the right half of the face were defective and the tongue deviated to this side. The deep reflexes on the right half of the body were brisker than those on the left, the right plantar gave an upward response and the abdominals on this side were diminished. Subsequent examination showed that there were profound changes in sensibility in the right upper and lower extremities and confirmed the supposition that the loss of power was to a great extent of afferent origin.

From the first his speech was jargon. He knew what he wanted to say, but his words poured out in phrases which had no grammatical structure and were in most cases incomprehensible. He could not repeat a sentence said to him and, when he attempted to read aloud, uttered pure jargon. He was unable to find names for common objects and yet his correct choice to printed commands showed that he was familiar with their usual nomenclature. Comprehension of spoken words was obviously defective and he was liable to be puzzled by any but the simplest oral commands. In general conversation he frequently failed to understand what was said and to carry on a subject started by himself. Spontaneous thought was rapid and his intelligence of a high order, but his power of symbolic formulation and expression was hampered by defects of internal speech. He undoubtedly comprehended what he read to himself, even in French, but any attempt to reproduce it aloud resulted in jargon. Single words were for the most part more easily written than spoken and, when at a loss, he could frequently write something which conveyed his meaning. But he was unable to read what he had written, and this, together with his difficulty in forming phrases, made it impossible to compose a letter or coherent account of something he wished to convey. He could copy perfectly, but wrote badly to dictation, because of the rapidity with which he forgot what had been said to him. He added and subtracted without difficulty and enjoyed solving financial problems. He could not name a single coin, but recognised their relative value. He played the piano, read the notes correctly and evidently recognised the constitution of a chord and the changes of key.

Major X, aged 42, was wounded on May 18th, 1915, either by a fragment of shell casing or by shrapnel. An operation was performed, probably on the following day. No official details came through to us, but we learnt from one of his friends, who saw him in France, that his temperature was constantly raised and that on May 28th he suffered from a series of epileptic fits.

He arrived in London on June 4th, 1915, and I was asked to see him the next day. His temperature was 102° F. (39° C.) and he was drowsy but conscious. He could scarcely say a word, although he seemed to understand what was said to him. He showed all the signs of a right hemiplegia with paresis of the lower part of the face and deviation of the tongue to the right.

His temperature fell to normal on June 8th and his mental state rapidly improved. Fuller examination on June 29th showed the following condition.

The original wound was represented by a granulating surface 2 cm. by 1·5 cm. just above the insertion of the left ear and 1 cm. behind the interaural line. It corresponded in level with a point 16 cm. backwards from the root of the nose and was 11 cm. from the middle of the scalp. The total nasion-inion measurement was 35 cm. (Fig. 8, Vol. 1, p. 449). This unhealed patch was surrounded on three sides by a horse-shoe-shaped incision, which had healed firmly. Within this lay an irregularly quadrilateral area, where the bone had been removed; this was covered by normal skin, except over the site of the original wound.

His speech was the most extraordinary jargon. There could be little doubt that he knew what he wanted to say, but the words poured out in phrases which had no grammatical structure and were in most cases incomprehensible. In many instances the words themselves were well formed, but they had no meaning as they were uttered. Occasionally, however, sufficient words were correctly placed to make his meaning clear. He could not repeat a sentence said to him and, when he attempted to read, he uttered pure jargon.

These difficulties in speech made him extremely angry. He was normally a man of somewhat impatient temper and inability to express his wants drove him to fury. This greatly hampered my observations, as I was always obliged to arrange my tests in such a way as not to excite his anger.

He suffered from no headache or vomiting and had not had any convulsions since May 28th. The optic discs were normal. The pupils reacted well and eye movements as such were unaffected. There was some weakness of the lower half of the face on the right side and the tongue deviated to the right, when he could be got to protrude it to command. The deep reflexes on the right half of the body were brisker than those on the left and the plantar gave an upward response. The superficial reflexes from the right half of the abdomen were greatly diminished compared with those from the left.

He was a right-handed man, who prided himself on being ambidextrous; but inability to carry out movements to order made it extremely difficult to determine exactly the loss of motor power. Told to touch his nose, he made no attempt to do so. If I touched my nose with my forefinger and then, after closing his eyes, gripped the index of one or other hand saying, "Do it," he could carry out the movement; but the right hand was obviously ataxic.

Sometimes he protruded his tongue to command; more often he licked his lips or cheek. Asked to show his teeth, he placed his left hand into his mouth and touched his upper denture. When he was told to hit me, in order to test the extensor power of his arm, he struck himself on the chest.

But in spite of these difficulties in examination, I was able to determine that there was no absolute paralysis of the right upper or lower extremity. Even isolated movements of the fingers were possible; but there was great incoordination both of the right arm and leg. If the hands were held out in front of him and the eyes closed, the right fell away unconsciously from the horizontal position showing defective recognition of posture. There was no obvious increase or diminution in tone, involuntary movements were absent and the limbs were not wasted.

No sensory measurements could be carried out at this stage; but all the signs pointed to considerable loss of recognition of posture in both upper and lower extremities of the right half of the body. When the six geometrical figures were placed in front of him and a duplicate was given into his left hand, he never failed to select the right one, using the right hand as an indicator. But if one of them was placed in the right hand, he made gross mistakes, such as selecting the cylinder instead of a sphere or the ovoid for a cube. As soon as it was transferred to the left hand he corrected his previous mistake, saying, "Yes, oh! yes."

Condition between September 12th and November 4th, 1915 (*from 117 to 170 days after he was wounded*).

On July 30th, 1915, he was transferred to a hospital under my care; he continued to improve rapidly, and between September 12th and November 4th I was able to make a more extended series of observations with the following results.

The wound had healed entirely and he suffered from no headache, epileptiform attacks or other seizures. Vision was normal and the discs unaffected. There was no gross hemianopsia or limitation of the visual field; finer perimetric observations were, however, impossible. Hearing was somewhat diminished in both ears, but he said he had always been slightly deaf. His pupils reacted normally and spontaneous eye movements were well executed, although they were carried out badly to command. There was now little if any difference between the movements of the two halves of the face and no paresis of the tongue. Arm-jerks, knee-jerks and ankle-jerks were normal on the two sides and both plantars gave a downward response. The reflexes obtained from the right and left halves of the abdomen were equal and brisk.

He could now walk considerable distances without a stick; but the behaviour of the right half of the body was obviously different from that of the left. He did not lift the right hip, but negligently cast the whole leg forwards in contrast with the orderly advance of the left lower extremity. The foot was placed clumsily on the ground; there was, however, none of that lack of dorsiflexion so common in hemiplegia of motor origin. The right shoulder was not dropped, but was quiescent, firmly approximated to the side, whilst the left arm swung freely.

All isolated movements of the fingers and thumb were possible, but the grasp of the left hand was somewhat stronger than that of the right. Movements of this upper extremity were somewhat clumsy and the incoordination was increased on closing the eyes.

Movements of the right lower extremity could be performed powerfully against resistance, though they showed considerable incoordination, increased by closing the eyes. He could stand on the left foot both with the eyes open or shut; he was unsteady on the right foot, but could not stand at all with his eyes closed.

I could find no signs of motor apraxia. Although the movements of the right hand were clumsy, he brushed his hair, shaved himself, struck a match and blew it out again after lighting a cigarette. He undid his buttons, but could not do them up again, with the right hand; when tying his pyjamas, he held the string in his right hand and made with the left all the movements of forming a knot.

Obviously at this stage of recovery his lack of motor power was mainly due to defective postural recognition. This view was borne out by the rough clinical methods of examination, although his loss of linguistic capacity made accurate measurements impossible.

Symbolic Formulation and Expression.

Before he was wounded he had been an unusually intelligent, highly educated man, interested in scientific pursuits and actively engaged in managing his large ancestral estates. His temper had always been somewhat hasty; this made it difficult to carry out a long series of observations, especially if he failed to respond coherently or to carry out the task set him. He would throw down the pencil, tear up the paper on which he was writing, or wave his hand to indicate that he was not going to try again.

In spite of the gross defects of symbolic expression from which he suffered, his general intellectual power was remarkably high. Day by day he followed the operations at the Front on large military maps; these he would spread upon his bed and, with a pencil, mark out some recent advance or outline our position, saying, "There, there you see."

During one of our sittings he touched the depressed part of the wound, within the area of bony defect, and then wrote "Forest branche." As I failed entirely to understand his meaning, he made me fetch from the cupboard in his room a book on forestry; he turned the pages until he came to a picture of a wood with undergrowth to which he pointed, saying, "branch," at the same time touching his head. He succeeded by this means in communicating his fear that, when he walked through a coppice, the branches might injure his wound. He was at once satisfied when I told him we would cover it with an aluminium shield.

The following incident shows how accurate were his powers of observation at this time in spite of grave inability to express his thoughts. He was walking in Kew Gardens with the medical officer in charge of the hospital, when he pointed out a new variety of heath. The doctor said "Scotch," to which the patient answered "No, no, you and me." It was a rare Irish heath, newly acquired by the botanical gardens, and both the patient and his companion were Irishmen.

He succeeded in conveying to a friend, who was visiting him in hospital, a piece of information not generally known. The visitor asked "Who told you that?" and, as the answer he received was incomprehensible jargon, he suggested "Was it the Admiralty?"; "No, no," was the reply. "Was it the War Office?" The patient repeated "No, no," and seizing a pencil wrote "Lansdowne." This greatly puzzled the friend until he remembered that the Marquis of Lansdowne had once been the Head of the Foreign Office; he therefore enquired, "Was it the Foreign Office?" "Yes, yes," replied the patient, who had employed the familiar name of a previous Foreign Minister to represent the department over which he no longer presided.

Articulated speech. His voluntary utterances consisted of a flood of jargon, containing occasional good and apposite phrases; but the sounds seemed to bear little direct relation to the form of words he wished to employ.

He could say "yes" and "no" correctly and answered "come in" to a knock at the door. He was extremely intelligent in the way in which he used the few words at his voluntary disposal to explain a map, a book, or a picture. He accompanied his lively gestures by "there, there," "down there," "up there" and similar indicative expressions. For instance, on one occasion, our interview was disturbed by an outburst of operatic singing; I asked what it was, and he swung round in bed and pointed correctly to the position of the neighbouring school, saying, "There, up there, over there, you know."

He could not say after me simple phrases, nor could he repeat exactly what he had just uttered voluntarily.

He was unable to find names for common objects of daily use; and yet his correct choice to printed commands showed that he was familiar with their usual nomenclature. In the same way he could not tell the time aloud, but set the clock correctly when the order was given in print.

Moreover, the following observations, made during the compass tests, show that the difficulty in naming was due to want of symbolic expression and not to any lack of nominal discrimination. When the compasses were applied to the normal hand in the usual way, his jargon made it impossible to conclude whether he appreciated them correctly. I therefore placed on his bed-table two sheets of paper; one bore the figure 1, the other a large 2. I then found that, whenever he was touched with one or with two points, he could place his finger without fail on the appropriate number.

Comprehension of spoken words. This was obviously defective and physical examination was hampered by his want of understanding and inability to carry out oral commands. Told to look to the right or to the left he rarely did so, although he followed my fingers perfectly in all directions. Sometimes he protruded his tongue to command; more often he licked his lips, thrust it into his cheek or touched it with his fingers.

He chose common objects of daily use on the whole correctly, though with considerable hesitation, provided the command was given in one word; but he was liable to be puzzled if the order was given in the form of a phrase such as "Hand me the pencil." When these objects were replaced by geometrical figures, he made several mistakes, although his choice was perfect to printed commands.

Time after time in general conversation he failed to understand what was said. He was reading an account in French of Napoleon's Russian campaign and wanted to tell me how closely the dates coincided with the retreat of the Russians, which was then taking place (September, 1915). He took the book in his hand, pointed to the words "15 Septembre," saying, "Now, just the same, there, yes, over there." I answered, "Yes, that was also a beautiful summer and the snow came early." He replied, "Yes, oh! did it, oh! yes." He showed so much interest in the similarity of the two events, that I asked him when Napoleon first had difficulty with the snow; but he turned the pages of the book aimlessly. I then questioned him as to the date on which Napoleon reached Moscow (September 14, 1812), the starting point of our conversation, but he shook his head and could not answer. Spontaneous thought was rapid and correct though the power of comprehension and symbolic expression in answer to questions was evidently defective.

Reading. He picked out an object without fail in answer to its printed name and set the clock or executed the complicated movements of the hand, eye and ear tests correctly to printed commands. Shown a paragraph about the taking of eight thousand prisoners, he uttered with great rapidity "yes, oh yes, no, one, two, three, four, five, six, seven, eight, eight," nodding his head on the last word. He followed the events mentioned in the newspaper and certainly understood the French book on Napoleon, which he was reading at this time. Thus, there can be no doubt that he comprehended the significance of printed symbols.

But any attempt to reproduce them aloud was followed by incomprehensible jargon. Asked to read the commands of the hand, eye and ear tests, he uttered a series of sounds which bore no relation to the text, although the movements were executed perfectly and without hesitation.

Writing. The power of writing suffered less than external speech, because the defect was essentially one of balance and rhythmic utterance. Thus, when asked to name a set of common objects, he made unintelligible sounds; but in fifteen out of eighteen attempts the names he gave them in writing were recognisably correct. Single words were so much more easily written than spoken, that he always carried about with him paper and a pencil to help him in his conversational difficulties. When at a loss, he would write something sufficient to convey his meaning to his puzzled auditor.

But he was unable to read what he had written, and this, together with his difficulty in forming phrases and sentences (vide infra, 1916, p. 226), made it impossible to compose a letter. One day, during a set of observations, he said, "Funny thing, this worse, that sort of thing." Then he seized his note-book and wrote "as, at"; I asked, "You mean conjunctions and prepositions?" and he replied, "Yes, that sort of thing."

He could write his signature correctly with the right hand. To this he appended his age and the address of one of his estates; but this was shortened, as if for a telegram, and one letter was omitted from the middle of the most important word.

He could copy print into cursive handwriting perfectly. But he wrote badly to dictation because of the rapidity with which he forgot the phrase that had been said to him; after writing one word correctly he would ask, "What is it?" unable to continue to the next. (See the hand, eye and ear tests, Table 4, p. 224.) On one occasion, asked to write "An enemy air-raid," he produced "A raidare air enemy."

Arithmetic and the value of money. He was able to add and subtract without difficulty. He kept his bank-book and could act correctly on the financial questions put to him by his banker and steward, provided they were patient enough to understand his answer. He enjoyed these problems, which did not disturb his equanimity.

He could make out a cheque correctly if the action was carried out spontaneously. But, when told to fill it in for a certain sum, he was liable to insert numbers in the place of words, although the actual amount was correct.

He could not name a single coin, but had no difficulty in determining their relative value, provided he did not have to express it in a phrase.

He set out a row of dominoes without a single mistake, rapidly placing all the doubles across in the usual way.

Music. This patient was musical and played for me on the piano Chopin's Largo (Op. 20), very slowly, reading the notes and giving the change of key correctly. The right hand was clumsy owing to the incoordination; but he succeeded in bringing his fingers on to the right notes of the chord and, if he was wrong, immediately corrected his error. Keeping his eyes on the music, he recognised by ear when he had struck a false note and that it did not correspond with the text of the music. He played to me other pieces, correcting the faults due to the clumsiness of his right hand; but the slow pace of the Largo was in his favour, whilst the complexities of the change in key showed how clearly musical notation conveyed to him the notes intended.

Serial Tests.

I have placed under one heading all my observations made during the period from September 12th to November 4th, 1915. But, before I had completed the serial tests, he left the hospital for urgent private reasons at the end of September and did not return to my care until November 1st. His condition mental and physical was, however, unchanged and I have therefore reported the results of these experiments together.

(1) *Naming and recognition of common objects.*

Table 1.

	Oral commands	Printed commands	Naming an object indicated	Writing name of object indicated	Copied from print	Object in left hand out of sight: Pointing to similar one on table	Object in left hand out of sight: Writing the name	Object in left hand out of sight: Naming
Matches	Correct	Correct	"Stres, miss, ness"	Match	Perfect	Correct	Match	Impossible
Pencil	,,	,,	"Miss, cow, stace"	peccot	,,	,,	Pencil	,,
Key	,,	,,	"No"	"No, I can't"	,,	,,	Key	,,
Scissors	,,	,,	"Sticken, stuck, stee"	,,	,,	,,	—	,,
Penny	,,	,,	"No"	penny	,,	,,	penny	,,
Knife	,,	,,	"I can tell you, I think so" [tried to write name]	Knife	,,	,,	—	,,
Key	,,	,,	Pure jargon	"Did I?"	,,	,,	Key	,,
Pencil	,,	,,	,,	pencil	,,	,,	pencil	,,
Knife	Penny	,,	,,	Knife	,,	,,	—	,,
Penny	Correct	,,	,,	penny	,,	,,	penny	,,
Matches	,,	,,	,,	Match	,,	,,	Match	,,
Scissors	,,	,,	,,	"What are they?"	,,	,,	Scissors	,,
Penny	,,	,,	,,	penny	,,	,,	penny	,,
Key	,,	,,	,,	Key	,,	,,	Key	,,
Scissors	,,	,,	,,	"What is it?"	,,	,,	Scissors	,,
Matches	,,	,,	,,	Match	,,	,,	Match	,,
Pencil	,,	,,	,,	picus; "No, I can't"	,,	,,	Pincel	,,
Knife	,,	,,	,,	Knife	,,	,,	Knife	,,

When the command was given orally, he chose with considerable hesitation; but to printed commands he was extremely quick and accurate.

He was unable to designate a single one of the common objects and the jargon he uttered did not seem to correspond in any way to the words he required; and yet he was obviously familiar with their names, for many were written correctly. In the same way, if an object was placed in his normal hand out of sight, he could indicate the corresponding one on the table before him, designated it correctly in writing on fifteen out of eighteen occasions, but was entirely unable to utter a single name.

He copied the printed words in cursive handwriting without mistake or hesitation.

(2) *Choosing geometrical figures to tactile, oral and printed commands.*

Table 2.

	Duplicate placed in left hand out of sight	Oral commands		Printed commands
		Command given	Choice made	
Sphere	Correct	"Sphere or ball"	Correct	Correct
Cube	,,	"Cube or square"	Cylinder	,,
Ovoid	,,	"Egg"	Pyramid	,,
Cone	,,	"Cone"	Correct	,,
Cube	,,	"Cube"	Cylinder	,,
Pyramid	,,	"Pyramid"	Correct	,,
Cylinder	,,	"Cylinder"	,,	,,
Cube	,,	"Cube"	Cylinder	,,
Cone	,,	"Cone"	Correct	,,
Sphere	,,	"Sphere or ball"	Cylinder	,,
Cylinder	,,	"Cylinder"	Cone	,,
Ovoid	,,	"Egg"	Correct	,,
Pyramid	,,	"Pyramid"	,,	,,
Sphere	,,	"Sphere or ball"	Cone	,,
Cube	,,	"Cube or square"	Cylinder	,,
Ovoid	,,	"Egg"	Correct	,,
Cone	,,	"Cone"	Pyramid	,,
Cube	,,	"Cube"	"I get con...no"	,,
Pyramid	,,	"Pyramid"	Correct	,,
Cylinder	,,	"Cylinder"	,,	,,
Cube	,,	"Cube"	,,	,,
Cone	,,	"Cone"	,,	,,
Sphere	,,	"Sphere or ball"	Cube	,,
Cylinder	,,	"Cylinder"	Correct	,,
Ovoid	,,	"Egg"	,,	,,
Pyramid	,,	"Pyramid"	,,	,,

This was a remarkable series of observations demonstrating the uncertainty with which he executed orders given by word of mouth. He chose rapidly and with certainty, when a duplicate was placed in his normal hand, or in response to the printed word. Oral commands were, however, badly carried out and he frequently selected the wrong figure; the choice was sometimes extraordinarily wide of the mark. I used the word "egg" in place of ovoid, which he did not seem to understand; but even this simple name did not lead in every instance to a correct response.

(3) *The clock tests.*

He set the clock quickly and accurately in simple imitation or to printed commands. But he found extreme difficulty in executing them, when given orally, and was totally unable to tell the time aloud.

When he attempted to write down the time shown on the clock he used a remarkable method. First he wrote in figures the number of minutes past the hour and then the hour, a sort of inverted railway nomenclature; he showed, however, that he fully appreciated the significance of the position of the hands.

When he wrote to dictation he adopted the usual manner of writing railway time. But the series came to a sudden end because, on making a mistake, he refused altogether to continue.

Table 3.

	Imitation	Oral commands	Printed commands	Telling the time	Writing down the time	To dictation
20 minutes to 6	Correct	Set 8.25. "No, how is it?" Corrected	Correct	"Six...six"	20.6	6.40
20 minutes past 11	,,	Correct	,,	"No"	20.11	11.20
25 minutes to 3	,,	Set 7.15. "No, I couldn't with here"	,,	"No"	25.2	11.40
A quarter to 9	,,	Correct	,,	Impossible	45.8	8.45
10 minutes past 8	,,	,,	,,	,,	10.8	8.10
Half-past 2	,,	,,	,,	,,	15.2	2.30
20 minutes past 9	,,	Correct; doubtful	,,	,,	20.9	9.10
5 minutes to 2	,,	Correct	,,	,,	55.1	1.55
5 minutes past 8	,,	"What was it now?"; set 4.50	,,	,,	5.8	8.10
Half-past 1	,,	Correct	,,	,,	30.1	1.30
20 minutes to 4	,,	Set 3.45. "I can't exactly; I forgot"	,,	,,	40.3	3.40
10 minutes past 7	,,	Correct	,,	,,	10.7	
20 minutes to 6	,,	Set 8.50	,,	,,	40.5	
10 minutes to 1	,,	Correct	,,	,,	50.12	
A quarter to 12	,,	Set 11.55	,,	,,	45.11	

(4) *Hand, eye and ear tests.*

Table 4.

	Imitation of movements made by the observer	Pictorial commands	Oral commands	Printed commands	Reading aloud and executing printed commands		Copying from print	Writing to dictation
					He said	Movement made		
R. hand to R. eye	Correct	R. hand to L. eye; then correct	Correct	Correct	"Rain, been to, no, no"	Correct	Perfect	Correct
L. hand to R. ear	,,	Correct	,,	,,	"Raca, bre, no and reets no"	,,	,,	L. hand to R. *eye*
R. hand to L. eye	,,	,,	R. hand to L. *ear*; then eye. "Which is it?"	,,	"Read and bac to and leave and black een"	,,	,,	Correct
L. hand to L. ear	,,	,,	Correct	,,	"Brack and two, daf and een"	,,	,,	L. hand to L. *eye*
L. hand to R. eye	,,	,,	,,	,,	"Brack, hack, bleak and blacking"	,,	,,	Correct
R. hand to L. ear	,,	,,	,,	,,	"Yes, barry ee, barry ee"	,,	,,	R. hand to right
L. hand to L. eye	L. hand to R. *ear*; L. hand to R. eye; then correct	L. hand to L. *ear*; "No, no"; then correct	L. hand to L. *ear*; "Which?"	,,	"Back and back and black and green"	,,	,,	L. hand to left
R. hand to R. ear	Correct	Correct	Correct	,,	"Brack and..."	,,	,,	L. hand to R. *eye*
L. hand to R. eye	,,	,,	L. hand to R. *ear*	,,	"Yes, two, brack and..."	,,	—	—
R. hand to L. eye	,,	,,	R. hand to L. *ear*	,,	"No, the wack and two green"	,,	—	—

Printed commands were carried out perfectly, although he was entirely unable to read them aloud. With oral commands he was slow and uncertain; he made several mistakes and said, "Its rather to the hear." I asked whether it was difficult, and he answered "Yes."

Direct imitation of my movements and orders given in the form of pictures were accurately carried out and, although he responded somewhat slowly, he was definite in his answers.

He could copy the printed orders in cursive handwriting, but was very inaccurate to dictation, repeatedly demanding "What is it?"

Subsequent Progress.

On December 20th, 1915, he came into the house before luncheon and suffered from a sudden lapse of consciousness; he remembered nothing until he found himself in his bedroom, about half an hour later, washing his hands. Similar attacks occurred on January 22nd, February 13th and March 25th, 1916.

On April 20th, 1916, he was found unconscious on the floor of his bathroom, and on May 27th he had another almost exactly similar seizure. On this occasion, whilst preparing his bath, he evidently felt ill, but succeeded in returning to his room, where he was found unconscious on his bed. A minute sinus had opened in the centre of the wound, from which a fragment of bone, measuring 0·6 cm. by 0·5 cm., was extruded shortly after this fit.

When I saw him again on June 8th, 1916, the scar was depressed and pulsating; a recent scab covered a small opening in the centre. We therefore determined to explore the wound and, on June 16th, small fragments of bone were removed from a pocket in the new dural tissue just under the sinus. Some of the dense fibrous tissue was removed, but the brain was not exposed at any point. On June 25th, the sinus had closed and the surgical incision had healed by first intention.

He succeeded in conveying to me, partly in speech and partly in writing, that the seizures began with a hot feeling down the right arm and leg accompanied by a gradually increasing taste and smell. This was associated with a state of mind which he could not describe in comprehensible terms; but he wrote in explanation, "Indistinct of the foliage of a minute." During his efforts to convey the nature of these prodromal symptoms he scrawled on paper the following words, "In mouth two minutes there is bad taste," "Heat is before," "Clofer" (erased and evidently intended for chloroform), "Ether, mouth." Then he drew a diagram with lines and dots, appending the description, "legs lapse, arms, mind, mouth, face."

On June 21st, Dr Riddoch watched an attack from start to finish. The patient was answering questions in his usual manner, partly in writing, when the pencil suddenly dropped from his hand, which fell powerless on to the bed. He ceased talking for nearly three minutes, but did not seem to be completely unconscious; he was not convulsed. Later he explained that a tingling feeling passed down the right side and he lost power in the arm and leg. At the same time he could not speak and found he was powerless to think. The smell and taste he had experienced in previous attacks were absent on this occasion.

On September 7th, 1916 (one year and sixteen weeks after he was wounded), I was able to make my last consecutive series of observations.

The wound was firmly healed and the scar depressed. He had suffered from no further seizures or headache. The discs were normal. Movements of the face were almost equally well executed on the two sides and the tongue deviated very slightly on protrusion.

He was not apraxic and could carry out all the usual tests; he tied a true reef-knot, pulling on the two ends to show me it had been formed correctly. He could now walk five miles with ease and his gait did not resemble that usually seen in hemiplegia. There was no motor paralysis or change in tone, and coordination was greatly improved; but he still used his left hand by preference.

The reflexes were equally brisk on the two halves of the body; the abdominals were easily obtained and the plantars gave a downward response.

He was quiet and rational, much less liable to outbursts of irritability. His speech had somewhat improved, but still consisted of isolated words or jargon. Asked to blow his nose, he found he had no handkerchief in his pocket and exclaimed, "No, funny thing, must buy, I don't know why, but..."

He could not repeat what was said to him and still had some difficulty in obeying oral commands.

Isolated words were written down to fill in the gaps in his conversation. Thus he wrote "axe" to indicate that he was ambidextrous, "buy a" to express his want of a handkerchief, "lot" or "number of persons" to show that his speech was worse in company. Left to himself he wrote spontaneously, "I am gong to London seeing a Doctor. In night the darkness is very funny. The weather is good for the corn and not now spoiled." But he could not read a word he had written and, when I asked him what it contained, he answered, "I can't, I know, I suppose in time, not now, funny thing why."

He could not write consecutively to dictation. Thus "I am very much better" became "I am very better," and, when I dictated "My leg and my arm are much better," he wrote "I an" and said, "No, I can't, that's it." A few minutes later he snatched the paper from me and began "Our legs," but ceased, saying, "No, that's funny."

From this time onwards he progressed favourably and his speech somewhat improved. During the years 1917 and the early part of 1918 he showed conspicuous business ability and became extremely clever in circumventing his difficulties of speech.

He was not known to have had any further fits or attacks until June 10th, 1918, when he was found dead with the upper part of his body in the bath and his legs hanging over the edge. Evidently he had been caught by a seizure as he was stepping into the water.

No. 15

A case of Syntactical Aphasia, due to injury by a rifle bullet, which traversed the left temporal lobe from before backwards to make its exit behind the ear.

The left eye was destroyed; but the right showed loss of vision over the upper and outer quadrant of the field due to a lesion of the extreme lower fibres of the optic radiations. A fortnight after he was wounded there was a little weakness of the right half of the face and the tongue deviated slightly to the right. There was no loss of motion or sensation in the body or limbs. The deep reflexes were somewhat greater on the right than on the left side, the right plantar gave an upward response and the abdominals on this side were diminished. All these signs, except the quadrantic hemianopsia, passed off within five months.

He gradually developed attacks consisting of a "nasty smell" which nauseated him. Six years after he was wounded this aura culminated for the first time in an epileptiform seizure, accompanied by loss of consciousness and characteristic chewing movements.

His speech was a perfect example of jargon due to disturbance of rhythm and defective syntax. He did not use wrong words and, if the subject under discussion was known, it was not difficult to gather the meaning of what he said. He tried to "rush" his phrases and it was difficult to hear the prepositions, conjunctions or articles; these parts of speech were frequently omitted. The same errors marred his attempts to repeat what was said to him or to read aloud; even when reading to himself, he became confused by internal jargon and lost the significance of all but the simplest phrases. His power of naming was preserved, although his nomenclature was sometimes unusual; he could also state the time correctly. On the whole he understood what was said to him, unless he was compelled to repeat it to himself. Simple oral commands were well executed, but he hesitated and made several errors over more complex tests. His spontaneous writing was poor and he had little power of reproducing in written words the contents of a paragraph he had apparently read with understanding. He wrote equally badly to dictation, but could copy perfectly. In the earlier stages, before the full development of the fits, he experienced little or no difficulty in counting and solved simple problems in arithmetic. He could name coins, knew their relative value and made no mistakes in the use of money. He evidently appreciated the full meaning of pictures, but found extreme difficulty in describing them in spoken or written words. He drew a spirit lamp both from the model and from memory, but failed to represent an elephant correctly. Orientation was unaffected and he drew a perfect ground-plan of a familiar room.

Private Frank Edward S., aged 25, was admitted to the London Hospital on March 2nd, 1915, with a gunshot wound of the head. He was incapable of giving any account of his injury, and the sole information sent with him was a card stating that he was "admitted to No. 2 Stationary Hospital on February 2nd, 1915, with an operation wound on the head" and that "mentally he has improved steadily since admission; no further operation performed."

A rifle bullet had entered just to the left of the inner canthus of the right eye, and had made its exit directly above the insertion of the left ear. The wound of entry was represented by a minute perfectly healed white scar. On the other hand, its exit consisted of an irregular opening in the bone and tissues of the scalp, and through this protruded a small suppurating hernia cerebri, which pulsated. Bone had been removed over an irregularly quadrilateral area about 3 cm. in vertical and the same distance in horizontal extent; below, this opening reached the level of the insertion of the ear, and above it was about 13 cm. from the middle line of the scalp. The nasion-inion measured 35 cm., and the anterior border of loss of bone corresponded to a point 13 cm. along this line, whilst the posterior edge was 3 cm. behind it. Above the wound was a large horse-shoe-shaped surgical incision, which had healed completely. (Cf. Figs. 8 and 9, Vol. 1, pp. 449 and 451.)

He did not as a rule say anything spontaneously; but in answer to questions his speech was jargon. When he wanted to ask if he might smoke, he said, "Want treat Christian"; but the intended meaning of the words became obvious when he put an imaginary cigarette into his mouth and pretended to light it.

The left pupil was fixed and the cornea insensitive; the lid drooped and he was unable to move the globe in any direction except downwards. This eye was blind from rupture of the choroid and atrophy of the optic nerve. Evidently the bullet had caused gross damage to the left eye as it passed backwards in the direction of the temporal lobe.

The lower portion of the right half of the face moved slightly less than the left, and the tongue was protruded a little to the right of the middle line. Arm-jerks and knee-jerks were brisker on the right than on the left side and there was a tendency to clonus at the right ankle-joint. The right plantar reflex gave an upward response, whilst the left was normal. Over the left half of the abdomen the responses were unaffected; but on the right side no reflex could be obtained from the lower segment, whilst that from the upper part of the abdomen was evidently diminished. Motor power, muscular tone and coordination were unaffected and sensation appeared to be normal.

CONDITION IN JUNE 1915 (*eighteen weeks after he was wounded*).

By June 5th, 1915, the cerebral hernia had entirely disappeared, the wound was firmly healed and he was up all day, busy and helpful in the ward. During the following week a complete series of observations was made with the following result.

He had suffered from no fits or seizures during his stay in hospital, and was free from headache and vomiting. The left globe was shrunken and had subsequently to be removed. Vision of the right eye was $\frac{6}{6}$, but there seemed to be some restriction of the upper and outer quadrant of the visual field, although the right fundus showed no definite changes. He was somewhat deaf in the left ear, but he thought that the tuning-fork placed on the forehead was heard better on this side. No gross changes could be seen on otoscopic examination, though apparently the bullet on making its exit had in some way injured the auditory apparatus of the left ear. Smell and taste were certainly unaffected. There was still a little weakness of the lower portion of the right half of the face, and the tongue was protruded slightly to the right of the middle line. Arm-, knee- and ankle-jerks were brisker on the right side than on the left, but there was no ankle clonus. The right plantar reflex gave an upward response, whilst the left great toe went downwards. The lower segment of the right half of the abdomen now responded to stimulation, but the reflex was diminished and was less than that obtained from any other portion. There was no paralysis or paresis and sensation was not affected.

Symbolic Formulation and Expression.

He was cheerful and willing, laughed when he was successful in performing the task set him, and did not become irritable, though he failed to express himself intelligibly. When he recognised that his jargon was incomprehensible, he dropped his head and sometimes showed the beginning of a blush; he did not then care to make another attempt to express those particular thoughts. He was intelligent and useful in the work of the ward, provided he was not compelled to express himself in speech. For example, he would go about serving the patients, washing up, laying the cloth correctly; but as soon as he attempted to formulate his wants, such as that he required a purge, he became confused, not only in utterance but in thought.

Articulated speech. He said little spontaneously, but answered questions readily; once started, his speech was rapid and voluble. He tried to "rush" his phrases and not uncommonly was brought to a standstill by pure jargon. It was extremely difficult to hear the prepositions, conjunctions or articles, and these parts of speech were frequently omitted. Thus, asked what he had done since he came to the London Hospital, he said: "To here; only washing; cups and plates." *Q.* "Have you played any games?" *A.* "Played games, yes, played one, daytime, garden." *Q.* "What did you play?" *A.* "We had four bowls each; big bowls; about four each. Always chuck to a small white 'un; try to hit it. Round one, flat one; chuck it on to flat bit of wood. Me and another try to play it, see who could get the most numbers." Asked about his wound he said, "When I woke straight in bed; I couldn't say it. I knew what it was, but couldn't say it. I couldn't say, France nobody was; but I couldn't say it."

He did not use wrong words, and if the subject under discussion was known, it was not difficult to gather the sense of what he said. Thus, when I was testing his taste, and placed some quinine upon his tongue, he said: "Rotten to drink it.

Something medicine or that. Make you drop of water after it, so to take out of your mouth." The rhythm of the words and the balance of each phrase was mainly affected. Syntax was gravely disordered.

He could say the alphabet and the months correctly and in order.

Understanding of spoken words. He seemed to comprehend what was said to him, and carried out simple oral commands correctly; thus he chose without fail a common object or colour named by me. But, as soon as the order of necessity took the form of a group of words or a short phrase, it was executed more slowly and with some hesitation; when setting the hands of a clock, he was liable to confuse "to" and "past" the hour, and he made several mistakes with the hand, eye and ear tests.

Reading. He was asked to select something from the daily paper to read aloud, and chose the following large block type heading on the front page: "Mr Lloyd George says Red Tape must go. The Truth about Przemysl. Russians evacuate Galician town after removing guns and stores. Success in the North. German lines pierced and prisoners taken." These he read rapidly as: "Mr Lloyd George says red take, take must go. The troop about towns, what lost 'em. Russ-ns exclose some big town after refunded...re...refunded guns and stories...stoppies. Success in the north. German binds prisoners and prisoners taken."

I then said: "You have just read me something; what was it about?" He answered: "What looking at paper?" "Yes." He then continued: "Germans what lost big town and the Americans...Germans have already won it. Some of the prisoners on its road, its country...prisoners over it. Mr Lloyd George says, Act beer something." The substitution of "Red take must go" for "Red tape," when he read the headings aloud, evidently confused him, and, on attempting to reproduce the meaning, he substituted legislation about beer, much discussed at this time.

He chose a common object or colour, and set the hands of a clock quickly and accurately to printed commands; but he carried out the hand, eye, and ear tests slowly and with several errors. So long as the order was given in a single word, his response was prompt; on the other hand, a phrase, which he was compelled to repeat to himself silently before he performed the movement required, was liable to lead to confusion.

He understood not only the details but also the general meaning of pictures, though he had extreme difficulty in formulating aloud what he had learnt from them.

Shown a picture of two Belgian gunners explaining the mechanism of a field-gun to a British Red Cross woman worker at the Front, he said: "It's the ladies... come on the hospital...come to see how men work it." *Q.* "What sort of men are they?" *A.* "Till France...the men come from France...the France men... she might come from England...lady." *Q.* "What are they showing her?" *A.* "A gun...a 75 isn't it?"

He was then told to read the legend aloud, which he did as follows: "Belgian gunners explode...no, explay...the max-stick something...of their wetton...to a Red Cross...worker, worker...She belongs to the British nursing...some corps" (Belgian gunners explaining the mechanism of their weapon to a Red Cross worker. She belongs to a British Nursing Yeomanry Corps.)

I then asked: "What is the picture now?" and he answered: "It's a guns belongs to Belgian...She a hospital lady from England...comes from England... The Belgians just telling what it's made of...the different names, the works and..."

Writing. Asked to write his name and address, he did so rapidly as Frank Edwe Sams, 203 Parkhurst Road, Manor Park, E.; but when he attempted to do the same for his mother with whom he lived, he failed entirely. I said to him: "Now write your mother's address"; he hesitated and asked: "What, her name before?" To this I replied: "No, her name now; as if you were going to direct a letter to her." He wrote "S"; then after a pause: "Sams," and, saying "Susie," gave up the attempt. Urged to try again, he wrote "S. Sams 203," and said: "No, I can't, you mean her address? No, I can't."

In response to a request to write a letter, he produced the following: "My dear Sister I now write to you that I hame getting the best of hearl, and I am getting to walk to the garden to play a lot of game and I hame the all of." Asked to read aloud what he had written he said: "My dear Sister I now write to you that I am now getting the best of health, and I getting to walk to the garden to play a lot of games, and I have the whole of...I've forgotten now what I was going to say."

He spent much of his time on the balcony reading the newspaper and I asked him to choose some passage, which was of interest, and to write down for me what it conveyed to him; for he told me he liked reading, "but I can't say it." The result was as follows: "the men of the rich we have been fiching for a day and we have gorn 200 yard of and we will go a..." I then enquired, "What did you want to write?" and he answered, "Our division was firing...was firing all day...was fighting all day and all the regiment...all the regiment had moved...at night all the regiment moved on...two hundred yards all our regiment."

The alphabet was written as follows: *a b c d e f g h i j k l m n o p u r s t*[1] *u y w x y z*, and when dictated, *a b c d e f g h i j k l m n o p* Q R S T U X *w z y z*.

Numbers and coins. He named every coin correctly throughout a series of twenty-one tests, and had no difficulty in expressing the relative value of any two of them to one another. Simple addition and subtraction were carried out perfectly. The coin-bowl test evidently presented no difficulty and the various movements were executed without mistake both to oral and printed commands.

[1] Probably an uncrossed t.

Drawing and pictures. Asked to draw a spirit-lamp placed before him on the table, he produced an excellent picture, and said, "I was good drawder...drawer ...at school." The model was removed and ten minutes later he was asked to draw it from memory; the result was an almost exact reproduction.

Then I said to him, "Draw me an elephant." He replied, "Yes I seen them... up other end...India." He then produced the following figure (Fig. 27).

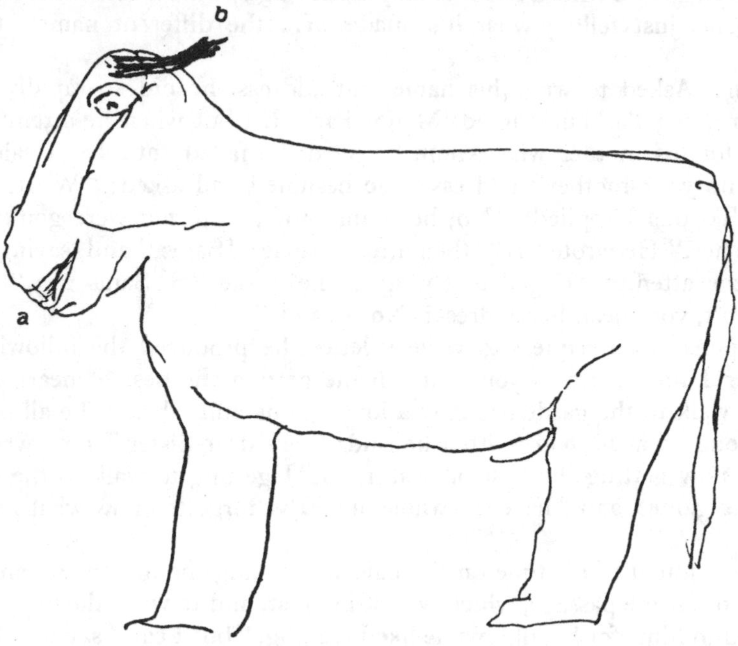

Fig. 27. Attempt by No. 15 to draw an elephant to command. When drawing in the region marked (*a*) he said "mouth"; then uttering the words "irons," "highons," he added in the region marked (*b*) structures evidently intended for horns.

When drawing (*a*) he said "mouth," and then uttering the words "irons," "highons," he added to the picture what were evidently intended for horns. After he had finished I asked, "What has an elephant got in front?" He answered, "They carry big trees...tied round a bit of an iron thing." I then said, "Behind you have given him a tail, what has he in front?" He replied, "He has a big one, quite straight, about a yard long." *Q*. "What is it called?" *A*. "Same what you drive water with." *Q*. "Has your elephant got a trunk?" *A*. "He's lost it" and at once he wanted to add the missing part. I then pointed to the horns he had drawn on the head of his figure, asking, "Has an elephant got horns?" He replied, "Yes silver what you stick out" (pointing to the corner of his mouth and placing his pencil into the position of a tusk). *Q*. "What are they made of?" *A*. "Kind of a white bone one, what grows in the mouth, on the roof, on the edge of the mouth." Evidently he had been confused by saying the jargon words representing horns, and impulsively added them to the figure; but he was finally able to explain his error by gestures, giving a correct interpretation of his intention.

Games. He played a perfect game of dominoes and was excellent at bowls.

Serial Tests.

(1) *Naming and recognition of common objects.* All these tests were carried out correctly, but on two occasions he called a pencil "black lead" or "blacking"; otherwise his nomenclature was accurate, and he was quick in selecting the object named orally or in print.

(2) *Naming and recognition of colours.*

Table 1.

	Pointing to colour shown	Oral commands	Printed commands	Naming colours shown	
				1st series	2nd series
Black	Perfect	Perfect	Perfect	Correct	Correct
Red	"	"	"	"	"
Orange	"	"	"	"Can't say it"	"
White	"	"	"	Correct	"
Green	"	"	"	"Gur...green"	"
Violet	"	"	"	"Vilet[1]"	"Volley"
Blue	"	"	"	Correct	Correct
Black	"	"	"	"	"
Red	"	"	"	"	"Blue"
Orange	"	"	"	Slow, correct	"Vilet"
White	"	"	"	Correct	Correct
Green	"	"	"	"Blue"	Slow, correct
Violet	"	"	"	"Volley"	"Volley"
Blue	"	"	"	Correct	Correct
Black	"	"	"	"	"
Red	"	"	"	"	"
Orange	"	"	"	"Can't think of it"	"More like a yellow one"
White	"	"	"	Correct	Correct
Green	"	"	"	"	"
Violet	"	"	"	"Vilet[1]"	"Bluey"
Blue	"	"	"	Correct	Correct

[1] Probably, as a Londoner, his normal pronunciation was "vilet."

Here again he chose correctly to oral or printed commands, but the names he applied were less accurate and he was specially troubled by violet and orange.

(3) *The man, cat and dog tests.*

He read these short phrases aloud without difficulty, but wrote them down inaccurately, not infrequently reversing the order or substituting one noun for another. Exactly the same trouble occurred when he wrote to dictation. He could, however, copy these simple phrases perfectly.

Table 2.

	Written to dictation	Copied in cursive handwriting from the printed cards[1]	Reading aloud from the printed cards and writing what he had read	
			(a) Read aloud	(b) Wrote
The dog and the cat	The dog and the cot	Perfect	Perfectly	The dog and the cat
The man and the dog	The men of	,,	,,	The dog and the men
The cat and the man	The cot and the men	,,	,,	The cat and the men
The dog and the man	The dog and the men	,,	,,	The dog and the men
The dog and the cat	The dog and the cat	,,	,,	The dog and the cat
The man and the dog	The men and the dog	,,	,,	The men and the dog
The cat and the man	The cat and the dog	,,	,,	The men and the dog
The dog and the man	The dog and the cat	,,	,,	The men and the cat
The dog and the cat	The cat and the dog	,,	,,	The dog and the men
The man and the dog	The men and the dog	,,	,,	The man and the cat
The cat and the man	The cat and the men	,,	,,	The cat and the men
The dog and the man	The dog and the men	,,	,,	The dog and the man

[1] The handwriting was much better than in the written tests (1) or (3).

(4) *The clock tests.*

Table 3.

	Telling the time	Oral commands	Printed commands	Direct imitation	Writing down the time shown on a clock face	Printed commands read aloud and executed
10 minutes past 7	"Ten past seven"	Correct	Quick, correct	Perfect	10 minutes past 7	Both correct
20 minutes to 6	"A quarter to six"	,,	,,	,,	20 minutes to 6	,,
10 minutes to 1	"Ten to one"	Slow, correct	,,	,,	10 minutes to 1	,,
A quarter to 9	"Quarter to nine"	Correct	,,	,,	45 to 9	,,
20 minutes to 4	"Twenty to four"	4.20	,,	,,	20 to 4	,,
5 minutes to 2	"Five to two"	Correct	,,	,,	5 to 2	,,
20 minutes to 6	"Twenty to six"	,,	,,	,,	20 to 6	,,
Half-past 2	"Half-past two"	,,	,,	,,	30 past 2	,,
20 minutes past 11	"Twenty past eleven"	,,	,,	,,	20 past 11	,,
Half-past 1	"Half-past one"	,,	,,	,,	30 past 1	,,
5 minutes past 8	"Five past eight"	7.55	,,	,,	5 past 8	,,
25 minutes to 3	"Twenty-five to three"	2.40	,,	,,	25 to..."I forget"	,,
20 minutes past 9	"A quarter to four... nine twenty"	Correct	,,	,,	20 past 9	,,
10 minutes past 8	"Ten past eight"	Slow, correct	,,	,,	2 past 8	,,

He set one clock in exact imitation of another and told the time accurately. Printed orders were well executed, but oral commands were carried out somewhat slowly, and in two instances he mistook "to" and "past" the hour. He could write down the time on the whole correctly although his nomenclature was peculiar. Thus a quarter to nine became "45 to 9" and ten minutes past eight was written as "2 past 8" because the long hand, standing at ten minutes past the hour, pointed to the number 2.

(5) *The hand, eye and ear tests.*

He imitated my movements, when we sat face to face, correctly, though somewhat slowly, and executed pictorial commands with three slight errors only. When reflected in the mirror, these tests were carried out perfectly and without hesitation. His response to oral and printed commands was slow and in both cases he made several mistakes; but throughout it was easier for him to execute printed orders than those given by word of mouth.

Six weeks later he was readmitted. The observations on his speech were confirmed, but the physical signs had changed for the better. There was now no weakness of the right half of the face and the tongue was protruded straight; the reflexes were equal on the two halves of the body and both plantars gave a downward response. Motion and sensation were unaffected.

Table 4.

	Imitation of movements made by the observer	Imitation of movements reflected in a mirror	Pictorial commands	Pictorial commands reflected in a mirror	Oral commands	Printed commands
L. hand to R. eye	Correct	Perfect	Correct	Perfect	Reversed	Correct
R. hand to R. ear	,,	,,	,,	,,	R. hand to R. ear; then *eye*	R. hand to R. *eye*
R. hand to L. eye	Slow, correct	,,	,,	,,	Correct	Correct
L. hand to R. ear	Correct	,,	,,	,,	,,	L. hand to R. *eye*
R. hand to R. eye	,,	,,	L. hand to R. eye	,,	R. hand slowly to R. *ear*	Correct
L. hand to L. ear	,,	,,	L. hand to L. *eye*; then ear	,,	Correct	Slow, correct
L. hand to L. eye	,,	,,	Correct	,,	,,	,,
R. hand to L. ear	,,	,,	R. hand to L. *eye*; then ear	,,	,,	Correct
L. hand to R. eye	,,	,,	Correct	,,	,,	,,
R. hand to R. ear	,,	,,	,,	,,	,,	Very slow, correct
R. hand to L. eye	,,	,,	,,	,,	,,	Correct
L. hand to R. ear	,,	,,	,,	,,	,,	,,
R. hand to R. eye	,,	,,	,,	,,	,,	,,
L. hand to L. ear	,,	,,	,,	,,	,,	,,
L. hand to L. eye	,,	,,	,,	,,	,,	L. hand; then R. hand to L. eye
R. hand to L. ear	,,	,,	,,	,,	Very slow, correct	Correct
L. hand to R. eye	,,	,,	,,	,,	,,	,,
R. hand to R. ear	,,	,,	,,	,,	Correct	,,
R. hand to L. eye	,,	,,	,,	,,	,,	,,
L. hand to R. ear	,,	,,	,,	,,	,,	,,
R. hand to R. eye	,,	,,	,,	,,	"No, I can't"	,,
L. hand to L. ear	,,	,,	,,	,,	L. hand to R. ear	,,
L. hand to L. eye	,,	,,	,,	,,	Correct	Slow, correct
R. hand to L. ear	,,	,,	,,	,,	R. hand to L. *eye*	Very slow, correct

CONDITION IN OCTOBER 1920 (*five years and nine months after he was wounded*).

The scar was in perfect condition, deeply depressed and not pulsating. It was not tender and gave him no discomfort. He suffered from no headache or vomiting, but complained that occasionally a "smell of gas" came into his mouth, which turned him from his food. This was not associated with any external manifestations, and passed unnoticed by his wife and parents. He was not unconscious, even for a few moments, but he complained, "Sometimes smell of gas coming out of my mouth; taste or something. Want to be sick and can't. Nasty smell comes out of the mouth. Feel I want to be sick; stop me eat, eat up half my dinner and can't."

The left globe had been extracted and the socket was in perfect condition. Vision of the right eye was $\frac{6}{6}$, but careful perimetric examination under favourable conditions showed that there was distinct limitation of the upper and outer portion of the visual field. The boundaries were difficult to define and seemed to shade gradually into parts where the sight was preserved. On ophthalmoscopic examination the inner half of the disc was somewhat pale, but its edges were clear, and there were no signs of optic neuritis.

Hearing of the right ear was normal, and a watch could be appreciated at a distance of 4 ft. With the left ear he said he could not hear the watch on contact, but a tuning fork was audible at about 4 in.; when placed on the forehead it was said to be heard better in the right than in the left ear. The left membrane was somewhat withdrawn and thickened.

Symbolic Formulation and Expression.

He was married and lived on his pension; neither he nor his wife did any work, but they spent most of their time walking about London in the parks and wherever there was anything to be seen. Mentally he was in the same state as before; to direct examination he was an excellent subject and his answers were remarkably constant, but, when he attempted to narrate his introspective experiences, he became confused and frequently gave up trying to make himself understood.

Articulated speech. He still talked jargon, which was usually comprehensible if the subject of conversation was known. Thus, wanting to explain to me about a hernia, which had developed since he had left the hospital, he said, "I got that rupture, after left hospital, when dark, no lights, when airships came over. Couldn't see, smashed the wall, the house like, smashed into wall, couldn't see. Had a pain, saw doctor, pushed it to. If it should come up, press it up and use what you call 'em. When it do go up, pain inside."

He could repeat single words or even simple phrases, such as those of the man, cat and dog tests, without difficulty. But, when asked to repeat short sentences, which he had not heard before, his defective syntax became evident. For example, "I have not suffered from headache lately" became "I have not suffered headache"; "I am afraid there is going to be a coal strike" was repeated as "I afraid there is going to be a coal strike," and "It was difficult to find your house to-day," "It's difficult to find your house again." I then asked him to repeat together the three sentences he had said, but he answered, "There is a coal strike. I can't think."

Understanding of spoken words. He had no difficulty in choosing a common object or colour named by me, or in setting a clock to oral commands. Even the complex hand, eye and ear tests, though slowly executed, were carried out with two mistakes only.

But there was no doubt that he occasionally failed to comprehend exactly what he was told to do in the course of general conversation. An order given in the form of a single word or short phrase led to a prompt response. But his father, who was a builder, said that it was impossible to employ him, because of his unexpected lapses of memory; thus, told to fetch a ladder, he would bring a short plank, although he seemed at first to appreciate the nature of the order. On testing him carefully this seemed to depend on want of power to reproduce exactly a phrase or sentence he had heard; so long as the order was comprised in a single word, it was performed without hesitation.

Reading. He had no difficulty in reading single words or the various combinations of the man, cat and dog tests. But he failed badly when made to read aloud a paragraph from the newspaper (vide infra). He said, "It's all right these small words: thick ons can't understand 'em."

He chose a common object or colour and set the clock correctly to printed commands: single words, or small verbal groups, seemed to give him no trouble. But he carried out the hand, eye and ear tests slowly and inaccurately.

Writing. His signature was written perfectly and he no longer had any difficulty with the name and address of his mother. Single words used as names were badly spelt and his handwriting was poor. Simple phrases, such as those of the man, cat and dog tests, when dictated, were extremely well written, though he failed badly in his attempts to reproduce a series of descriptive sentences in writing (vide infra).

Numbers, etc. He could count perfectly and solved correctly the six simple arithmetical problems usually set. He had no difficulty with money or with the names and relative value of coins.

Drawing and pictures. Told to draw an elephant he produced an inadequate figure without a trunk or tusks.

I then asked him to point to the various parts of the beast, and he said: "Zisis ear" (this is his ear); "Head" "Nose" (Trunk), "Legs," "Tail," "Body," "Eye," "Mouth." I said, "Have you left out anything?" *A.* "No." *Q.* "From his mouth?" *A.* "Bonezinks" (Bone things).

General understanding of words and pictures. To test his power of speech, reading, writing, together with the understanding of words and pictures, he was shown a photograph of a railway station during the war, where a collecting box had been placed for flowers to be sent to the wounded. Beneath was printed the following description: "This box has been placed on the platform at Snaresbrook Station as a receptacle for flowers for the wounded. Many of the passengers contribute nosegays daily from their gardens and these are sent to the Bethnal Green Infirmary." This he read silently and, on attempting to describe in writing what he had read, got no further than "Fres flours for wooded solders for sail." The passage was dictated to him and he wrote: "The box has been on the platform at s slaton at for for the woȯded many of the pas...c...no get dail for ther and to the...infom." He then read the legend aloud as follows: "This box has placed on the...platform at...can't name either...station...at a...no sir...for flowers for the wounded. Any of the...passengers can't stand (understand) that letter...nosegay...daily...for the gardens...and these are sent...to the Befnal Green...Infirm." I then asked him to show me the different objects in the picture and he pointed them out, saying, "Two ladies" "buying flowers," "flowers for wounded soldiers," "box" "at Bethnal Green"; then reading the words on the box "Firmry." He evidently had not comprehended exactly what he had read, and was misled by his first statement that the flowers were "for sail"; for pointing to the station master he said, "He's selling 'em." Then he was told to copy the description and did so perfectly; but asked to narrate what he had just written he said, "Flowers for sale; selling at stations. At Bethnal Green, at Bethnal Green station."

Serial Tests.

(1) *Naming and recognition of common objects.*

Table 5.

	Pointing to object shown	Oral commands	Printed commands	Naming an object indicated	Writing name of object indicated	Duplicate placed in hand out of sight
Knife	Correct	Correct	Correct	"knife"	knif	Correct
Key	,,	,,	,,	"kay"	key	,,
Penny	,,	,,	,,	"penny"	Pennie	,,
Matches	,,	,,	,,	"matches"	match	,,
Scissors	,,	,,	,,	"scissors"	cissis	,,
Pencil	,,	,,	,,	"pencil"	pencle	,,
Key	,,	,,	,,	"key"	key	,,
Scissors	,,	,,	,,	"scissors"	cissis	,,
Matches	,,	,,	,,	"masses"	match	,,
Knife	,,	,,	,,	"knife"	knif	,,
Penny	,,	,,	,,	"penny"	pennie	,,
Matches	,,	,,	,,	"matches"	match	,,
Scissors	,,	,,	,,	"scissors"	sissor	,,
Pencil	,,	,,	,,	"pencil"	pencle	,,
Penny	,,	,,	,,	"penny"	pennie	,,
Knife	,,	,,	,,	"knife"	knif	,,
Key	,,	,,	,,	"key"	key	,,
Pencil	,,	,,	,,	"pencil"	pencle	,,
	very quick					very quick

Oral and printed commands were carried out perfectly, and he named the various objects on the table before him correctly, apart from slight errors of pronunciation. This verbal deformation, with perfect nomenclature, was still more evident when he attempted to write the name of an object shown him.

(2) *Naming and recognition of colours.*

Oral and printed commands were accurately executed, and most of the names given to the colours were rightly pronounced. But if he attempted to write them down the words were deformed, although the nomenclature was obviously correct. Even when he was allowed to say the names aloud, he wrote them equally badly.

Table 6.

	Pointing to colour shown	Oral commands	Printed commands	Naming colour shown	Writing down name of colour shown	Naming colour shown and writing down the name	
						He said	He wrote
Black	Correct	Correct	Correct	Correct	Correct	Correctly	Correctly
Red	,,	,,	,,	,,	,,	,,	,,
Blue	,,	,,	,,	"Bē-lue"	,,	,,	,,
Green	,,	,,	,,	Correct	gren	,,	gren
Orange	,,	,,	,,	,,	orgen	,,	orgen
White	,,	,,	,,	,,	whit	,,	what
Violet	,,	,,	,,	"Vilet"	viren	Vilet	vorat
Yellow	,,	,,	,,	"Yeller"	dewor	Yeller	yerow
Red	,,	,,	,,	Correct	Correct	Correctly	Correctly
White	,,	,,	,,	,,	whit	,,	what
Yellow	,,	,,	,,	"Yeller"	lemon	Yeller	yerow
Blue	,,	,,	,,	Correct	Correct	Correctly	Correctly
Green	,,	,,	,,	,,	gren	,,	gren
Black	,,	,,	,,	,,	blak	,,	blak
Orange	,,	,,	,,	,,	orgen	,,	orgon
Violet	,,	,,	,,	"Vilet"	viron	vilet	vorat

(3) *The man, cat and dog tests.*

Table 7.

	Reading aloud	Reading from pictures	Writing from dictation	Writing from pictures	Repetition	Reading what he had written
The dog and the cat	Correct	"Cat Dog"	The dog and the cat	dog and cat	Correct	Correct
The man and the dog	,,	"Man Dog"	The man and th dog	man and dog	,,	,,
The cat and the man	,,	"Man and cat"	The cat and the man	man and cat	,,	,,
The cat and the dog	,,	"Dog and cat"	The cat and th dog	dog and cat	,,	,,
The dog and the man	,,	"Man and dog"	The dog and the man	man and dog	,,	,,
The man and the cat	,,	"Man and cat"	The man and th cat	man and cat	,,	,,
The dog and the man	,,	"Man and dog"	The man and th dog	man and dog	,,	,,
The cat and the man	,,	"Man and cat"	The cat and the mam	man and cat	,,	,,
The dog and the cat	,,	"Dog and cat"	The dog and th cat	dog and cat	,,	,,
The man and the dog	,,	"Man and dog"	The man and the dog	man and dog	,,	,,
The cat and the dog	,,	"Cat and dog"	The cat and the dog	cat and dog	,,	,,
The man and the cat	,,	"Man and cat"	The man and th cat	man and cat	,,	,,

These simple phrases were read aloud and repeated after me correctly. But as soon as he was asked to read or write from pictures, a curious tendency to reverse the order of the two nouns became apparent. Thus, shown two pictures, a cat to the left and a man to the right, he both said and wrote "man and cat." Yet this was not universal, for on the next occasion the same combination was given correctly. Reversals of this kind also occurred when the phrases were written to my dictation; it seemed as if he found difficulty in repeating the words to himself in the correct order.

(4) *The clock tests.*

Table 8.

	Direct imitation	Clock set to oral commands	Clock set to printed commands	Telling the time	Writing down the time shown on the clock
5 minutes to 2	Perfect	Correct	Correct	"Five to two"	five to 2
Half-past 1	,,	,,	,,	"Half-past one"	half past 2
5 minutes to 8	,,	,,	,,	"Five to eight"	five to 8
20 minutes to 4	,,	,,	,,	"Twenty to four"	20 to for
10 minutes past 7	,,	,,	,,	"Ten past seven"	Ten past 7
20 minutes to 6	,,	,,	,,	"Twenty to six"	20 to six
A quarter past 12	,,	,,	,,	"Quarter past twelve"	¼ past 12
10 minutes to 1	,,	,,	,,	"Ten to one"	Ten to one
A quarter to 9	,,	,,	,,	"Quarter to nine"	¼ to 9
Half-past 2	,,	,,	,,	"Half-past two"	half past 2
20 minutes past 11	,,	,,	,,	"Twenty past 'leven"	20 past 11
25 minutes to 8	,,	,,	,,	"Five and twenty to eight"	25 to 8
A quarter past 6	,,	,,	,,	"Quarter past six"	half past 6
25 minutes to 3	,,	,,	,,	"Five and twenty three"	25 to 3
10 minutes past 4	,,	,,	,,	"Ten past four"	10 past 4

He set the clock to oral and printed commands and told the time correctly. When he attempted to write down the time shown on a clock set by me, the words were deformed, but the nomenclature was accurate.

(5) *Hand, eye and ear tests.*

Table 9.

	Imitation of movements made by the observer	Imitation of movements reflected in a mirror	Pictorial commands	Pictorial commands reflected in a mirror	Oral commands	Printed commands	Printed commands read aloud and executed		Writing down movements made by the observer
							He said	Movement executed	
L. hand to L. eye	Correct	Perfect	Correct	Perfect	Slow, correct	L. hand to L. *ear*	Correctly	L. hand to L. *ear*	Correct
R. hand to R. ear	,,	,,	,,	,,	,,	Slow, correct	,,	Correct	,,
R. hand to L. eye	,,	,,	,,	,,	,,	,,	,,	,,	,,
L. hand to R. eye	,,	,,	,,	,,	,,	,,	,,	,,	L. hand to L. eye
L. hand to L. ear	,,	,,	,,	,,	,,	,,	,,	,,	Correct
R. hand to R. eye	,,	,,	,,	,,	,,	,,	"R. hand to R. *ear*, eye"	R. hand to R. *ear*	,,
L. hand to R. ear	,,	,,	,,	,,	,,	,,	Correctly	Correct	L. hand to R. *eye*
R. hand to L. ear	,,	,,	,,	,,	,,	,,	,,	,,	Correct
L. hand to L. eye	,,	,,	,,	,,	L. hand to L. *ear*	L. hand to L. *ear*	,,	,,	,,
R. hand to R. ear	,,	,,	,,	,,	Slow, correct	Slow, correct	,,	,,	,,
R. hand to L. eye	,,	,,	,,	,,	,,	,,	"R. hand to L. *ear*, eye"	R. hand to L. *ear*; corrected	,,
L. hand to R. eye	,,	,,	,,	,,	L. hand to R. *ear*	R. hand, then correct	Correctly	Correct	,,
L. hand to L. ear	,,	,,	,,	,,	Slow, correct	Slow, correct	,,	,,	L. hand to L. *eye*
R. hand to R. eye	,,	,,	,,	,,	,,	,,	,,	,,	R. hand to R. *ear*
L. hand to R. ear	,,	,,	,,	,,	,,	,,	,,	,,	L. hand to R. *eye*
R. hand to L. ear	,,	,,	,,	,,	,,	,,	,,	,,	Correct

He imitated my movements, sitting face to face, and carried out pictorial commands without mistakes of any kind; but he was much quicker and more certain when either of these orders was reflected in a mirror. Both oral and printed commands were executed slowly and imperfectly. He made several mistakes in writing down the nature of movements made by me, although he could imitate them without fail.

CONDITION IN DECEMBER 1922 (*seven years and ten months after he was wounded*).

He was in excellent general physical health. But the hallucinations which he described as "Nasty smell in mouth; make you sick like" had recurred about every fortnight. In April, 1921, they were followed by a definite epileptiform attack in which he became unconscious; further similar seizures occurred in August and November, 1921, and in October, 1922. The last of these was seen from start to finish by his parents. He was sitting on the sofa, when he lost consciousness and fell back struggling; he did not wet himself or bite his tongue, but the attack was accompanied by characteristic chewing movements. He complained that each seizure was preceded by the "nasty smell" and, when I enquired whether he had been troubled by vomiting, he replied, "Dirty, like be sick, makes me like sick and I can't; comes out of my mouth and nasty smell of it." *Q.* "What comes out of your mouth?" *A.* "Nasty smell. Try to be sick and can't. It might be two weeks, perhaps three weeks, might get 'em two, three days. The strength of my leg goes out of my leg when I'm like that."

He had suffered occasionally from pains in the head, and he pointed to the left half of the forehead and around the left eye. It was extremely difficult to discover their character, except that they made his head "thick"; he said, "Get out, lay down, go to sleep, sometimes goes away. If sit in kitchen, moving about working makes me getting worse on it."

Vision in the right eye was $\frac{6}{6}$, but there was no doubt that it was lost in the upper outer quadrant of the field. This scotoma had no definite boundaries, merging into parts where vision was defective. Disc and fundus were not abnormal.

Hearing was defective; a watch could be heard at a distance of 5 ft. on the right side, whilst in the left ear it was not even appreciated on contact. He said he heard a tuning fork, placed in the centre of the forehead, on the right side only; but over the left mastoid it was certainly audible, although the duration was shortened in comparison with the right.

Smell was grossly defective in both nostrils and he did not even react to ammonia.

Taste was good when the tongue was withdrawn into the mouth, but not when it was extended. This is not abnormal in an habitual smoker.

The pupil reacted well, there was no ocular paralysis, and face and tongue moved equally well on the two sides. The reflexes were normal, including the plantars and abdominals. There was no paresis, incoordination, tremor, change in tone, or any other motor affection. Sensation was perfect; appreciation of posture and passive movement, discrimination of two points, localisation, recognition of differences in intensity, size, shape and weight, were equally good on the two sides.

Symbolic Formulation and Expression.

He was not in any way mentally defective; but a long course of idleness and inability to work had rendered him intellectually lazy. He lived on his pension in two rooms with his wife and child; she apparently talked to him very little and took no interest in his difficulties of speech. He never read a book or a newspaper.

Though he was still a willing witness and anxious to be examined, he was much more taciturn and less easily roused to say what he felt. He obviously recognised his disability in speaking and had grown used to remaining silent; but during our talks he became perceptibly brighter and more lively.

Articulated speech. His speech was difficult to understand without the most careful attention. He was liable to begin with some odd sound and frequently passed on without attempting to pronounce the word correctly; he probably failed to recognise that it was incomprehensible to his auditor. I have given above several examples of this jargon, and his condition so closely resembled what it was during his first stay in the London Hospital that I formed the opinion he was degenerating in consequence of the epileptiform attacks.

He repeated certain sentences after me as follows: "I have suffered from some headache lately" became "I have suffered from headache"; "On Saturday I had an attack," "On Sat-day I had attack"; "I find it difficult to speak," "I find it diff-cut speak...I find to speak." I then asked him to say them over once again all together, and he replied, "I had headache on Saturday...I can't zinc of thother" (the other). It was not so much the act of repetition which was at fault, but the power of retaining a phrase accurately in his memory sufficiently long to reproduce it.

Understanding of spoken words. He certainly understood what was said to him and could carry out oral commands, although he was a little uncertain with the complex hand, eye and ear tests. But there was no doubt that he occasionally failed to follow something said by me in the course of general conversation in answer to one of his remarks, and his father still found it impossible to employ him for this reason.

Reading. He chose a common object of colour and set the clock correctly to printed commands, but had more difficulty with the hand, eye and ear tests.

He could read aloud the simple phrases of the man, cat and dog tests, but had profound difficulty with a consecutive paragraph (vide infra); his jargon became particularly evident when he attempted to read aloud, and this led to great want of comprehension of the meaning of printed matter.

Writing. He wrote his name and address together with that of his wife fairly well, although Emma was written "Emme" and Colchester Avenue shortened to "Colchester Ave."

The following letter written spontaneously to me was certainly worse than his previous efforts:

"Dr. Head

just a line to you know I an allrigt as you ore the same. I for now Frank."

(This was evidently intended to be "Just a line to let you know that I am all right as I hope you are the same. I am for the present yours, Frank.")

He wrote badly to dictation but copied a long paragraph without a single mistake.

Printed paragraph read silently or aloud, written and narrated. I somewhat modified the procedure adopted in 1920, in order to make this test more specific. I gave him the following printed legend without its accompanying picture: "During the War a box was placed on the platform at Snaresbrook Station as a receptacle for flowers for the wounded. Many of the passengers brought nosegays daily from their gardens and these were sent to the Bethnal Green Infirmary." This he read silently and could tell me only, "During the War...there was some flo-wens at Station...Horspedl, I think...some green...No, can't zinc no more."

He read it through again to himself and wrote, "Do the war ther was fowers for the hoseple at the at the Gren."

He took the paper into his hand again and read aloud: "Durin the war...a box...was placed on...on the plaf-orm...at...can't memb' it...station...as a...no sir, can't get it...for flowers...for the...woun-ed...many of the...passengers...brought...no-gays...daily...from the gardens...and those were sent...to the...Bet-nel Green...In-fir-mary."

I then said, "Tell me what you have understood?" He replied, "Some flowers for the wounded...in the Hospedl...the Hospital...No, sir."

To my dictation he wrote, "Doing the war a box was Place on the plapfon at slaion as a resel for flers for the wooded. Many of the stition brout nos-gays daily from thir garnen lhes (these) wer sent to the Belnol Gren Infemer."

But, when asked to copy this paragraph in cursive handwriting, he carried out the task perfectly without a single mistake.

Asked, however, what he had understood he could only reply, "Got to the stashn...for some flowers...for the wounded Horpedls...at Burnel Green... ain't it...Bur-nal Green."

Numbers and arithmetic. He counted slowly and deliberately up to 30, and I noticed no defects of pronunciation until he came to "thirty-tree" (thirty-three). He continued correctly up to 39, but, instead of saying "forty," began the thirties over again, reaching 44 without a mistake. From this point he became uncertain, saying, for instance, "62, 64, 66, 57, 58, 59, 60"; he was perpetually thrown out of his stride and tempted thereby into some false sequence. At 70 he broke down altogether, saying "No, I can't think more."

Addition.			Subtraction.		
215	238	385	234	281	512
324	424	638	123	168	389
429 (wrong)	6312 (wrong)	91113 (wrong)	111	124 (wrong)	3 (Then gave up)

Coins and their relative value. All the coins were named correctly and their relative value was given without fail, though rather slowly. When shopping he had no difficulty with change, as far as I could gather from his relatives.

Drawing. He drew a good picture of a spirit-lamp both from the model and subsequently from memory. Asked if he could "see the lamp," when drawing from memory, he replied, "See whole lamp and glass...and glass...bit of string to light it" (the wick). But he drew an extremely poor representation of an elephant, without trunk or tusks.

His ground-plan of the room in which we worked was on the other hand accurate in every particular.

Serial Tests.

It is interesting to notice how closely these observations bore out the results obtained more than two years earlier, a testimony to the trustworthiness of the methods employed.

(1) *Naming and recognition of common objects.*

Table 10.

	Pointing to object shown	Naming	Oral commands	Printed commands	Writing name of object indicated
Knife	Perfect	Correct	Correct	Correct	kinfe
Key	,,	,,	,,	,,	key
Penny	,,	,,	,,	,,	Pomey
Matches	,,	,,	,,	,,	Mahey
Scissors	,,	,,	,,	,,	Cyses
Pencil	,,	,,	,,	,,	ponsel
Key	,,	,,	,,	,,	key
Scissors	,,	,,	,,	,,	Cyses
Matches	,,	,,	,,	,,	Mayes
Knife	,,	,,	,,	,,	knefe
Penny	,,	,,	,,	,,	poney
Matches	,,	,,	,,	,,	Moyes
Scissors	,,	,,	,,	,,	Cyses
Pencil	,,	,,	,,	,,	ponsel
Penny	,,	,,	,,	,,	Poney
Knife	,,	,,	,,	,,	knefe
Key	,,	,,	,,	,,	key
Pencil	,,	,,	,,	,,	ponsel

All these tests were carried out perfectly except when he attempted to write the name of an object indicated; then his spelling became worse than might have been expected from the state of his education and the words were curiously malformed.

(2) *Naming and recognition of colours.*

Table 11.

	Pointing to colour shown	Naming	Oral commands	Printed commands	Writing name of colour indicated
Black	Perfect	Correct	Correct	Correct	Block
Red	,,	,,	,,	,,	Red
Blue	,,	"Bĕ-lew"	,,	,,	Bue
Green	,,	Correct	,,	,,	Gran
Orange	,,	,,	,,	,,	Oren
White	,,	"Whide"	,,	,,	whit
Violet	,,	"Brown"	,,	,,	Velen
Yellow	,,	"Yeller"	,,	,,	Yolow
Red	,,	Correct	,,	,,	Red
White	,,	,,	,,	,,	whit
Yellow	,,	,,	,,	,,	Yolow
Blue	,,	,,	,,	,,	bue
Green	,,	,,	,,	,,	Grem
Black	,,	,,	,,	,,	Blok
Orange	,,	,,	,,	,,	Oren
Violet	,,	"Brown"	,,	,,	Valen

His choice to oral and printed commands was excellent, but his pronunciation of the names was not perfect and, on attempting to write them down, the words were badly formed. Throughout, the more abstract colours gave him greater difficulty than the concrete names of common objects.

(3) *The man, cat and dog tests.*

Table 12.

	Reading aloud	Repetition	Reading from pictures	Writing from pictures	Writing from dictation	Copied from print in cursive script	Reading aloud and writing	
							He read	He wrote
The dog and the cat	Correct	Correct	"Cat...dog"	Cat and dog	The dog and cat	Perfect	Correctly	The cat and dog
The man and the dog	,,	"Man and dog"	"The dog and the man"	man and dog	The man and dog	,,	,,	The man and the dog
The cat and the man	,,	"Cat and the man"	"Cat and the man"	Man and Cat	The man and cat	,,	,,	the cat and man
The cat and the dog	,,	"Cat and the dog"	"Dog and the cat"	Cat and dog	The cat and dog	,,	,,	the cat and dog
The dog and the man	,,	Correct	"Dog and the man"	Dog and man	The dog and man	,,	,,	the dog and cat
The man and the cat	,,	,,	"Cat and the man"	Man and cat	The cat and man	,,	,,	the man and cat
The dog and the man	,,	"Dog and the man"	"Man and the dog"	Man and dog	The dog and man	,,	,,	the man and dog
The cat and the man	,,	Correct	"Man and the cat"	Man and cat	The cat and man	,,	,,	the cat and man
The dog and the cat	,,	,,	"Dog and the cat"	Dog and cat	The dog and man	,,	,,	The cat and dog
The man and the dog	,,	"Man and the dog"	"Man and the dog"	Man and dog	The man and dog	,,	,,	the Man and dog
The cat and the dog	,,	"Cat and the dog"	"Cat and the dog"	Cat and dog	The cat and man	,,	,,	The cat and dog
The man and the cat	,,	"The man and a cat"	"Man and the Cat"	Man and cat	The man and cat	,,	,,	The man and dog

He read aloud and copied these simple phrases perfectly and made no definite mistakes in repeating the words after me. But, with every other form of this test, he showed the same extraordinary tendency to alter the sequence of the two nouns, which was so apparent in previous observations. On reading from pictures he frequently went from right to left instead of in the usual direction, and this reversal occurred even when he wrote the words to my dictation. Similar mistakes in writing occurred after he had read each phrase aloud; for, although he said exactly what was put before him in print, he made many errors in the sequence of the words he wrote.

(4) *The clock tests.*

Table 13.

	Direct imitation	Telling the time	Oral commands	Printed commands (both ordinary nomenclature and rail-way time)	Writing down the time shown on a clock
5 minutes to 2	Correct	"Five to two"	Correct	Correct	Five to to
Half-past 1	,,	"Half past one"	,,	,,	half pas one
5 minutes past 8	,,	"Fi pās eight"	,,	,,	Five pas Eigt
20 minutes to 4	,,	"Twenty to four"	,,	,,	temy to fur
10 minutes past 7	,,	"Ten past seven"	,,	,,	Ten pas sevn
20 minutes to 6	,,	"Twenty to six"	,,	,,	temy to sex
10 minutes to 1	,,	"Ten to one"	,,	,,	Ten to One
A quarter to 9	,,	"Qūār to nine"	,,	,,	45 to nie
20 minutes past 11	,,	"Twenty pās leven"	,,	,,	Temy past 11
25 minutes to 3	,,	"Twenty five to three"	,,	,,	35 to tre

He set a clock to oral and printed commands and told the time correctly: his only faults were those of pronunciation. When he attempted to write down the time, his spelling was remarkably bad and he tended to adopt an abnormal nomenclature, such as "45 to 9" instead of "a quarter to nine."

(5) *The hand, eye and ear tests.*

He imitated my movements slowly, when we sat face to face, and made a few mistakes in executing pictorial commands; but he was extremely quick and accurate if either form of order was reflected in a mirror. He wrote down imperfectly movements made by me, sometimes reversing the order of hand and eye or ear. Oral and printed commands were also carried out somewhat slowly, and in these tests he made several errors.

Table 14.

	Imitation of movements made by the observer	Imitation of movements reflected in a mirror	Pictorial commands	Pictorial commands reflected in a mirror	Oral commands	Printed commands	Writing down movements made by the observer	Copying printed commands in cursive script
L. hand to L. eye	Correct	Perfect	Correct	Perfect	Correct	Correct	Left eye hand left	Perfect
R. hand to R. ear	,,	,,	,,	,,	,,	,,	Rigt ere Rigt	,,
R. hand to L. eye	Very slow, corrected	,,	Reversed	,,	,,	,,	Rigt eyr Rigt	,,
L. hand to R. eye	Slow, correct	,,	Corrected	,,	,,	,,	left Rigt Eye	,,
L. hand to L. ear	,,	,,	Slow, correct	,,	,,	,,	left Ere left hand	,,
R. hand to R. eye	,,	,,	,,	,,	R. hand to R. *ear*	,,	Rigt Eye Rigt hand	,,
L. hand to R. ear		,,	,,	,,	Correct	L. hand to L. ear	left hand left Ere	,,
R. hand to L. ear	,,	,,	,,	,,	,,	Correct	Rigt hand left Ere	,,
L. hand to L. eye	,,	,,	R. hand to L. eye	,,	,,	,,	left hand left Eye	,,
R. hand to R. ear	,,	,,	Correct	,,	,,	,,	Rigt hand Right Ere	,,
R. hand to L. eye	,,	,,	,,	,,	,,	R. hand to L. *ear*	Rigt hand left Eye	,,
L. hand to R. eye	,,	,,	,,	,,	,,	Correct	left hand left Ege	,,
L. hand to L. ear	,,	,,	,,	,,	L. hand to R. ear	,,	left hand left Ere	,,
R. hand to R. eye	,,	,,	Reversed	,,	R. hand to R. *ear*	,,	Right hand Rigt Eye	,,
L. hand to R. ear	,,	,,	Correct	,,	Correct	L. hand to *R. eye*	Rigt hand Rigt Ere	,,
R. hand to L. ear	,,	,,	,,	,,	,,	Correct	Rigt Ere Rigt hand	,,

No. 17

A case of Verbal Aphasia, due to a gun-shot injury of the left hemisphere, extending between the inferior precentral and the lower third of the post-central fissures. About ten days afterwards a rifle bullet was removed from the brain and this operation was followed by the formation of an abscess. When he came under my care five months later, the wound was represented by a sinus from which exuded a considerable quantity of pus; this healed completely in three months.

At first he suffered from Jacksonian attacks in the right hand associated with a temporary increase in the loss of speech. These ceased entirely after healing of the wound.

He showed gross spastic hemiplegia in the right arm and leg with some weakness of the same half of the face and tongue. This was associated with profound changes in sensibility. All the deep reflexes on the right half of the body were exaggerated, the abdominals were absent and the plantar gave an upward response. Vision was in no way affected.

He showed characteristic difficulty in finding words to express his thoughts and said that at first he had no more than a "twenty word vocabulary." Words were uttered singly or in short groups, isolated by pauses of varying length, and a single word of many syllables was liable to be slurred. Even a year after the injury he could not say the alphabet perfectly and had much difficulty in counting. He was able to repeat the content of what was said to him, but had the same difficulty in word-formation as during spontaneous speech. He named objects shown him after considerable effort; this was due to defective power of verbal formation rather than to ignorance of their nomenclature. He seemed to understand completely what he heard and oral commands were executed with accuracy. But he confessed that, for a fortnight after he was wounded, he had difficulty in understanding things said to him, unless they were "very simple and said very slow." He carried out printed commands correctly, but could not read to himself with comfort, nor could he be certain that he understood exactly what was in the book before him. When he read aloud, his articulation showed the faults evident during voluntary speech, though to a less degree. He wrote slowly and with great effort, using the left hand. His spelling was preposterous considering his education and the form of the written words showed the same defects that were manifested in spontaneous speech. Similar errors were present when he wrote to dictation, but he copied the same passage from print without mistakes in cursive script. He counted slowly and with effort, yet he showed remarkable powers of arithmetic. If he uttered a wrong number, as when scoring at Bridge, he was not misled, but brought out a correct total. He drew excellently with his left hand. Orientation was not affected and he constructed a perfect ground-plan of his room at the hospital. He played card games well and enjoyed puzzles.

Lieut. W. L. W. first came under my care for a bullet wound of the brain on May 10th, 1915. He was then twenty-five years of age and up to the outbreak of war had been a medical student.

On December 13th, 1914, he was wounded with a rifle bullet, which penetrated the brain in the left Rolandic region. He fell, was not unconscious, but from the first moment suffered from "motor aphasia." He was entirely unable to speak and found it extremely difficult to write, but insists that he could understand what was said to him; when he tried to tell the surgeon in writing that he had taken a quarter of a grain of morphia, he was unable to do so, although he could write the word "opium."

During the week he spent at the clearing hospital his temperature ranged between 99° and 103° F. (37·2° to 39·4° C.); he was semi-conscious and the right hemiplegia became complete in face, arm and leg. He was then transferred to the base, where, about ten days after he was wounded, the bullet was removed from the brain through a trephine opening.

He was evacuated to an officers' hospital in England on January 16th, 1915, and both his power of speech and movement improved to such an extent that he was sent for convalescence to the country. Here he began to suffer from headache and had an epileptiform seizure, which necessitated his return to London. Shortly afterwards the small sinus at the site of the wound was opened up and two loose fragments of bone were removed (April 21st, 1915); but the local condition was not satisfactory and his temperature ranged between normal and 102° F. (38·8° C.).

When he first came under my care, on May 10th, 1915, the flap turned down at the original operation had healed and the wound was represented by a sinus from which issued a considerable quantity of pus. This opening was situated 16 cm. backwards along the nasion-inion line in the centre of an irregular area, from which bone had been removed; this measured 4·5 cm. vertically and 6 cm. horizontally, and extended between two points 13 cm. and 19 cm. posterior to the nasion. The upper border of this bony opening lay 6 cm. from the middle line of the scalp (Fig. 7, Vol. 1, p. 445).

He showed gross loss of power in the right arm and leg with some weakness of the same half of the face, and the tongue was protruded to the paralysed side. All the deep reflexes on the right half of the body were exaggerated, the abdominals were absent and the plantar gave an upward response. The reflexes on the left side were normal.

His subsequent progress can be divided into two periods. The first of these comprised the events directly due to active sepsis in the wound, whilst the second followed the healing of the local manifestations and was occupied with detailed examination of his speech defects and of the physical signs due to coincident destruction in the central nervous system.

The first stage can be dismissed in a few words; for although it was associated with many points of surgical interest, the condition of the patient at the time precluded the application of extensive and serial tests. Throughout the first month after admission to the London Hospital, the sinus continued to discharge pus; but his general condition improved and he seemed to be progressing slowly until June 8th, when he had an epileptiform seizure. This began with abnormal sensations accompanied by movements in the right hand, which spread to the whole upper extremity and ended in a general convulsion accompanied with loss of consciousness.

On June 16th the wound was therefore explored; a flap was turned down and this exposed an area of brain about 5 cm. in diameter which was uncovered by dura mater. Several fragments of bone were removed from a small pocket in the brain substance, which in turn communicated with a definite abscess cavity. This was evacuated and drained by a tube passed through the flap.

Whenever an attempt was made to discontinue this tube, his headache reappeared and he suffered from minor Jacksonian attacks, consisting mainly of "sensations" in the right hand. Finally a vaccine was prepared from the pus (staphylococci) and this was injected once a week from July 14th to August 21st. On August 5th the tube was removed successfully, and by August 19th the wound had healed completely. From this time onwards the local condition ceased to be of any importance in the clinical picture.

CONDITION DURING DECEMBER 1915 (*one year after he was wounded*).

During September, 1915, I was able to make a full neurological examination and to determine roughly the extent of his aphasia; but no complete series of observations on speech were possible until later in the year. As, however, the physical signs remained unaltered, I shall give an account of his condition between December 15th and 28th, 1915, when he was readmitted to hospital for investigation.

His mental state was extremely good; bright, cheerful and intelligent, he evinced keen interest in the tests to which he was exposed, and his comments were often of the greatest value.

He suffered from no headache unless he was over-fatigued; when it occurred at the end of a tiring day, the pain was both general and situated in the neighbourhood of the wound. It passed away entirely after sleep.

There had been no epileptiform seizure since July 21st. But about once in ten days he tended to suffer from "dizziness," which came on suddenly and was usually accompanied by tingling in the right hand. This was not associated with loss of consciousness or any convulsive movement. "I can read through the dizzy attack," he said, "but I can't speak so well for about ten minutes afterwards; I can speak, but not so well. I can understand what I read, but it is an effort." These attacks were diminishing in frequency and severity for at least six weeks before he was readmitted to hospital, in spite of the fact that he was taking no drugs.

Vision was $\frac{6}{6}$, the fields were normal and the discs showed no changes. Hearing, smell and taste were excellent. His pupils reacted normally; there was no ptosis, ocular paralysis or nystagmus. The lower half of the face on the right side moved slightly less than normal and the tongue was protruded definitely to the right.

The arm-, knee- and ankle-jerks were greatly exaggerated on the right side, the abdominal reflexes were absent and the plantar gave an upward response. All the reflexes from the left half of the body were normal.

On the right half of the body he showed the characteristic signs of a spastic hemiplegia. His grasp was feeble and isolated movements of the fingers were impossible. He possessed considerable power at the elbow and shoulder but the movements were clumsy. The whole limb was hypertonic; there were, however, no organic contractures.

The right lower extremity showed extreme extensor rigidity both at the knee and foot with considerable loss of power of dorsiflexion; plantar extension could be performed strongly. He could walk and stand alone but his gait was profoundly hemiplegic though without much ataxy.

He complained that the right hand felt as if it was covered with a glove and as if he had an extra pair of trousers on his right leg. He was always conscious of the existence of his arm and leg as somewhat numb; during the Jacksonian seizures, however, the right hand, and to a less extent the forearm, seemed to disappear, but returned to consciousness immediately the attack was at an end.

There was profound loss of recognition of passive movement and posture in the right hand and foot; elbow and ankle were also somewhat affected. With this was associated gross loss of appreciation of the vibrating tuning fork, inability to discriminate the compass points, poor localisation and defective sensibility to contact with the test-hairs over the hand and, to a less degree, over the sole of the foot. The response to prick and thermal stimuli was not demonstrably affected; but all power of recognising differences in weight, size and shape was lost in the right hand.

Symbolic Formulation and Expression.

When he was originally admitted to the hospital under my care, he spoke with characteristic slowness, finding his words with difficulty. He could not name objects to command, nor could he read aloud. He wrote his name and address and the telephone number of his temporary home, but could not transmit in writing the description of a consecutive series of events. He took an intelligent interest in all that went on around him, understood what was said, and executed oral commands of a simple order correctly.

He was not, however, in a suitable condition for complete examination; but, by December, 1915, he had so greatly improved both in general health and in his powers of speech, that I was able to make an extensive series of observations, which can be summarised as follows.

Articulated speech. He showed characteristic difficulty in finding words to express his thoughts. Left to himself he could laboriously describe his symptoms and was quite clear about what he wanted to say. He talked very slowly in a staccato manner and frequently was at a loss for a word. "I want to say a word, but it is at the back of my mind; I can't just...dig it up." Descriptive expressions such as "dig it up," for "remember," recurred frequently in his speech, especially when he showed some hesitation in expressing his meaning; but he steadily improved, both in the number of words at his disposal and in the ease with which he could use them. He confessed, "At first I don't think I had more than a twenty word vocabulary," and added, "I know I'm wrong, when I use an adjective. A few days ago I said a person was 'strong willed' and 'strong headed.' I knew it was not what I wanted to say and, about a day and a half afterwards, I said 'you wanted to say head-strong.'"

The alphabet was said as follows: "A B C D E F G H...H I J K L M...M ...O P Q...S T U V W X Y Z." He then began again at L, "L M M...L M N ...O P Q...R S T...U V W X Y Z." He said, "When I had trouble with R, it wasn't because I didn't know it, but because I had to think of the pronunciation. I wanted to say 'A' instead of 'R' because I was thinking of A R E."

The months were said in their correct order but January was called "Jun-ury" and February "Feb-urary."

Words were uttered singly or in short groups, isolated by pauses of varying length, and a single word of many syllables was liable to be slurred. Syntax and the grammatical structure of a phrase was not affected, except that he was often unable to complete it in accordance with the way in which it began. "I sometimes ...have to...alter the whole...to alter the sentence...because...I...have... difficulty...in finding...the word."

He was vividly conscious of his mistakes, even if he was unable to correct them. "I am always sure when I am wrong in what I say. If I am not certain of a thing I write it down and see; I may write it wrong, but when I see it I know it's wrong."

He could repeat the content of what was said to him correctly, but had the same difficulty in word-formation as during spontaneous speech, although the words were better formed and more easily pronounced.

But he suffered from more than a loss of articulatory power; his difficulty consisted in finding the words he required. I asked him to recite the chorus of a popular music hall ditty; this he did with great effort, much hesitation and very imperfectly. When I set the tune going on a gramophone, he sang the words with considerably greater ease; but many were omitted or slurred in his attempt to keep pace with the music. If, however, in addition I placed in his hand the printed words, he sang the chorus almost without hesitation, omitting nothing. His enunciation became perfect as soon as he had not to find the words and was supported by the tune.

Understanding of spoken words. He seemed to understand completely what was said and took a most intelligent interest in all that went on around him. He listened to our discussions over his bed as to his condition or treatment and would correct or assent to the statements made by house physician or nurse. Oral commands were executed quickly and accurately. But he confessed, "The first fortnight... I could not understand...things said to me...but very simple and said very slow...difficulty in fathom...fathom...words...digging them up. Now it's... only...mechanical...my tongue does not go right...I know it's not...the correct ...pronunciation...I don't always...corret it...because I shouldn't get it right ...in five or six times...unless someone...says it for me...I very often get the tense wrong...but I always know...it's the wrong tense."

Reading. He carried out printed commands correctly, even those of the complex hand, eye and ear tests. But he could not read to himself with comfort, nor could he be certain that in the long run he understood what was in the book before him. "I can't read a book to myself," he said, "because I'm bothered, when I say the words to myself. I can get the meaning of a sentence, if it's an isolated sentence, but I can't get all the words. I can't get the middle of the paragraph; I have to go back and start from the preceding full stop again."

He read aloud slowly, but with less hesitation than in speaking and the words were pronounced more correctly. Moreover, reading aloud evidently helped him to retain the meaning with greater certainty than when he read to himself.

Asked to read aloud the opening paragraphs of the *Vicar of Wakefield*[1] he did so slowly and with evident difficulty; but he then dictated from memory the following excellent account of what he had read: "I was always of the opinion that a man who was married and bred a large family, he was more use to the state than a man who was single and only talked of population. So when I took orders, I...I looked about for a wife and found one good-natured natural woman and though her gown was not...fine...it had the property...wedding gown, it had the property of wearing well. She...could read an English book without much spelling and as for her breeding no country lady could show better. But as for the pickling and cooking they were eslent (excellent). She prided herself on her housekeeping but I never found we were much in pocket over her...her...thrift...or her...

[1] "I was ever of opinion that the honest man, who married and brought up a large family, did more service than he who continued single, and only talked of population. From this motive, I had scarce taken orders a year, before I began to think seriously of matrimony, and chose my wife as she did her wedding-gown, not for a fine glossy surface, but such qualities as would wear well. To do her justice, she was a good-natured notable woman; and as for breeding, there were few country ladies who could show more. She could read any English book without much spelling; but for pickling, preserving, and cookery, none could excel her. She prided herself also upon being an excellent contriver in housekeeping; though I could never find that we grew richer with all her contrivances."

I want another word, but I can't get it." Six months later he explained that the word he strove to recall was "economy."

Writing. When he first came under my care he could write his name, address and telephone number, but not a consecutive sentence. Within a year of his wound, and four months after it had healed, he was able to write a short letter. But he wrote slowly and with great effort, saying, "I always have to spell out every word even the little ones; I have to say 'of'—I know it's a preposition, but then I have to think is it 'to' or 'from' or 'of.' Prepositions are always a bother to me." He complained, "It's no use my trying to spell out the words, when I am blocked for a word. But if I can visualise it I am alright, visualise the word as it is written. It's not the long words that stop me. Some words have gone; it may be words of four or five letters. It's not specially the long words that are the trouble. My spelling of Latin derivatives is better than that of other words. When I was puzzled over a word like 'help,' I had difficulty in knowing if l or p came last. My bankers are Holt and Co. At first I had difficulty in knowing whether the l or the t came last. Now I've written to them so often I've learnt it; I know the t comes last."

On another occasion he said, "I can't spell, I think I can write if I have tries on the blotting paper. I have difficulty, a little, in finding the words because I speak the thing out, when I write it. When I write a letter hurriedly, I hurry on and leave out lots of 'to's' and 'at's' and words. The easiest way for me to correct is to get somebody to read aloud and I say, wait a minute, I want to put in an 'of' or 'to.'" He continued as follows: "I'm teachable...If I spell a word...wrong... wrong...my wife tells me...I get it right...when I wrote...to my Bank man-ger ...I always spelt...'man' and 'ger'...She told me that...now I get it...right." But it is interesting to notice that this exactly expressed his pronunciation of the word "manager" at that time.

After reading to himself the opening paragraphs of the *Vicar of Wakefield*, he attempted to write down what he had gathered from them. But the effort was so great that he gave up the attempt after the first sentence. He wrote, "I was alway of the openion that a man who married and bred a large family was doing more for the State than a single man who only was the need of populisation."

He could copy a passage accurately from print in cursive handwriting; the letters were better formed and the script more legible than under other conditions.

To dictation his writing showed the same kind of mistakes, in word-formation and spelling, present when he wrote spontaneously. I dictated, "Lieutenant General Sir William Robertson, now chief of the General Staff, will become Chief of the Imperial General Staff with the temporary rank of General. No man ever better deserved it by ability, hard work and honesty of purpose." He wrote as follows: "Lieut.-General Sir Wm Robertson now chief of the general Staff will become chief of the imperial General Staff with the temporary rank of general. No man ever better deserved by a ability, hard work, and honesty of pupose."

The actual formation of the letters gave him no trouble and he wrote the alphabet consecutively without fault though somewhat slowly.

Numbers and arithmetic. He could count up to ten, a month after he had been wounded, and by December, 1915, could reach twenty slowly without error. He then went to thirty and stopped; when encouraged, he succeeded in counting up to a hundred, but ninety was called "nineteen."

He could solve simple arithmetical problems although he had considerable difficulty in expressing himself correctly in numbers. "When I am scoring in a game I say 28, when I mean 41. But that makes no difference to my score; I count 41 though I say 28. I do the sum right, but get the figures wrong." "When I first began to look at reference books, like the Army List, I couldn't say it was 982, when I looked a page up; but if I didn't try to say it, I could look up the page without any difficulty. If I tried to say it, I would say different numbers and then I would muddle myself and have to look it up again. Silent thought was easy, but vocal thought was muddling."

He kept accounts, checked his bank-book and was acutely alive to his financial position.

Drawing. He could draw excellently with his left hand from a model or from memory and produced a recognisable portrait of himself with the help of a mirror.

Orientation, etc. He had no difficulty in finding his way or in describing any familiar route accurately and minutely. His ground-plan of the private room he occupied in the hospital was perfect in every particular.

Visual images. He had a remarkable power of recalling visual impressions and relied upon them in his answers to the various tests. Thus, when drawing a ground-plan of his room he described the appearance of each object as it was inserted in its place and gave the colour of the curtains and walls correctly, saying, "I always did visualise in my work."

Appreciation of pictures. He recognised at once both the detailed and general significance of pictures and his comprehension of pictorial jokes was perfect.

Music and singing. Asked to say the words of the chorus of a popular song, his utterance was slow, his articulation defective, and he made several mistakes. He could, however, sing the melody alone correctly. I then set the tune with the words going on the gramophone and, though he found them more easily, they were still imperfectly pronounced. Finally, when I gave him the written words and started the melody again, he sang freely with little or no hesitation.

Thus, his difficulty was not in articulation, but in finding the words he required. The music helped him greatly to do this, and, if at the same time he was allowed to read the words, he could enunciate them almost perfectly.

Games, etc. He played a good game of Bridge and enjoyed putting together jigsaw puzzles.

Serial Tests.

Naming and recognition of objects. At first he could not find words in which to name objects in front of him. But he improved so greatly that, by the time he reached a condition in which full examination was possible, I used geometrical shapes in place of the usual common objects.

He selected with extreme ease and certainty the figure corresponding to that which he had been shown or held in his left hand out of sight, and he could indicate perfectly the one mentioned by me orally or printed on a card. He was even able to name them correctly, though with difficulty, if he was allowed to say "globe" for sphere and "egg" for what he once succeeded in calling "elliptical ovoid." Sometimes he called a pyramid "a solid I-soos-les (isosceles) triangle," but the nature of the object he was striving to name was never in doubt.

Asked to write the names of these solid figures, his nomenclature was correct, but his difficulty in spelling became manifest; pyramid became "pymared," sphere was written "shere," and he inserted the p afterwards. Throughout he was slow, pausing in the middle of writing a word; not infrequently he said the name aloud and then continued his laborious efforts to form the letters. When each word was finished, he looked it over and frequently corrected the defects; but "pymared" was missed until he had completed the whole series and the sheet had been removed. Then he suddenly said, "I'm sure pyramid was wrong; y should come before r, like this," and he wrote the word correctly on the blotting paper.

The clock tests. None of these tests gave him any difficulty at the stage of recovery when he could be systematically examined. He set the hands to oral or printed commands, told the time correctly and wrote down each position of the clock without fail. He said, "It's child's play to me. I could tell the time a fortnight after my wound. But a week after I was hit I was shown a watch; it was a quarter to two; but I couldn't say it I couldn't write it down and it did not convey anything to me. I didn't know it was time for lunch."

The hand, eye and ear tests. (Table 1.) These observations were of interest mainly on account of his explanatory remarks. He had not the slightest difficulty in executing oral or printed commands. When he sat opposite to me and imitated my movements, he twice began with the wrong hand, but on both occasions corrected himself and finished the series without even this trivial form of error. Pictorial commands were carried out with one error and two corrections on his part. But as soon as either my movements or the pictured attitudes were reflected in the glass he imitated them with great rapidity and certainty.

Alluding to imitation of my movements face to face and to the execution of pictorial commands, he said, "It doesn't make much difference to me except the first time or two. I think, if you use that hand (pointing to my left), I shall have to use this (holding up his left) and then I am ready. As soon as I have learnt my lesson I can go easily; I never say it to myself, I know. I have rehearsed it whilst you are getting ready and I don't say it. Before I commence I say 'if he does it with that hand (my right) it is this hand (his right).' I've done a lot of signalling." "I've always said it is like translating a foreign language which I know but not very well; it's like translating from French into English."

During the series of pictorial commands he began to hesitate and made a false set of movements; he said, "That was my concentration going," pulled himself together, and the last seven tests were carried out perfectly.

Table 1.

	Imitation of movements made by the observer	Imitation of movements reflected in a mirror	Pictorial commands	Pictorial commands reflected in a mirror	Oral commands	Printed commands (silently)
L. hand to L. eye	Correct	Correct	Correct	Correct	Correct	Correct
R. hand to R. ear	,,	,,	L. hand to L. ear; then correct	,,	,,	,,
R. hand to L. eye	L. hand; then correct	,,	Correct	,,	,,	,,
L. hand to R. eye	R. hand to L. eye; then correct	,,	,,	,,	,,	,,
L. hand to L. ear	Correct	,,	Reversed	,,	,,	,,
R. hand to R. eye	,,	,,	Correct	,,	,,	,,
L. hand to R. ear	,,	,,	,,	,,	,,	,,
R. hand to L. ear	,,	,,	,,	,,	,,	,,
L. hand to L. eye	,,	,,	L. hand to R. *ear*; then correct	,,	,,	,,
R. hand to R. ear	,,	,,	Correct	,,	,,	,,
R. hand to L. eye	,,	,,	,,	,,	,,	,,
L. hand to R. eye	,,	,,	,,	,,	,,	,,
L. hand to L. ear	,,	,,	,,	,,	,,	,,
R. hand to R. eye	,,	,,	,,	,,	,,	,,
L. hand to R. ear	,,	,,	,,	,,	,,	,,
R. hand to L. ear	,,	,,	,,	,,	,,	,,

CONDITION IN JANUARY 1919 (*four years after he was wounded*).

He was in excellent general health and had suffered from no epileptiform seizures since February, 1918, when he was greatly worried about the birth of his child. The spastic hemiplegia was unchanged and all the accompanying physical signs were exactly as before, except that he had developed some arthritis of the right knee.

Articulated speech. He talked slowly, with frequent pauses, evidently unable to find the words he required; but the sequence of his remarks was strictly logical and the phrases were coherent. Thus, he described to me in the following words how he had consulted a surgeon on account of the secondary affection of his knee: "Well...I went by...taxi...and saw him...and explained...er...er...to him

...er...how I had...er...er...osteo-arthritis in this knee...and...er...er... spasticity...er...had made a...hallux valgus...er...er...the toe-joint...the toe-joint...er...creaks...I can hear it, you know..."

Although he had evident difficulty in producing the right word, he had no defect in naming objects placed before him; thus, with geometrical shapes he always succeeded in finding some appropriate designation. Shown a pyramid he replied, "I should call it a solid i-soos-les triangle" (isosceles triangle), and with a sphere he said, "That's a globe...or a hemisphere...a hemispherical globe."

He repeated words and phrases correctly after me, but his articulation showed the same faults as were evident in spontaneous speech.

Understanding of spoken words was perfect and he carried out even the complex hand, eye and ear tests without fail.

Reading. On reading aloud his articulation was astonishingly better than when he talked spontaneously. He no longer hesitated and, on the whole, the words were well pronounced, except that a few, such as "going," were slurred and reduced to a single syllable.

Printed commands were perfectly executed and he was no longer confused when he read to himself; he enjoyed reading to a degree impossible in earlier stages of his recovery.

Writing. He had acquired a remarkable facility with the left hand, although the words were inaccurate and he expressed himself with difficulty. Asked to read a short story and write down what he had gathered, he produced a coherent account, logical, detailed and without omission of a single point. But he failed to spell many of the smaller words correctly; thus "help" was written "held," "utilised" became "utisised" and there were many other mistakes of a similar character. When he finally read over as a whole what he had written, he corrected all these mis-spelt words.

To dictation his writing was distinctly better, and he could transcribe print into cursive script slowly, but accurately.

All the *serial tests* were executed perfectly and even the complex hand, eye and ear movements were carried out with ease.

This patient began as a severe example of verbal aphasia, but steadily improved to such an extent that the only serious defect was shown in power to discover the exact form of the words in which to clothe his thoughts. This appeared, not only in pronunciation during spontaneous speech, but also when he expressed himself in writing.

No. 18

A case of Semantic Aphasia, produced by a gun-shot injury in the region of the superior parietal lobule on the left side, combined with subcortical destruction due to an abscess in the substance of the brain.

When first he came under my care a month after he was wounded, no operation had been performed and there was a small stellate fracture which exposed the surface of the brain. In the centre of this opening was a minute sinus leading down to fragments of bone. These were subsequently removed and an abscess evacuated. This operation was followed by slight Jacksonian attacks in the right hand which ceased entirely on healing of the wound, eight months after its infliction.

My observations, made when he was first under my care in 1915, *did not differ materially from those six and a half years later, and they can therefore be summarised together.*

He suffered from no fits or seizures of any kind after the wound was finally healed. There was complete right hemianopsia and the pupils did not react to light thrown on to the blind half of the retina. There was no hemiplegia; face and tongue moved equally on the two sides. Individual movements of the digits could be carried out perfectly with the eyes open; but, when they were closed, the fingers of the right hand performed such finer movements clumsily. These digits were slightly atonic. The power of recognising posture and passive movement was diminished. The compass test, localisation, tactile sensibility and discrimination of shape, weight and texture were unaffected. All the reflexes, including the plantars and abdominals, were normal and equal on the two sides.

The defects of symbolic formulation and expression consisted in want of ability to recognise fully, to retain firmly and to act logically in accordance with the general meaning of a situation. Details could be appreciated correctly, but were not uniformly coordinated with certainty to form a total impression.

No abnormality could be noticed in the course of ordinary conversation, beyond a certain hesitancy and diffidence in expression. Intonation, the distribution of the pauses and the syntax of each phrase was perfect; and yet there was a tendency for his talk to die out before it had reached its full logical conclusion. He named correctly and repeated everything he heard with ease. He understood what was said to him and could carry out simple orders, although more difficult oral commands confused and puzzled him. He could read silently or aloud and understood the meaning, if it was not complex. He wrote his name and address correctly, but when he attempted to write down the gist of what he had been told or read to himself, he was liable to make curious errors. The act of writing was extremely rapid, as if he was afraid of forgetting what he wanted to express and, even to dictation, he was liable to omit important words. He found difficulty in writing the alphabet, although he could say it correctly. Simple arithmetical exercises were badly performed; in fact he started in each instance from left to right. It was not the detailed significance of numbers that was at fault, but the general conception of the acts of addition and subtraction. Once this had been rectified in his mind, the same problems were easily solved. In spite of the fact that he named coins and stated their relative value correctly, he was greatly puzzled by monetary transactions in daily life. Orientation was not so grossly affected as in some other patients of this group, but he did not like to go out unattended. The plan he drew of the room in which we worked was defective, although he could indicate orally the relative position of its salient features. He understood straightforward pictures; those which demanded composition of detail or the simultaneous comprehension of a printed legend usually failed to convey to him their full meaning. He had the greatest difficulty in formulating the general intention of some act he was about to perform spontaneously or to order; but he was able to copy simple actions with ease, provided they did not demand recognition of several alternatives. Oral, pictorial and printed commands suffered to an almost equal extent. He could not put together the parts of a piece of furniture he had made under guidance and was unable even to lay the table with certainty. He could play no games with pleasure, and disliked puzzles, which confused him.

Private W. W., aged 23, was wounded by shrapnel at Neuve Chapelle on March 15th, 1915. He remembered being hit, but rapidly became unconscious, waking to find himself in a hospital at Boulogne. No operation was performed.

On April 15th he was admitted to the London Hospital under my care without records of any kind. There was an irregularly shaped wound in the left parieto-occipital region, with a small stellate fracture of the underlying bone. The granulating patch was 7 cm. in length and, at the point of impact of the missile, was 2 cm. in breadth; this central portion lay about 22 to 23 cm. back from the root of the nose and 1·5 cm. to the left of the middle line of the scalp. The total nasion-inion measurement was 35·5 cm. and this was cut, at 15 cm. from the root of the nose, by the interaural line (Figs. 12 and 13, Vol. 1, pp. 460 and 461).

He had not suffered from epileptiform attacks, headache or vomiting and the optic discs were normal. But from the first he had noticed a tendency to collide with objects to his right and perimetric examination revealed a complete right hemianopsia. Hearing, smell and taste were unaffected. The pupils reacted normally, except when the light was thrown on to the blind half of the field. Movements of the eyes, of the face, and of the tongue were carried out perfectly. All the reflexes were normal. Even the finer movements of the fingers could be executed, although there was a distinct want of coordination in the right hand with a tendency to fall away when the eyes were closed. The lower extremities were unaffected. The right hand seemed "numb" and sensibility to passive movement and to vibration was diminished in the fingers; the compass test and localisation were not materially affected at this time. Size, shape, weight and texture were correctly appreciated, although he was quicker and said it was "easier" with the left hand than with the right. The threshold for the tactile hairs seemed to be slightly raised over the fingers of the affected hand, and he was conscious that they seemed "different" from those of the normal side. Sensibility to pricking, to heat and to cold was unchanged.

He was an intelligent young man, who had succeeded in reaching the highest standard in an elementary school at thirteen years of age, in spite of the fact that he was compelled by his parents to earn money for them by working on a bowling green. He said he had always been particularly good at arithmetic and drawing.

During his stay in the London Hospital he was unusually bright and willing. He took kindly to the tests I set him, smiling when he succeeded and showing no anger if he failed. He helped in the work of the ward, carrying out simple orders well; but he found difficulty in laying the table for meals and was liable to become confused with regard to his intentions.

There was no apraxia; he could strike a match and extinguish it after lighting a cigarette, brushed and combed his hair, and dressed himself perfectly. Moreover, he performed all these acts perfectly in pantomime.

He did not talk much, but preferred to sit quietly by himself, looking at pictures or with a book.

Condition between May 31st and June 11th, 1915 (*eleven to thirteen weeks after he was wounded*).

Symbolic Formulation and Expression.

At this time his condition did not differ materially from that found six and a half years later; I shall, therefore, indicate shortly the results obtained at this early stage, in order to dwell with greater detail on the many illuminating observations made at a time when he had long been in a stable condition physically and mentally.

Articulated speech. Articulation, intonation and the syntax of his phrases was unaffected. He had no difficulty in finding names for common objects, but he was liable to become confused when attempting to express himself in ordinary conversation. Words said to him were correctly repeated.

Understanding of spoken words. He understood and carried out simple orders perfectly.

Reading. He could read to himself, but complained that he had become very slow and found difficulty in understanding exactly what it was about. "I've been a fortnight in reading this book; but I'd have read it in three days, reading the time I do." Printed commands were carried out well. He had no difficulty in reading aloud, but, when asked to say what he understood, he tended to abbreviate the story considerably.

Writing. He wrote his full name and address and that of his mother correctly. A short letter written spontaneously was intelligible and fairly well expressed although calligraphically inferior to phrases copied from print. Asked to write the months he omitted October, but otherwise reproduced them correctly, and, on reading over what he had written, noticed his error.

The alphabet. He was able to say and to repeat the alphabet rapidly and correctly. But, although he ultimately succeeded in writing the letters in their correct order, he did so slowly and with hesitation. He complained, "I seem alright starting off, but half way through I get mixed up; I seem to forget what letter comes next; I'm alright if I can get straight at it. I forget the shape of the letters." This exactly expressed what I observed whilst he was writing; after F he had difficulty in finding the form of G, and the same thing occurred with S and X, although finally the alphabet was reproduced correctly.

Numbers and arithmetic. He counted up to a hundred and wrote the numbers in correct sequence to twenty and thence onwards by decades.

When asked to work out simple arithmetical exercises he failed entirely; he began in each case from left to right and finally became gravely confused.

Addition.

215	284	595	
323	516	868	
538	7011 (wrong)	3614 (wrong)	He said, "That makes three thousand six hundred and fourteen"

It is interesting to notice that, although he worked these sums the wrong way, he carried over the digits correctly from column to column.

Subtraction.

586	816	
214	357	
372	56	He then said, "I'm not much good there; I can't take a seven from a six"

Drawing. He said that he was fond of drawing when at school, but his attempts to reproduce the outlines of a spirit-lamp, placed on the table in front of him, were feeble and ineffective. From memory he made a somewhat fuller drawing, describing the details correctly as he drew them. He produced a much better figure of an elephant to command than might have been expected considering his disability; all the salient parts were correctly named and indicated.

General comprehension of meaning and intention. There was no doubt that he understood the significance of pictures, provided the meaning was displayed in the details of the drawing; but he frequently failed to carry out a command given in the form of a diagram.

When in the army, he had been a waiter at the officers' mess and was familiar with the details of laying a table. But in the London Hospital he complained, "Several times, laying the dinner here, I've laid knives and forks wrong, knives where forks ought to be; I've given two spoons and nurse asked 'where are all the spoons gone.'"

On another occasion he said, "If I pay too much attention, I get wrong with what I've got to do."

Serial Tests.

Geometrical shapes were named correctly and chosen to oral and printed commands. He could name colours and select them to verbal orders spoken by me or presented in print. The man, cat and dog tests were read aloud without fault, were well written to dictation, and especially when he was allowed to copy the short phrases from printed cards. The coin-bowl tests were also executed correctly. Observations with the clock and the hand, eye and ear tests alone revealed faults of execution.

The clock tests. He could tell the time on a clock set by me, but had considerable difficulty in placing the hands in the correct position to oral or printed commands. He tended to mistake the hands and to confuse "to" and "past" the hour.

The hand, eye and ear tests. Here he made many mistakes, when imitating my movements sitting face to face, or when carrying out pictorial orders. But he succeeded perfectly to oral or printed commands, whenever either my movements or the diagrams were reflected in a mirror.

On June 14th, 1915, he was sent to a convalescent hospital. The wound had healed except for a minute opening, the mouth of a small sinus, which was drained by means of a thin strip of gauze. The importance of this exit was not recognised and it was allowed to close; he began to suffer from headache, became depressed and moody, and one day, when out for a walk, took the train to his home, where he remained for two days. This was treated as a disciplinary offence and he was sent back to the London Hospital on August 4th.

Pus had obviously accumulated owing to the closure of the sinus and was then pouring from the wound. It soon became evident that a foreign body was lying in the brain about 1·5 cm. from the surface, and we succeeded in extracting a small piece of bone. On August 25th, Mr Walton exposed the track by a linear incision, removed several long bony fragments and inserted a small tube with a glycerine wick.

All seemed to be going well until September 4th, when the patient complained of a "curious feeling in the right hand." He lost his power of speech, but kept on saying, "You know what I mean." After a few minutes, twitching began in the right hand. This ceased after a few minutes and consciousness was preserved throughout. A quarter of an hour later, whilst I was talking to him, he had another attack, which began with a "funny feeling" in the right hand, followed by clonic movements in the fingers and arm, lasting in all just under a minute. Face, tongue and leg were not affected and there was no loss of consciousness. Subsequently, from time to time, he suffered from transitory difficulty in speaking and curious sensations in the fingers of the right hand; but he had no further convulsions or attacks of any kind.

The wound became reduced again to a minute sinus, extending for 8 cm. directly downwards, forwards and inwards into the substance of the brain. By November 15th, 1915, it had entirely healed and he was completely free from headache and abnormal symptoms, except those connected with speech.

A full examination carried out in the middle of November, 1915, revealed no new features. He showed the same complete hemianopsia of the right half of the visual field; the movements of the face and tongue were normal and the reflexes unaffected. He still had difficulty in executing the clock tests and in performing the hand, eye and ear movements; arithmetic was faulty and he could not occupy himself with games or puzzles.

CONDITION BETWEEN OCTOBER 21ST AND NOVEMBER 4TH, 1921 (*six years and eight months after he was wounded*).

I kept in touch with this patient at his home in the country and in October, 1921, he was again placed under my care in order that I might report on his condition. In the light of my riper experience, I was then able to make a complete and exhaustive examination.

Physical Examination.

The site of the wound was occupied by a firm deeply depressed scar covering a roughly quadrilateral area, where the bone had been removed. This measured 2 cm. in either direction; it extended between two points 22·5 cm. and 24·5 cm. along the nasion-inion and lay 1·25 cm. from the middle line of the scalp.

There was no pulsation in the vertical position, or if he lay quietly propped with pillows on a couch. But, when he stooped as if to lace up his boots, I could feel distinct pulsation at the bottom of the scar and he became conscious of "a heavy beating and thumping."

He suffered from occasional headaches, usually situated over the vertex, but occasionally occupying the whole of the head, including the occipital region. This pain was always worst "over the crown of the head" to both sides of the middle line and not over the site of the wound; when it was severe, the hair became so tender that he could not brush it.

This headache could be evoked by any violent movement, by lifting heavy weights, or by riding in a motor omnibus, but was no longer produced by a journey in the train. It disappeared in half an hour, if he lay on his back or left side, although it could be brought on by lying on the right.

Physical fatigue did not at once produce this headache and, if he could sit down and sleep for a few minutes, he recovered entirely; but after it had lasted for some time he felt intensely tired and took a long while to recover. Intellectual effort, especially reading, was liable to cause this pain; a visit to a cinematograph produced a violent headache in a few minutes and anything which confused him evoked it immediately.

This headache was not associated with nausea or vomiting. But, when it became violent, he had a feeling as if he had lost some of the power in the right arm and leg and his speech became more confused. This passed away when the headache was relieved.

He had not suffered from any form of seizure or attack since he left the London Hospital in November, 1915.

Vision was $\frac{6}{6}$ imperfectly, with either eye, but the hemianopsia was as definite as before. He could not appreciate movement, form, white or colours over the whole of the right half of the field, excepting within a small zone extending less than $5°$ to this side of the middle line. Here movement alone was recognised and he was blind to form and colour.

The discs and fundi were in every way normal.

Hearing, smell and taste were unaffected.

In low artificial illumination the right pupil was smaller than the left. Both reacted to light, except when the beam was directed so that it fell on to the nasal half of the right retina, or the temporal side of the left. Ocular movements were well executed and there was no nystagmus.

Face and tongue moved equally well on both sides.

He was a strongly right-handed man, who threw in the usual manner, and could not cut with the loose jointed scissors held in the left hand.

The right grasp was somewhat stronger than the left and individual movements of the digits could be carried out perfectly with the eyes open; but, when they were closed, the fingers of the right hand performed these finer movements more clumsily and less perfectly than the left. He touched the tip of his nose less accurately with the right forefinger and said he thought this test was "easier with the left hand." Moreover, the fingers of the affected hand seemed to me to be slightly atonic in comparison with those of the normal one.

He said that the right lower extremity appeared to him "all right," unless he had a severe headache; then "the power seems to go out of it and it feels as if it was made of ice." At that time the right arm also became numb and cold. I could discover no paralysis or alteration in tone, but he had distinct difficulty in finding the right great toe with the left heel and could not stand on the right foot with the eyes closed.

On sensory examination he undoubtedly appreciated passive movement less easily in the thumb, index and other digits of the right hand; on the left side he responded perfectly to 1°, whilst in the right hand he required an excursion of from 3° to 5°. The wrist was slightly affected, but I could find no defect at the elbow-joint. There was no difference between the measurements obtained from any part of the two lower extremities.

The compass test, localisation, tactile sensibility and discrimination of shape, weight and texture were unaffected.

All the reflexes, including the abdominals and plantars, were normal and equal on the two sides.

Symbolic Formulation and Expression.

He was intelligent, cheerful and a most willing witness. During our numerous quiet sittings his spontaneous comments revealed considerable powers of observation and furnished me with much introspective information.

Articulated speech. No abnormality was noticeable in the course of ordinary conversation, beyond a certain hesitancy and diffidence in expression. Intonation and the distribution of the pauses were not otherwise affected and the syntax of each phrase was perfect; and yet there was a tendency for his talk to die out before it had reached its full logical conclusion. He gave the correct names of common objects or of colours and could repeat accurately anything he had heard, provided it was not extremely complicated.

Understanding of spoken words. He understood what was said to him and could carry out simple orders; but the more complex oral commands of the hand, eye and ear tests confused and puzzled him.

Reading. He could read to himself and occupied his leisure with the newspaper, rarely reading a book; for he was easily confused and, if he grew puzzled, became tired and headache supervened.

He read aloud perfectly; intonation and articulation were unaffected, but he had difficulty in reproducing the full significance of what he had read aloud.

Writing. He wrote his name and address correctly. When, however, he was asked to write down the gist of something he had read, he was liable to make curious errors and to fail in composition; he would begin a new sentence after a full stop with a small letter and scattered capitals throughout the text unnecessarily. He wrote with great rapidity as if fearful of forgetting what he wanted to express. To dictation, and even when copying a printed text, his writing tended to exhibit the same faults.

The alphabet. He could say the alphabet spontaneously and repeat it correctly. Asked to write it down, he complained that the shape of the letters "bothered" him; "I know what to put down, but I forget the shape of the letters." This exactly corresponded to what I observed during the act. He paused at f, finally producing a figure ("ȣ") which corresponded closely with the one he employed for j. At the first attempt z replaced s, but was erased and written correctly; y gave him considerable trouble and he hesitated over the shape of x, though in the end all the letters were written in recognisable form and accurate sequence. To dictation, he wrote in capitals and yet found the same trouble with the form of F J and X. He copied capital letters with ease, but found some difficulty in transcribing them into cursive handwriting; f and j again resembled one another and he "could not think of the small letter for Q and X."

A printed paragraph. I selected the following account of the sinking of the Lusitania, which interested him greatly. It consisted of a series of definite details united together by a coherent general meaning, and evoked from the patient valuable introspective observations on the nature of his disabilities. The passage ran as follows:

"The great Cunard steamer Lusitania was torpedoed by a German submarine and sunk off the south coast of Ireland on May 7th, 1915. She was within a few hours of harbour. There were nearly two thousand persons on board and of these between 500 and 600 were saved and landed at Queenstown. There were many hospital patients amongst the passengers and several of these have since died."

After perusing the paper for several minutes in silence, he said, "It's about the sinking of the Lusitania. The Lusitania was sunk by a German submarine off the coast of Ireland...near Queenstown." I asked if he could remember anything more and he answered, "There were 600 persons drowned."

He again took up the paper and read the sentences through to himself. Then he wrote "The Liner Surtania was sunk by torpodoe off the South Coast of Ireland." He complained, "I know some more, but I can't get what's between." He then began lower down on the paper and wrote "there between 500 and 600 persons saved." I asked, "What is your trouble?" and he replied, "I seem to get my mind on one thing and forget the remainder. When I first read it, I got the 500 persons saved wrong; I knew afterwards it must be wrong and this seemed to fix it in my mind. When I came to write it, this kept recurring in my mind and seemed to prevent me remembering the other part of it; this seemed the most important part."

He read the whole account aloud perfectly; no words were omitted, badly pronounced, or wrongly stressed. He then reproduced its substance as follows: "The Cunard liner Lusitania was sunk off the west coast of Ireland near Queenstown. There were nearly two thousand people on board. Between five and six hundred were saved." After a pause he added, "Something about hospital patients ...and some have since died."

To dictation he wrote as follows: "The great Cunard Steamer was torpedoed by a German submarine and sunk off the South Coast of Ireland on May 7th, 1915. She was within a few hours of harbour there were nearly 2,000 persons on board and of these between 500 and 600 were saved and landed at Queenstown there were many Hospital patients among the passengers and several of these have since died." He then pointed to the broken lines saying, "I see I shouldn't have made a break there at all."

He read what he had written with complete ease and as if it were in every way perfect, even inserting the name of the Lusitania, which he had omitted.

When I then said to him, "Don't tell me the story; write down as many things as you can remember," he produced the following series:

"Great Liner Lusitana"
"Torpedoed"
"2000 persons on Board"
"between 500 and 600 saved"
"many hospital cases."

I then prepared a list of the main features of the story and wrote them in sequence, one below the other. "Cunard steamer. Lusitania. Torpedoed. South coast of Ireland. May 7th, 1915. Close to harbour. 2000 persons on board. 500 to 600 saved. Landed at Queenstown. Hospital patients. Several since died." This he read silently and reproduced as follows: "Great Liner. Lusitania. Torpedoed and sunk. May 15th, 1915. 2000 persons on Board. between 500 and 600 saved. Landed at Queenstown. many have since died."

This test revealed his capacity to remember detail, if it was formulated for him, and is in remarkable contrast to his defective powers of spontaneous composition.

On writing the date ("May 15th, 1915") he said, "I couldn't make it out. I seemed to think it was later than 1915, but I seemed to have to write 1915. I couldn't make that out; if I'd stopped to consider, I should have put 1916. But I must have remembered what I'd read on the paper, I must have been following the paper though without thinking. I really didn't intend to put 1915 down." This conflict threw a vivid light on the habitual confusion of his mind. He surmised rightly that 1916 was the correct date, but was compelled by what he had read to write 1915; so strong was the impulsion to write "15" that he also changed the day of the month from the 7th to the 15th, for which there was no excuse. The number "15" was evidently over-stressed on the level of execution, whilst logically he wanted to change the date to 1916.

Finally he copied the printed matter as follows in cursive handwriting: "The great Cunard steamer Lusitania was torpedoed by a German Sutmarine and sunk off the south Coast of Ireland on May 7th 1915 there were nearly 2'000 persons on board and off these between 5,00 and 6,00 were saved and landed at Queenstown there were many hospital Patients amongst the passengers and several of these have since died."

Numbers and arithmetic. He counted and wrote the numbers with ease, and could enumerate the decades from 20 to 200 correctly.

Addition.			Subtraction.		
354	468	586	958	862	921
625	324	965	432	428	458
979	7812 (wrong)	4511 (wrong)	526	44	5

With each of these simple arithmetical problems he started from left to right. This made no difference to the first addition; but, when he came to the third term of the second sum, he said, "I can't put down twelve; something is wrong." Finally he wrote 12, saying, "I know that's wrong somehow, but I don't know how." At the end of the third addition he wrote 11 after great hesitation and repeated his complaint that he could not tell what was wrong.

He fell into the same confusion over the subtraction sums. With the first example his method of working from left to right made no difference; but with the second he said, "I can't take eight from two," and with the third, "Take the five from twenty-one, but I can't take it from the two and I don't know what I'm going to do with the eight." He added, "They seem to go alright until I have to come to a stop and it's plain it can't be done."

Later, in the course of the same morning, he suddenly exclaimed, "I've discovered where I went wrong in the sums. I started from the wrong end. I've been wondering what I had to do with the figures at the end, with the figures I had over and didn't know what to do with. I wondered and it suddenly struck me that I hadn't started right. I think I could get them right this time. I was always good at arithmetic before I was wounded."

I therefore laid the same problems before him again and he solved them all correctly, working from right to left. When he came to the first subtraction he started to add, and on my saying, "That's subtraction," replied, "Oh, yes, I didn't notice that," and at once corrected his procedure.

Here it was not the detailed significance of numbers that was at fault, but rather the general conception of the acts of addition and subtraction. Once this had been corrected in his mind the problems were solved easily.

Coins and their relative value. Every coin was named without hesitation and the relative value of any two of them was correctly stated.

But in spite of this obvious recognition of their value, he had difficulty in ordinary life with the computation of change. "If it's odd coppers I don't trouble to reckon it. It confuses me." "It's usually with half a crown I get mixed up. If I went in for two small articles and had half a crown, I should get puzzled. If one were threepence and the other fourpence halfpenny, I should never try to reckon the change, unless they tried to give me no change for half a crown; but I shouldn't add the two together and reckon the change from half a crown. With a shilling it's alright. Above a shilling I should expect to get some coppers and if they looked right I should take them. I shouldn't reckon them unless they looked wrong."

Drawing. He made a remarkably good drawing of a spirit-lamp placed before him on the table, and reproduced it later from memory with a considerable amount of correct detail. His drawing of an elephant was distinctly above the average; he did not however block out the figure, but built it up detail by detail. He added, "I don't see the picture before my mind at all."

Orientation and plan drawing. He said he could find his way, but did not like to go out unattended. Within the walls of the hospital he seemed to gain confidence and made no obvious mistakes.

Asked to draw a ground-plan of my consulting room, familiar to him from our many sittings, he produced first of all an irregular quadrilateral figure on too small a scale for the purpose. He then took another sheet of paper and traced an oblong with openings for the two doors, a recess for the fireplace, and within this space he indicated many details, such as chairs and tables, in their correct position. But he gave the room a single window instead of the two with which it was provided and omitted the large couch, one of its most prominent features.

He described from memory the situation of each salient object in accurate relation to the place where he sat when we were at work; he not only indicated the doors, fireplace and articles of furniture, but also pointed out correctly the relative position of each window in turn, although they had been reduced to one on the plan. I asked if he could see both of them at the same moment and he replied, "No, there is a break; I can throw my mind straight from one on to the other, but I can't seem to catch the two at the same moment, it doesn't matter how hard I try."

Significance of pictures, etc. Any picture, which contained the direct representation of some act or scene with no ulterior significance, was appreciated perfectly. Details were recognised and given their proper value; in fact, looking at pictures of this kind was one of his principal amusements.

But he was liable to be puzzled, if it was necessary for complete comprehension to unite a series of pictures into a coherent whole or to add the meaning of a printed legend. I showed him a sequence of thumb-nail sketches showing a man in evening dress, who, arriving late at a theatre, inadvertently stripped himself to his shirt-sleeves to the horror of the surrounding spectators. He said he saw the joke and proceeded to explain it as follows: "It's about a man who goes into a theatre late. He gets in everybody's way, when he's taking his coat off, and he disturbs them, when he's seated. I couldn't exactly say what was making them so excited. After looking a long time I saw it was him laughing." This explanation satisfied him completely until I said, "Don't you see he has taken off both coats; he is in his shirt sleeves." He then looked at the picture again and replied, "I can see it now; I thought it was because he was laughing so loud."

This difficulty in uniting the significance of details into a coherent whole was still more evident if full comprehension of a picture depended on some more or less elaborate legend. The majority of printed jokes were, therefore, incomprehensible to him, even when he read the printed matter aloud.

Comprehension of ultimate meaning. The curious divergence between his power of understanding details and lack of comprehension of their general significance was exhibited by the following test. I put together a series of simple sentences bearing on the vexed question of the relative advantages of "Summer-time" and handed them to him in print.

"Summer Time is now at an end and there has been much correspondence in the papers regarding its value. Some say it is a great boon to working people whilst others say it is useless or even harmful. The truth seems to be that it has added greatly to the pleasure of those who live in towns. But since the cows and other animals regulate their life by the sun and not by the clock, it can make no difference to those who work in the country, for they cannot rise earlier to any advantage."

He took the paper in his hand, read it through carefully, and, when he said he had finished, we had the following dialogue:

Q. "Tell me what you have read?"

A. "It starts with a question as to whether official summer-time is any advantage to the people. They say there is to a man in the town and that it's not to a man in the country, because it makes no difference to the habits of cows."

Q. "What happens to the clocks in summer-time?"

A. "They are altered an hour."

Q. "Which way?"

A. "I don't know. It's always a puzzle; I've given up thinking about it."

Q. "Why does it make a difference to the people in the town?"

A. "It gives them an hour extra daylight."

Q. "Why doesn't it make any difference to the people in the country?"

A. "I can't see that, unless it's because they can't alter the habits of the animals. The animals expect to be fed at a certain time in the morning and the people would be an hour *late*, feeding them or going out to milk them. I fail to see myself how it would make any difference at all. If the time were altered an hour late, they would be an hour late expecting their feed; they would forget it and it would make no difference."

He then added, "I never hold an argument on any subject. I've once or twice been proved wrong so I've given up. If there is anybody arguing with me they go too fast for me to follow. I can't follow it with any clearness at all."

Formulating the general intention of an act. Since his discharge from the army several attempts have been made without success to train him for some useful employment. He complained, "I have difficulty in following out whatever I am doing; it makes me very confused. They put me on a course of sign-writing. I was an absolute failure at that. You've got to keep your eye on a certain spot whilst you're doing a letter. I used to put the brush perhaps between the lines where I should be working." "They put me to cabinet making. I used to work from drawings. I could not follow the drawings; even before I started to work I could not follow the drawings. They were too complicated for me; I could not sort them out at all. I could have made an article if they had given me one and said 'make one like that.' I could put together a chest of drawers from the bits; but I used to take a very long time over it." I then asked, "What bothered you?" He replied, "I used to catch hold of a piece and then I had to think a long time where it had to go. Perhaps I'd get hold of the wrong piece. A piece of furniture has to go together in a certain order; that is the easiest way if you get it in the correct order. I used to go the wrong way about for the commencement; before now I've put the frame of a cupboard door together and then had to take it all to pieces again to get in the panels. Several times I hinged a wardrobe door so that the hinges came on the wrong side."

I placed at hand all the necessary utensils and asked him to lay the table for breakfast. He set the saucer in front of him with the fork to the left, the knife to the right and the large spoon above; the teaspoon was laid alongside the knife. Then he became confused and gave up further attempts, leaving the cup, plate, salt-cellar and pepper-pot untouched. He added in explanation, "I've often gone wrong in this; it takes me a long time; they are getting used to me in the hospital giving one man two or three spoons and no knife."

He was slow in seeing the shortest method of performing an act, which he ultimately carried out perfectly. Thus, when he was given a clock and told to place the hands in the exact position shown on another one set by me, he tended to swing the hand he was setting round the whole face instead of moving it back a few points. For instance, I set my clock at a quarter to nine and he placed his hour hand exactly opposite 9; then he moved the minute hand into its proper position and instead of pushing back the other one for a minute fraction of the space between 8 and 9, he swung it all round the face until it reached the correct spot just short of the number 9.

Games, etc. He could not play any games with pleasure, and disliked puzzles, which confused him.

Mental images, etc. Whilst he was drawing the spirit-lamp from memory, he complained that he could "picture" some of the details, but could not see "the way they went; separately I can picture each part. In the hospital I can picture the hall. Then I must leave that behind and I can then picture the lift and the staircase.

Then you turn a corner into the passage; at the end of the passage is the ward. I couldn't picture the inside of the ward and the end of the passage. I couldn't think of any two patients, but I can think of each one all round the ward; but I mustn't think of two at a time, I can't do that. I could direct my picture from any one object back to any other one, but I can't hold the one whilst I did that; I must leave the one behind."

In the same way, when filling in the plan he had drawn, he said he could not hold two objects in his mind together. "I can pass from one to the other, but as soon as I catch the other, it goes straight out of my mind. As soon as I attempt to think of the other, before I seem to catch it in my mind, the first one has gone."

I then placed before him on the table a salt-cellar and a pepper-box. After he had looked at them carefully, they were removed from his sight and he said, "I don't see them together; I can see the tall one and then I can go to the short one and then the tall one is gone. I seem to have to go from the tall one on to the other one."

The salt-cellar was again placed before him and, after its removal, he drew it fairly correctly in outline; in the same way he produced a passable representation of the pepper-box. I then placed both objects together on the table and, on removing them, asked him to draw the two side by side. This task he executed correctly, and when I asked how he did it he replied, "I drew the one first, the salt-cellar; I forgot this one and then I drew the other. I had no thoughts of the salt-cellar, whilst I was drawing the pepper-box, I could think of the salt-cellar because I had got it (the drawing) in front of me and I could think about it. I couldn't picture the actual pepper-box and salt-cellar, but I could notice some connection between them and I could think about them together because I'd got the drawing straight in front of me."

I met with great difficulty in determining how much of this disability was natural to him and to what extent it had been produced by the injury. Most of my patients had been in the habit of visualising strongly and had recognised that their processes of thought were normally associated with the formation of "pictures in the mind." But in this man the power of forming visual images was in all probability never of this vivid character. Asked "Could you picture things in your mind before you were wounded?" he replied, "I never noticed; it was a surprise to me to find I couldn't picture them after you asked me. The first time I noticed it was when you asked me to picture an elephant and I couldn't; I began to think about it and I was surprised that I couldn't do it."

"I often wondered why I didn't dream. I used to dream a great deal before I was wounded. I used to see sorts of prehistoric animals, but never to be frightened of them. I used to dream I was at home, when I was far away. Since I was wounded all my dreams stopped and I often wondered why."

Asked if he could picture the place where he was now living, he answered,

"No, I can't even picture my own house; but I can describe it. It's three and a quarter miles from the centre of Worcester on the main road leading to...I know the next village beyond it, Grimley, but I don't know where it leads to after that. I know every little place we pass, but I don't know where it leads to."

I then asked him a number of direct questions, "Can you picture the ward in the hospital, your wife's face or figure, the colour red, the form of the cup out of which you drank your tea?" All of these he answered in the negative.

He was unable to recall smells, such as that of violets, tastes, for example sugar, or touch. He could not hear his wife's voice or imagine the sound of a church bell. But when questioned as to numbers, he said, "I can imagine numbers, but very, very slow; I was thinking of numbers on the door. I can picture the brass plate on your door."

I could not discover that pictorial images arose involuntarily and he complained, "If I fix my mind, I can't get anything."

To my enquiry, if he could think of himself turning the door-handle, he replied, "I know how I should turn the door-handle, but I can't think of myself doing it. I should just do like this," imitating the movement correctly.

Q. "Can you think of yourself putting on your hat?"

A. "No, I can't call it to mind."

Q. "How would you do it?"

A. "I should take it from the hook and put it on my head," at the same time he made the movements of lifting his cap from the wall and putting it on his head.

Thus, it is evident that his power of evoking visual images was feeble; but there is no reason to suppose that he ever visualised strongly. His memory was based mainly on the power to reproduce acts he had once carried out and to recall in orderly progression the manner in which he had arrived at any series of points in space. But, since his wound, this capacity of combining detail into a coherent sequence had suffered; for this reason his disability was in some ways severer than if his memory had depended normally more exclusively on visual imagery.

Serial Tests.

(1) *Naming and recognition of common objects.* He gave to each one its proper name and made a correct choice to either oral or printed commands. He wrote the names and copied them from print without difficulty. In fact this test revealed no obvious abnormality.

(2) *Naming and recognition of colours.* In the same way this set of observations failed to show any serious mistakes.

(3) *The man, cat and dog tests.* He could read these simple phrases aloud from print or from pictures. He wrote them perfectly to dictation or in response to pictures, and copied them in good handwriting. He repeated each sentence correctly and read what he had written with ease.

(4) *The clock tests.*

Table 1.

	Direct imitation	Oral commands	Printed commands: Ordinary nomenclature	Printed commands: Railway time	Telling the time	Writing down the time shown on a clock: Ordinary nomenclature	Writing down the time shown on a clock: Railway time
5 minutes to 2	Correct	2.5	2.5	Correct	Correct	Correct	2.5
Half-past 1	2.30	Long hand 1; short hand 6	Correct	,,	,,	Half past 2	Correct
5 minutes past 8	Long hand 8; short hand 1	Correct	,,	8.25 (long hand at 5)	,,	Correct	,,
20 minutes to 4	Correct	4.20	4.20	Correct	,,	,,	,,
10 minutes past 7	,,	10 *to* 7	10 *to* 7	Long hand 7; short hand 10	,,	,,	,,
20 minutes to 6	,,	6.20	Correct	Correct	,,	,,	,,
10 minutes to 1	,,	Correct	,,	,,	,,	,,	1.50
A quarter to 9	,,	,,	,,	,,	"Quarter to 8"	,,	Correct
20 minutes past 11	,,	,,	,,	,,	"20 minutes to 12"	20 to 12	,,
25 minutes to 3	,,	3.25	3.25	,,	Correct	Correct	2.25

Just as on every previous occasion, he failed to carry out these tests accurately. Even simple imitation was not exact and the hands were placed into position with abnormal slowness; he tended to swing the one he was setting round the whole face instead of moving it back a few points. When I set my clock at a quarter to nine, he placed his hour hand exactly opposite 9; then he moved the minute hand into the proper position and instead of pushing back the other for a minute fraction of the space between 8 and 9, he swung it all round the face until it reached the correct spot just short of the number 9. He showed a tendency to move the hands clock-wise, whatever position he intended ultimately to reach.

To oral and printed commands, he confused the significance of the hands and the meaning of "to" and "past"; moreover, there was no essential difference in the ease with which he set the clock, when the printed order was given in the usual nomenclature or in railway time. He could tell the time on the whole correctly; but he tended to become confused, because the hour hand had been set in strict proportion to the number of minutes. He wrote the time slowly, but with two mistakes only; he was, however, easily confused.

Finally, he complained, "I am always very bad at telling the time; it takes me a very long time. I always show my watch and enquire."

(5) *The coin-bowl tests.* These seemed to him "quite easy." He made his choice correctly to both oral and printed commands, whether fully expressed in words or given in numbers only.

(6) *The hand, eye and ear tests.*

During imitation of my movements, sitting face to face, and whilst carrying out pictorial commands, he made the following remarks: "After the motion I can see I am wrong sometimes; I change it. I don't follow it out; when I have done it,

Table 2.

	Imitation of movements made by the observer	Imitation of movements reflected in a mirror	Pictorial commands	Pictorial commands reflected in a mirror	Oral commands	Printed commands	Writing down movements made by the observer	Saying aloud and executing movements made by the observer		Reading aloud and executing printed commands	
								He said	Movement executed	He read	Movement executed
L. hand to L. eye	Correct	Correct	Correct	Correct	Reversed	Correct	Correct	Correctly	Correct	Correctly	Correct
R. hand to R. ear	Corrected	”	Reversed	”	”	”	”	”	”	”	”
R. hand to L. eye	R. hand to R. *ear*	”	Correct	”	Correct	”	”	”	Corrected	”	”
L. hand to R. eye	Correct	”	Reversed	”	”	Reversed	L. hand to R. *ear*	”	Correct	”	”
L. hand to L. ear	Reversed	”	Correct	”	Reversed	Correct	Correct	”	”	”	”
R. hand to R. eye	Correct	”	”	”	Correct	R. hand to R. *ear*; corrected	”	”	”	”	”
L. hand to R. ear	”	”	Reversed	”	Correct; very slow	Correct	”	”	”	”	”
R. hand to L. ear	Reversed	”	Correct	”	Correct	”	”	”	”	”	”
L. hand to L. eye	Correct	”	”	”	”	”	”	”	”	”	”
R. hand to R. ear	”	”	”	”	”	”	”	”	”	”	”
R. hand to L. eye	R. hand to R. eye	”	”	”	”	”	”	”	Doubtful	”	”
L. hand to R. eye	Correct	”	”	”	”	”	”	”	Correct	”	”
L. hand to L. ear	”	”	Reversed	”	Reversed	Corrected	”	”	”	”	”
R. hand to R. eye	R. hand to R. *ear*; corrected	”	L. hand to R. eye	”	Corrected; slow	Confused; finally correct	”	”	”	”	”
L. hand to R. ear	Correct	”	Correct	”	Correct	Correct	”	”	”	”	”
R. hand to L. ear	”	”	”	”	”	”	”	”	”	”	”

I can sometimes see where I've gone wrong; it's too late to change it. I know I went wrong because I did two movements the same; that must have been wrong."

When imitating either my movements or the pictures reflected in the glass, he said, "It seems very simple; I could see your movements and I had to follow. I feel just as if you showed me a thing and told me to repeat it and there was nothing extraordinary about it. The other one confused me being opposite."

Both oral and printed commands tended to confuse him in the same way. "It seemed as if I had to think what hand it was I had to use. Then it seemed as if there was a sort of break. I had to look again to see what I had to do." This was exactly what I observed; he looked at the card, raised his hand, and looked again to decide its destination. For this reason printed orders were better executed than those given orally.

The actual number of his mistakes, when he attempted to write down the movements made by me, did not express the difficulty he had in carrying out this test; he was slow and repeatedly looked back at the position of my hand, which I maintained until he had finished writing. He would sit and stare at me for many seconds before he could make up his mind to begin to write; then he looked back repeatedly for confirmation.

If he was asked to explain aloud the nature of the movements made by me, before he attempted to carry them out, the results were better than with direct imitation. But he complained, "That made my head spin; I seemed to have a lot to think about to get it correct."

When, however, he read the order aloud before executing it, the results were better and the whole process was carried out more easily. He said, "This is easier; there's no confusion about it. I simply did what was wanted without having to hesitate or wait." The difference was profound; the act of reading aloud seemed to start an immediate automatic response, whereas, when he described aloud the movements made by me, there was no impulsion to action on his part. The act on his side was completed when he had spoken the words aloud, and the demand for subsequent movement simply confused him; in many cases it required an actual verbal repetition by him of what he had previously said he before could evoke an impulse to make the movements. On the other hand, reading aloud in itself acted as a command requiring and setting free an immediate movement; hence his feeling of ease.

No. 19

A case of severe Verbal Aphasia, the result of being bombed from the air whilst riding a motor bicycle. There was no external wound and the injury was evidently situated deep in the substance of the brain.

The patient was unconscious for three weeks and recovered his senses to find that he was hemiplegic and was unable to say any word but "yes."

When he came under my observation three years and nine months after the accident, the hemiplegia had passed away, except for some weakness and clumsiness of the right hand and to a less degree of the toes of the right foot. He was almost completely speechless and could not find words to designate familiar objects and colours. But he recognised their names; for he selected without fail a card bearing the appropriate designation of the object or colour shown him. By this means he could name them correctly, although external verbalisation was almost impossible. He seemed to understand everything said to him and executed oral commands correctly. He showed remarkable power of understanding printed words, provided he did not attempt to read them aloud or to spell out the letters of which they were composed; printed commands were carried out perfectly. Writing was grossly affected. He could not write down unaided the names of objects or colours, the time shown on a clock, or movements made by me. But he succeeded better to dictation and copied correctly printed words in cursive script. He even found difficulty in constructing an alphabet out of block letters. He counted up to ten (with the exception of seven) and then continued, "One one" (eleven), "one two" (twelve), etc. up to one hundred, which was "One no no." He failed to solve several simple problems in arithmetic.

This case is an example of almost pure loss of verbalisation with no disturbance of the appreciation of verbal meaning. It shows that the power of forming words may be destroyed without loss of recognition of names.

Sergeant Arthur John H., aged 23, was sent to see me on December 1st, 1920, as a case of pure "motor" aphasia.

In February, 1917, he was riding a motor bicycle on the Salonica front, when he was bombed from the air. Many of his companions were killed; he was rendered unconscious and remembers nothing that happened to him for at least three weeks. He then found he was paralysed down the right half of his body and had lost his speech; the only word he could utter was "yes." The hemiplegia passed away rapidly and in three or four months he could walk with the help of a stick and use his arm slightly.

He reached England in the spring of 1917, and was discharged from hospital in November of the same year. He retired to the country on his pension, took a small cottage and allotment near his parents and then married. But the conditions of his life were not satisfactory; he worried greatly, lost his sleep, and on

January 10th, 1920, was sent for special treatment to the Tooting Neurological Hospital.

I owe the opportunity of studying his condition to the kindness of Colonel Percy Sargent, D.S.O., and the other authorities of this hospital, who did everything in their power to facilitate my observations.

When he was admitted on January 10th, 1920, two years and eleven months after the injury, he was almost completely aphasic, but could utter a few words and make his meaning plain by the addition of signs. He understood perfectly simple sentences said to him. He appreciated the meaning of single written words but not of sentences. He could write his name and address. He recognised objects shown to him and explained their use by signs, though he was unable to name them. He counted up to six and then from eight to ten, omitting seven; eleven was called "one one," twelve "one two," etc.

His memory for past events seemed to be good. He remembered people though he could not name them and he found his way about perfectly.

There was no history of fits or any similar attacks. Vision was perfect and the discs and fundi showed no changes. He was deaf on the right side to aerial, but not to bony conduction. His hearing was perfect in the left ear. The pupils reacted normally and the movements of the eyes were perfect. There was slight weakness of the right half of the face and tongue with considerable loss of power of the right arm and to a less degree of the leg. Both plantars gave a flexor response and the knee-jerks were not exaggerated.

Condition in December 1920 (*three years and ten months after the injury*), and also in March 1921 (*three months later*).

Owing to the courtesy of the Officer in Command of the Tooting Neurological Hospital, I was permitted to make two extensive sets of observations in the quiet surroundings of my consulting room. The first series was carried out between December 1st, 1920, and January 15th, 1921, and the second three months later from March 19th to 23rd, 1921. As the records were in striking accord, I shall deal with the results as a whole, emphasising any slight differences that threw light on the nature of his loss of speech.

Symbolic Formulation and Expression.

He was an unusually intelligent man, who had been a sergeant in the Royal Army Service Corps (Motor Transport) and was a most willing patient. He enjoyed the examination and frequently made suggestions which showed he had appreciated the significance of the tests. His memory was excellent. On several occasions he drove the motor ambulance in which he was sent to my house; it was then dismissed and he had no difficulty in finding his way back to Tooting. At first he got me to write down the address of the hospital and the number of the omnibus he must catch; but he soon dispensed with these precautions and found his way back alone without the slightest difficulty.

Articulated speech. He was almost wordless for voluntary expression, but his gestures were surprisingly apt and full of meaning. For instance, one morning on arrival he said, "I been good," moving his hands as if manipulating the steering wheel of a motor car, and added, "same come here." I asked if he had driven the motor and he answered, "Yes, good, I been good." To a further question, "Did you find it difficult?" he replied, "No, no." On another occasion he said, "Can I, you know, yes, like this," placing his hand over the lower part of his abdomen; I showed him the lavatory and he went in to pass water, saying, "Yes, thank you." Subsequently he used this gesture without words to express his desire to pass water.

The following conversation illustrated the manner in which, with sympathetic help on the part of the listener, he could triumph over his immense difficulties of expression. I asked him about his education and he was able to convey to me in numbers that he reached the 6th standard at an elementary school at the age of twelve. He added, "Then was going," and, lifting his left hand in the air, "you see?" I suggested, "To a higher school?" and he answered, "Yes. He something here," pointing to his chest, "he died." I asked, "Your father died?" to which he replied, "Yes. Not enough me go there," and raised both hands. I summed up, "You had not enough money to go to a higher school?" to which he assented, "Yes, yes."

He was quite unable to repeat words or sentences said to him. Sometimes the sounds he uttered gave an indication of the word he was struggling to reproduce; but on most occasions he simply shook his head.

Understanding of spoken words. He seemed to understand everything said to him in ordinary conversation and chose familiar objects and colours correctly to oral commands. He even set the hands of a clock and executed the complex movements of the hand, eye and ear tests without mistakes. But, when he was given a series of detailed directions by word of mouth, he was liable to forget some of them, if he could not recapitulate them to himself silently. Thus, told how to return from my house to the hospital, he did not remember exactly the number of the omnibus or its place of departure; but, when I wrote them down, he memorised them with ease and on the second occasion made the journey without the help of the written directions.

Reading. He showed remarkable power of understanding printed words, provided he did not attempt to read them aloud or to spell out the letters of which they were composed. He chose familiar objects and colours to printed commands and conversely selected the appropriate card bearing the name of any colour shown to him. In the same way, during the man, cat and dog tests, he not only picked out a card which bore a description of the two pictures he had seen, but also chose two pictures corresponding to the words on a card. The clock was set accurately to printed commands and the hand, eye and ear movements were performed without mistakes; here again he selected without fail a printed card with a description of the time shown on the clock or the movements made by me. Thus he was able to read to himself sufficiently well to understand printed orders and to pick out the appropriate word or phrase descriptive of some situation arising during the tests.

Yet he could not be certain of understanding anything he read in the newspaper, although he not infrequently recognised the meaning of the shorter and more simple headings. In the same way comprehension of what he read to himself was not sufficient to enable him to gather the full meaning of a short letter. Thus, on one occasion, I wrote asking him to come to my house; hour and day were correctly understood, but he did not recognise that I wished his wife to accompany him until the letter was read aloud to him by the medical officer of the hospital. Pictures as such were appreciated perfectly; but he was greatly hampered in arriving at their meaning if the printed legend was necessary for complete comprehension.

He was entirely unable to read aloud words or phrases which he understood with ease, such as the names of colours; with the man, cat and dog tests he could not evoke even these monosyllables either in response to print or pictures. Moreover, the struggle to articulate the words audibly tended to confuse him and he sometimes failed to execute a printed order, if he attempted to read it aloud, especially when he spelt it out letter by letter.

Writing. His power of writing spontaneously was grossly defective. He wrote his name and the full address of the farm where he worked during 1918 and 1919, saying in explanation, "We've finish that now." But he failed to write down the present home of his wife, where he habitually spent his days on leave; after writing "17 Gal Putney" (for 17 Galveston Road, East Putney), he pointed to Putney and said, "Can't...er...it's there...but I can't." Told to write his number, regiment and rank, he was unable to do so, although, when I said or wrote the various grades from private upwards, he invariably stopped me at sergeant and would accept no branch of the Service except R.A.S.C. (Royal Army Service Corps).

This patient yielded many examples of the way in which the extent of the disturbance of writing depends on whether the act is performed spontaneously, to dictation, or consists of copying print in cursive characters. Thus, although he was completely unable to write the name of a colour shown to him, he succeeded to dictation in producing a combination of letters which bore some definite relation to the words said by me, and he copied every one of them correctly from print. Tested in the same way with the more concrete names of familiar objects, he succeeded in writing something which corresponded more or less distinctly with the word he was seeking to reproduce. To dictation the results were decidedly better and he copied the names almost perfectly from print in cursive script.

He had profound difficulty in discovering the letters he required to form the word he was trying to put down on paper. This want of capacity to write was not strictly speaking of "motor" origin; for he was unable to compose out of a set of block letters the name of a colour shown to him or said aloud by me. The results were equally bad in either case.

The alphabet. He was unable to say the alphabet, making a few meaningless sounds and then giving up the attempt.

Asked to repeat each letter after me, A B C were correctly reproduced. For D he said "E...Te...De." E and F were perfect but G became "Ce." H was "Eight." I was correct. J became "Jes...Ded...Dej." K was "Key"; L "A... Hed...can't"; M "Lem...Leb"; N "Air"; O was correct. P became "B... Ber...Boo"; Q "You, you"; R "Ai, ai"; S "Cee"; T "Dee"; U and V were correct; W was "vavesee...fave...no"; X "Ace...ess"; Y was correct, and Z "Dezz."

When told to write the alphabet he succeeded up to F, but in spite of repeated attempts could go no further; after he had given up he suddenly wrote O W V Y S Q in order to show me that there were other letters which he remembered.

He was then given the block letters and asked to arrange them in the order of the alphabet. He placed in one row B C D E F, and in another N U. Another attempt produced A B C D E F, and I K N U L Q B W X S; he counted over those remaining on the table and said, "There's ten yet." Then he shuffled them all together and began again, A B C D E F; after several wrong letters he added G and then gave up entirely, saying, "I can't...get enough."

I then said each letter in order and he selected the corresponding one from the heap on the table. A B C D E and F were chosen correctly. For G he first chose H, but replaced it by G, and then added H. When I said "I" he repeated "Oi" and chose O; he then took I, and placed it with the O, finally removing the O, leaving the correct letter. J K L M were rightly selected, but for N he chose T; for this, N was substituted on repetition of the order. Q and P were correctly chosen, but when I said "Q" he repeated "You" and selected R, then taking Q into his hands said, "Is that 'un?" and placed it in its proper position. R S T and V were correct; for U he chose W. For W he said "Can't." X and Z were rightly selected, but with Y he said "Eye" and chose U.

When, however, he was asked to write the letters from dictation, he did so correctly; J and Z were made to face the wrong way and Q was replaced by U; but otherwise he made no mistake.

Told to read the alphabet aloud he produced the following sounds:

"Ai" (A); B and C correctly; "Ve" (D); "Ai" (E); "E" (F); "Aye, Ai, You" (G); "Bow" (H); I J K correctly; "E" (L); "Von, vow" (M); "No" (N); O correctly; "Vow" (P); "Ve, ai, von, yoo" (Q); "You" (R); "Vee, vee" (S); "Ai, ai, no" (T); U correctly; "Vent, vee" (V); "Ai, no" (W); "You" (X); "Yah, Vev" (Y); "Vev" (Z).

Counting. Except that he learnt to say "seven," his method of counting remained the same throughout the four months he was under observation. At first he ran up to six correctly, made a sign to show that he could not say the next number and went on rapidly from eight to ten. Then he said, "one, one," "one two" (or "one and two") up to "one and six," missed "one and seven," and ended with "one and nine," "two and oh." From this point he continued in the same manner, to end the decade with "two and nine," "three and oh." He counted on in this way until he came to "six and nine" (69), when he exclaimed, "Ah! you've got me," beating his head. I suggested "seven"; he replied, "I know, that's what I want...sed," and continued to count as follows, "Sed one, sed two, sed three, sed four, sed five, six six, six eight, siz...no, I can't. I can go right, only that one I can't." Started with the word "eight," he went on, however, to "nine nine" and "one no no" for 100; 102 became, "One no and two" and 110 was "one one no."

Arithmetic. He solved the three problems in simple addition correctly; but, with the most difficult of the series, tended to record the sum of each pair of numbers independently. He failed entirely to carry out the simplest subtraction, exclaiming, "Can't get no...can do other one"; he added, "Me when that..." (pointing to a height three feet from the ground) "could do...that."

Addition.			Subtraction.		
654	438	864	865	582	921
132	454	256	432	326	347
786	892	10 12 0			

Coins and their relative value. He could not name a single coin, but could give their relative value correctly. All the numbers above ten were given by naming the digits; thus, when shown a penny and a shilling he at once said, "one and two" (12). He could shop with accuracy and experienced no difficulty with change.

Drawing and pictures. He made an excellent drawing of a spirit-lamp placed on the table before him, and ten minutes later reproduced it accurately from memory. He then drew spontaneously, without a model, a watch with the numbers in the correct position on the face, an excellent representation of a vase with flowers and a horse in motion. Asked to draw an elephant, all the particulars were accurately indicated though the figure as a whole was somewhat clumsy.

He had no difficulty in understanding pictures, provided their significance did not depend on the printed legend. But his comprehension of pictorial jokes was often defective; for although he grasped the direct meaning of the incidents depicted, he not infrequently missed the secondary implication, which depended on due verbal appreciation.

Orientation and plan drawing. He could find his way well even through the complications of a journey across London. He had no difficulty in remembering the position of the salient pieces of furniture in my consulting room, where we worked, and was able to draw an excellent ground-plan showing their arrangement with regard to one another.

Games. He played a good game of dominoes and draughts and was fond of billiards. He also played cards well, provided he was not obliged to call the suit or number, which would have been impossible.

Serial Tests.

I have selected for comparison two sets of observations, one taken in December, 1920, and the other three months later in March, 1921. They illustrate, in spite of some variation in details, the constancy of his responses and the trustworthiness of the tests I have employed.

(1) *Naming and recognition of common objects.*

Table 1.

	Pointing to object shown	Oral commands	Printed commands	Duplicate placed in left hand out of sight	Naming	Writing name of object indicated	Writing name to dictation	Copying from print
Knife	Correct	Correct	Correct	Correct	"Bank, no"	Ki	Knine	Kme, Kneh, Kni
Key	,,	,,	,,	,,	"Bank, no; bore, no"	Key	Key	Key
Penny	,,	,,	,,	,,	"No; one, that's all"	One	penny	penny
Matches	,,	,,	,,	,,	"Bank, no"	Ma	Match Box	Match Box
Scissors	,,	,,	,,	,,	"Bank, no" (shook head)	Sissin	Scissin	Scissors
Pencil	,,	,,	,,	,,	"See-er; eye, eye"	i	pe	Pencil
Key	,,	,,	,,	,,	"Bank, no; poke, perk, no"	Key	Key	Key
Scissors	,,	,,	,,	,,	"Show; shere; show, no"	Sissin	Scissin	Scissors
Matches	,,	,,	,,	,,	"Shar, no"	Mal	Match Box	Match
Knife	,,	,,	,,	,,	"Pho; fi; for, no" [? fork]	Kni	Knive	Knive
Penny	,,	,,	,,	,,	"One, one"	One	penny	penny
Matches	,,	,,	,,	,,	"Fi; son; some; for"	Ma	Match Box	Match Box
Scissors	,,	,,	,,	,,	"Shar; shere"	Sissin	Scissin	Scissors
Pencil	,,	,,	,,	,,	"Yes, eye; eye"	i	pennel	Pencil
Penny	,,	,,	,,	,,	"One"	One	penny	Penny
Knife	,,	,,	,,	,,	"Peek; pink"	Kni	Knive	Knive
Key	,,	,,	,,	,,	"Bank; bunk"	Key	Key	Key
Pencil	,,	,,	,,	,,	"Eye; eye"	is	pennel	Pencil

He had no hesitation in selecting the object which corresponded with one shown to him, or that he held in his hand out of sight. His responses, though somewhat slower, were also correct to oral or printed commands.

When asked to name a selected object, he was unable to do so; but this was obviously due to a want of words and not to lack of nominal appreciation; for a "penny" was always called "one."

Repetition was also almost impossible and it is interesting to notice that although I said "penny" he repeated it as "one"; "key" was, however, repeated correctly.

The three writing tests brought out results exactly consonant with the comparative difficulty of the verbal task. He was unable in most instances to write the name of an object shown to him; dictation produced a better result, whilst he was able to copy perfectly the printed words in cursive handwriting. It is noteworthy that "penny," even when dictated, was written "one." "Key" gave him no difficulty throughout, and he said, "Yes, I can see..." waving his hand in the air.

Table 2.

	Pointing to object shown; oral commands; printed commands; duplicate placed in left hand	Naming	Repetition	Writing name of object indicated	Writing name to dictation	Copying from print
Knife	Correct	(Shook his head)	(Shook his head)	Kl	Kl	Knife
Key	"	"Bow"	"Key"	Key	Key	Key
Penny	"	"One"	"One"	One	One	Penny
Matches	"	(Shook his head)	(Shook his head)	Mal	Ma	Match Box
Scissors	"	(")	(")	Sicil	Siss	Scissors
Pencil	"	"Siven"	"Penky"	Pinn	Pinne	Penny
Key	"	"Dee"	"Key"	Key	Key	Key
Scissors	"	(Shook his head)	(Shook his head)	Sr	Siss	Scissors
Matches	"	"No"	(")	Mal	Mat	Match Box
Knife	"	(Shook his head)	(")	Kl	Kl	Knife
Penny	"	"One"	"One"	One	One	Penny
Matches	"	"No"	"No"	Mats	Mal	Match Box
Scissors	"	"No"	(Shook his head)	Src	Siss	Scissors
Pencil	"	"Penk"	"Pent"	Prnn	Pinn	Pencil
Penny	"	"One"	"One"	One	One	Penny
Knife	"	"No"	(Shook his head)	K	Kle	Knife
Key	"	"Aye; no"	"No"	Key	Key	Key
Pencil	"	(Shook his head)	"Menk"	Pinn	Pinn	Pencil

(2) *Naming and recognition of colours.*

Table 3.

	Pointing to colour shown	Oral commands	Printed commands	Naming colour shown	Writing down name of colour shown	Writing name of colour to dictation	Copying name of colour from print	Choosing a card bearing name of colour shown
Black	Perfect	Correct	Correct	"I can't"	Impossible	D	Black	Correct
Red	"	"	"	(Shook his head)	"	Red	Red	"
Blue	"	Violet	"	(")	"	Bo	Blue	"
Green	"	Correct	"	"No, no"	"	Geen	Green	"
Orange	"	Yellow	Yellow	"No"	"	(Wrote nothing)	Orange	"
White	"	Correct	Correct	(Shook his head)	"	White	White	"
Violet	"	Blue; doubtful	"	(")	"	Vin	Violet	"
Yellow	"	Correct	"	(")	"	Yeller	Yellow	"
Red	"	"	"	(")	"	Red	Red	"
White	"	"	"	(")	"	Wh	White	"
Yellow	"	"	"	(")	"	Yeller	Yellow	"
Blue	"	Violet; slowly	Violet	(")	"	But	Blue	"
Green	"	Correct	Correct	(")	"	Ge	Green	"
Black	"	"	"	(")	"	D	Black	"
Orange	"	Yellow	Correct; slow	(")	"	Y; "No, not that"	Orange	"
Violet	"	Blue	Correct	(")	"	Vin	Violet	"

Shown a colour and asked to say what it was, he was completely unable to do so. This was due to want of words in which to express himself and not to defective recognition of names; for he picked out with certainty from cards laid on the table that one which bore the name of the colour which had been shown him.

When a colour was named to him, either orally or in print, his choice was somewhat slow, and he tended to confuse violet and blue, yellow and orange; otherwise he made no mistakes. He was quicker and more certain when allowed to select a printed card corresponding to the colour indicated.

He could not write the name of a single colour, and, when first examined in December, 1920, made no attempt to do so. Three months later, however, he was able to write "Yeller" and indicated the first letters of black, white, green and orange. He had great difficulty in writing the colour names to dictation, but copied them perfectly in cursive handwriting from a printed card. The more nearly the task approached pure imitation, the more easily and correctly was it performed.

He could neither read aloud the names of the colours nor repeat them after me.

Table 4.

	Pointing to colour shown	Oral commands	Printed commands	Naming colour shown	Writing down name of colour shown	Writing name of colour to dictation	Copying name of colour from print	Choosing card bearing name of colour shown	Printed name read aloud	Name repeated after the observer
Black	Perfect	Correct	Correct	Impossible	B	Bla	Black	Correct	"Em"	"Mack"
Red	,,	,,	,,	,,	(Wrote nothing)	Yeller	Red	,,	"Lis"	"Lev"
Blue	,,	Violet	,,	,,	(,,)	Bu	Blue	,,	"Be, be"	"Deï"
Green	,,	Correct	,,	,,	(,,)	G	Green	,,	(Shook his head)	"Yon"
Orange	,,	,,	,,	,,	(,,)	O	Orange	,,	"Oh"	(Shook his head) "No"
White	,,	,,	,,	,,	W	Wi	White	,,	(Shook his head)	(Shook his head) "No"
Violet	,,	,,	,,	,,	(Wrote nothing)	Vi	Violet	,,	(,,)	(Shook his head) "No"
Yellow	,,	,,	,,	,,	Yeller	Yeller	Yellow	,,	"Lev, lev"	"Ed"
Red	,,	,,	,,	,,	(Wrote nothing)	R	Red	,,	(Shook his head)	"Dead"
White	,,	,,	,,	,,	We	Whi	White	,,	(,,)	"No"
Yellow	,,	,,	,,	,,	Yeller	Yeller	Yellow	,,	"Lev, lev"	"Yei"
Blue	,,	Correct; slow	,,	,,	(Wrote nothing)	Bu	Blue	,,	"Be, be"	(Shook his head)
Green	,,	Correct	,,	,,	G	G	Green	,,	(Shook his head)	(,,)
Black	,,	,,	,,	,,	B	Bla	Black	,,	"Lev...be, be"	"Dead"
Orange	,,	Yellow; corrected	,,	,,	O	Oro	Orange	,,	"Oh"	(Shook his head)
Violet	,,	Blue; corrected	,,	,,	(Wrote nothing)	Vioth	Violet	,,	"No"	(,,)

A most instructive set of observations was carried out in the following manner. Sufficient block letters to compose the names of all the colours were laid on the table, and he was asked on the one hand to indicate with them the colour shown to him and on the other to put together the words said by me. The results were almost identical. (Table 5.) The power of naming was obviously retained, but word-formation was defective, even when the isolated letters were given. On the other hand, he was able in this way to give some indication of the names of the colours, which was impossible in writing; the task was easier, for at any rate the letters were given to him and he was not compelled to think of their formation.

Table 5.

	Printed name read aloud by patient	Names repeated after the observer	Putting together out of letters the name said by the observer	Putting together out of letters the name of a colour shown to the patient
Black	"O, no, E C B"	"Can't"	D	D. "I know that...I can't"
Red	"O; let's see...O E, can't that one" (pointing to R)	"Hed...er...hed"	"I know that." R E R. He removed R. "Oh! I know. There you are," choosing D	R E D
Blue	"B B; no, I can't"	"Do...no"	B U I. "No," removed I. "No, that's same"; B I U	B I U E. "I didn't know whether that one, other one." (Is satisfied with B I U E)
Green	"E E O I O U; you, yoo. I can't know some"	"Dee...do...no"	G R E E G; removed G and replaced it by N. "Yes, yes"	G R E E. "Oh! yes, I know." N
Orange	"O O" (pointing to first letter). "Couldn't got no, that" (pointing to R)	"Oh! yes" (Shook head)	Y. "I know." E L L E G; removed G, placed N in its place. Removed N. "No, no"	Y E L L E R
White	"A O C P O...C C"	"No I can't. I know, but I can't"	W H I N; removed N. "I can't see"	W H I N. Shook his head. Removed N; replaced it by E. Not satisfied, but made no further move
Violet	"Pork, pear...I, I" (pointing to I) "O" (pointing to O) "E...C C"	"Good...bear"	Pointed to Y and said, "Not quite same." Chose V, "Yes, there you are." I, then gave up	V I O. "No"
Yellow	"O...I see now"	(Shook head)	Y E L L E R. "No, yes, that's right"	"Oh! yes" Y E L L E R
Red	"E" (pointing to E) "B C E" (again to E)	(Shook head)	R E D. "Yes, look"	R E D
White	"U...No, U U" (pointing to W)	"Oh! no"	W H I N I; removed I. Substituted E; removed E. "No," gave up	W H I N E; removed N. Chose L; rejected it. Chose E; rejected it. Chose T. "Oh yes!"
Yellow	"I U there. No U there. A O P. No, where's P?"	(Shook head)	L L. Then rapidly Y E L L E R	Y E L L E R
Blue	"B...No, there's no B. No I'm gone here. I've got it...and it's gone"	"Oh! no"	B U...B I U E	B I E...B U I E...B I U E. Completely satisfied and shuffled letters preparatory to starting again
Green	"E I O I. No...B, no"	"Q, N...no"	G E. Placed R between and then made G R E E N	G R E E N
Black	"B...I've got B. I've got that. B I"	"No"	D. "But then now...No"	D. Shook his head and said, "No"
Orange	"O O" (pointing to O) "I I, no"	(Shook head)	Y E L L E R	Y E L L E R
Violet	"I" (pointing to I) "O" (pointing to O) "B, no, U E...Where's E?"	(Laughed and shook head)	V. "Yes, that," I	V I O N; removed N. T; removed T. E T. "That's right?" Then spaced V I O L E. "It's not that." Then added T. V I O L E T. "It looks too much"

(3) *The man, cat and dog tests.*

Table 6.

	Reading aloud	Reading from pictures	Repetition	Choosing printed card from pictures	Choosing pictures from printed card	Copying from print	Writing to dictation	Writing from pictures
The dog and the cat	"No" Impossible	"No" Impossible	"No" Impossible	Perfect	Perfect	The Dog and the Cat	Dog and Cat	Dog and Cat
The man and the dog	,,	,,	,,	,,	,,	The Man and the Dog	Man and Dog	Man and Dog
The cat and the man	,,	,,	,,	,,	,,	The Cat and the Man	Cat and Man	Cat and Man
The cat and the dog	,,	,,	,,	,,	,,	The Cat and the Dog	Cat and Dog	Cat and Dog
The dog and the man	,,	,,	,,	,,	,,	The Dog and the Man	Dog and Man	Dog and Man
The man and the cat	,,	,,	,,	,,	,,	The Man and the Cat	Man and Cat	Man and Cat
The dog and the man	,,	,,	,,	,,	,,	The Dog and the Man	Dog and Man	Dog and Man
The cat and the man	,,	,,	,,	,,	,,	The Cat and the Man	Cat and Man	Cat and Man
The dog and the cat	,,	,,	,,	,,	,,	The Dog and the Cat	Dog and Cat	Dog and Cat
The man and the dog	,,	,,	,,	,,	,,	The Man and the Dog	Man and Dog	Man and Dog
The cat and the dog	,,	,,	,,	,,	,,	The Cat and the Dog	Cat and Dog	Cat and Dog
The man and the cat	,,	,,	,,	,,	,,	The Man and the Cat	Man and Cat	Man and Cat

As the results obtained in December, 1920, and in March, 1921, were almost identical, the former alone are given in tabular form (Table 6). This series of tests showed that he was completely unable to read aloud from print or from pictures, or to repeat even simple phrases made up of monosyllabic words. On the other hand, he had no difficulty in choosing either a printed card corresponding to two pictures shown him, or in selecting the appropriate combination of pictures from a printed card. He retained the power of recognising the names of objects depicted, although he lacked words in which to express them.

Another striking feature of these observations was the similarity of the results obtained when he wrote from dictation or from pictures. In both cases he left out unessential words, but never failed to select the appropriate names or to place them in the correct order. It obviously made no material difference whether the command was received through eye or ear.

When copying print in cursive script, he wrote slowly, looking frequently at the card in front of him; he evidently found difficulty in retaining the words without repeated reference to the copy. Asked if he found this test easy, he replied, "Yes... good...good...when they gone can't see...you know...can't see," making a movement as if the cards had been removed from the table. He was evidently attempting to indicate his fleeting memory for the words he copied correctly.

(4) *The clock tests.*

Here again it was obvious that words failed him rather than names; for he had no difficulty in choosing a printed card corresponding to the time shown on the clock face. He could even write the name correctly if he was allowed to use figures only. "Past" and "to" the hour were never confused and he did not mistake the significance of the two hands. Moreover, the hour hand was set at a point proportional to the position of the minute hand and was not placed directly opposite the figure mentioned orally or in print.

Provided care was taken to note exactly what he said, it was obvious, in spite of the paucity of his vocabulary, that he recognised the time shown on the clock. Thus, for half-past one he said "one, three and no" (1.30), twenty minutes to six was "five, four and no" (5.40), and a quarter to nine became "nine, nine."

Asked to indicate the time shown on the clock face by choosing one of a set of printed cards, he made no mistakes; and yet in one series of observations the

Table 7.

	Direct imitation	Oral commands	Printed commands	Telling the time	Writing down the time	Choosing a printed card corresponding to time shown on the clock
5 minutes to 2	Correct	Correct	Correct	"Five two"	11.2	Correct
Half-past 1	,,	,,	,,	"One and six"	1.30	,,
5 minutes past 8	,,	,,	Correct; slow	"Eight and five"	8.5	,,
20 minutes to 4	,,	"Four, four, eight" Set correctly	Correct	"Three four and oh"	3.40	,,
10 minutes past 7	,,	Correct	,,	"Ten and...I can't tell that"	7.10	,,
20 minutes to 6	,,	"Six and four" Set correctly	,,	"Can't that one"	5.40	,,
10 minutes to 1	,,	Correct	,,	"Five and two and oh. No, not that one. Five, four and oh"	12.50	,,
A quarter to 9	,,	"Nine to nine" Set correctly	,,	"Nine nine"	8.45	,,
20 minutes past 11	,,	"One, one and four" Set correctly	,,	"One, one, two and oh"	11.20	,,
25 minutes to 3	,,	"Three and seven" Set correctly	,,	"Two and I can't. That's three and five (35)"	2.35	,,

Table 8.

	Direct imitation; oral commands; printed commands	Telling the time	Writing down the time	Choosing a printed card corresponding to time shown on the clock	Copying print in handwriting
5 minutes to 2	Correct	"Five two"	2.5	Correct	Five minutes to two
Half-past 1	,,	"One, three and no"	1.30	,,	Half past one
5 minutes past 8	,,	"Eight five"	8.5	,,	Five minutes past eight
20 minutes to 4	,,	"Three and four no"	3.40	,,	Twenty minutes to Four
10 minutes past 7	,,	"Seven ten"	7.10	,,	Ten minutes Past Seven
20 minutes to 6	,,	"Five, four and no"	5.40	,,	Twenty minutes to Six
10 minutes to 1	,,	"Ten" (shook his head)	12.50	,,	Ten minutes to one
A quarter to 9	,,	"Eight, four and five"	8.45	,,	A quarter to Nine
20 minutes past 11	,,	(Shook his head)	11.20	,,	Twenty minutes Past Eleven
25 minutes to 3	,,	"Two, three and five"	2.35	,,	Twenty Five minutes to Three

legend was displayed entirely in words and in another in figures only. Moreover, when he was timed with a stop-watch, I could not discover that this difference materially influenced the rapidity of his choice.

He copied the words on the printed card laboriously but correctly, looking back repeatedly for each word or even part of a word; with numbers, such as "eleven," he re-examined each letter, although the whole was correctly transposed into cursive handwriting.

(5) *The coin-bowl tests.* He was able to carry out oral and printed commands perfectly. Moreover, it seemed to make no material difference to the time required for choice whether the printed order was given in figures or in words; in both cases he seized on the essential numbers and executed the order with great rapidity.

(6) *The hand, eye and ear tests.*

This was the only series of tests which showed material improvement between December, 1920 (Table 9), and March, 1921 (Table 10). At first he had difficulty in imitating exactly movements made by me, when I sat opposite to him, and he tended to confuse right and left, though he never made a mistake in eye or ear. To a less degree similar errors appeared, when the command took the form of a picture placed before him.

But, as soon as the task consisted of imitating the reflections in a mirror of my movements or of pictorial commands, he neither hesitated nor made a mistake, flinging up his hand rapidly as if for a smart salute. Pointing to the mirror he said, "Yes, that's nothing," to express the ease with which this task could be executed.

After he had acquired the power of carrying out the movements sitting face to face (Table 10), he attempted to explain to me in the following manner how it was done. He thrust one hand forwards and drew the other backwards at the same time; then he made similar movements in an opposite direction, to indicate that his actions and mine must be conversely related.

Oral commands given slowly and repeated at his desire were carried out well. Usually he first raised the hand corresponding to the one I mentioned; then he looked up questioningly and waited for me to repeat the order before he decided whether to touch his eye or his ear.

Printed commands were executed on the whole correctly, so long as he did not try to read the words; but if he attempted to spell the letters he tended to become somewhat less certain.

He found extreme difficulty in writing down the movements made by me and ended by recording solely the hand I had used and whether I had touched an eye or an ear. He simplified the problem by omitting one of the variable factors. But he could copy the printed order in cursive handwriting without fail; he wrote, however, slowly and repeatedly referred back to the legend displayed before him.

If the printed cards were laid on the table, he could choose correctly the one which bore a description of the movement made by me. He explained, "You see, here," pointing to his forehead, "something to get hold of there," placing his hand on the cards. He evidently intended to signify that the printed legend enabled him to express his thoughts.

Table 9.

	Imitation of movements made by the observer	Imitation of movements reflected in a mirror	Pictorial commands	Pictorial commands reflected in a mirror	Oral commands	Printed commands	Reading aloud and executing printed commands		Writing down movements made by the observer	Choosing printed card describing movements made by the observer
							He read	Movement executed		
L. hand to L. eye	Reversed	Correct	Correct	Correct	Correct	Correct	"No"	Correct	Lef	Correct
R. hand to R. ear	”	”	”	”	”	”	”	”	4 eal	”
R. hand to L. eye	L. hand to L. eye	”	”	”	”	”	”	”	4 eye	Reversed; slow
L. hand to R. eye	R. hand to R. eye	”	”	”	”	”	Silent	”	L-eye	Correct; slow
L. hand to L. ear	Correct	”	L. hand to R. ear; corrected	”	”	”	”	”	L ear	Correct
R. hand to R. eye	”	”	Correct	”	R. hand to L. eye	R. hand to R. *ear*	”	”	r eye	”
L. hand to R. ear	R. hand to R. ear	”	Reversed	”	Correct	L. hand to R. *eye*; corrected	”	”	L ear	”
R. hand to L. ear	Correct	”	Correct	”	”	Correct	"I don't know"	”	ra ear	Correct; slow
L. hand to L. eye	R. hand to L. eye	”	”	”	”	”	Silent	”	L. eye	Correct
R. hand to R. ear	Correct	”	”	”	”	”	"Yes"	”	ro ear	”
R. hand to L. eye	”	”	”	”	”	”	”	”	r eye	”
L. hand to R. eye	Reversed	”	”	”	”	”	”	”	Le eye	”
L. hand to L. ear	”	”	”	”	”	”	Silent	”	L ear	”
R. hand to R. eye	Correct	”	”	”	”	”	"Yes"	”	r eye	”
L. hand to R. ear	”	”	Reversed	”	”	”	"Oh! yes"	”	L ear	Correct; very slow
R. hand to L. ear	”	”	”	”	”	”	"Yes"	”	r ear	Correct

Table 10.

	Imitation of movements made by the observer	Imitation of movements reflected in a mirror	Pictorial commands	Pictorial commands reflected in a mirror	Oral commands	Printed commands	Reading aloud and executing printed commands		Writing down movements made by the observer	Choosing printed card describing movements made by the observer	Copying print in cursive handwriting
							He read	Movement executed			
L. hand to L. eye	Correct	Correct	Correct	Correct	Correct	Correct	"Eye, eye . . . left"	Correct	Le e	Correct	Lefe Hand to Lefe eye
R. hand to R. ear	,,	,,	,,	,,	,,	,,	"Lef, lef *eye*"	,,	Wrote nothing	,,	Correct
R. hand to L. eye	,,	,,	,,	,,	,,	,,	"Lef. . . eye"	,,	L—e	,,	,,
L. hand to R. eye	,,	,,	,,	,,	,,	,,	"Lef . . . er . . . eye. Can't. . . no"	,,	L—Eye	,,	,,
L. hand to L. ear	,,	,,	,,	,,	,,	,,	"Yes, yes"	,,	L—Ege	,,	,,
R. hand to R. eye	,,	,,	,,	,,	,,	,,	"Right, right"	,,	R—Eye	,,	,,
L. hand to R. ear	,,	,,	,,	,,	L. hand to L. ear	,,	"Lef, lef, *eye*. . . right. . . lef"	,,	L—Eae	L. hand to L. ear; corrected	,,
R. hand to L. ear	,,	,,	,,	,,	Correct	,,	"*Eye*. . . right. . . lef *eye*"	,,	R—Eea	Correct	,,
L. hand to L. eye	,,	,,	,,	,,	,,	,,	Silent	,,	L—Eye	,,	,,
R. hand to R. ear	,,	,,	,,	,,	Correct; slow	,,	,,	,,	R—Ear	,,	,,
R. hand to L. eye	,,	,,	,,	,,	Correct	,,	"Head, right eye . . . left eye"	,,	R—Eye	,,	,,
L. hand to R. eye	,,	,,	,,	,,	,,	,,	"Yes, yes"	,,	L—Eye	,,	,,
L. hand to L. ear	,,	,,	,,	,,	,,	,,	"Lef. . . lef *eye*"	,,	L—Ear	,,	,,
R. hand to R. eye	,,	,,	,,	,,	,,	,,	"Eye, left, no, eight, no"	,,	R—Eye	,,	,,
L. hand to R. ear	,,	,,	,,	,,	,,	,,	Silent	,,	L—Ear	,,	,,
R. hand to L. ear	,,	,,	,,	,,	,,	,,	,,	,,	R—Ear	,,	,,

Physical Examination.

He was a tall well-built active man who had always been strongly right-handed; even in his present condition, in spite of the remains of a right hemiplegia, he used his right hand in preference to his left.

There were no signs of motor apraxia. He could light a match and blow it out again, manipulating it with skill, and had no difficulty in tying two ends of a piece of string into any form of knot desired. He mimicked correctly such actions as lighting a cigarette or brushing his hair with no objects in his hands.

He had never suffered from fits or other attacks and was entirely free from headache in any form.

Vision was $\frac{6}{6}$ in the right eye, $\frac{6}{9}$ in the left. The fields were unaffected and the discs were normal.

Hearing in the left ear was good, but he was deaf on the right side. A watch was not heard on contact and a tuning fork placed over the right mastoid was heard by conduction on the left side only. Both membranes appeared to be normal and the deafness was probably of nervous origin.

Smell was evidently intact. Given peppermint he nodded his head; but with asafoetida he shook his head, saying, "No, that bad."

Taste appeared to be unaffected; for with quinine or tartaric acid he withdrew his head, whilst when saccharine was placed on his tongue he said, "Good, good; no good other."

His pupils reacted well and the eyes moved perfectly in all directions. I could find no inequality in the movements of the two halves of the face and the tongue was protruded straight; when retracted, however, it tended to curl a little to the left. The slight weakness of face and tongue, noticed in January, 1920, on his admission to the Tooting Neurological Hospital, had passed away.

I could find no definite difference between the deep reflexes obtained from the two upper extremities; perhaps the right wrist-jerk was obtained a little more easily than the left, but neither was excessive. Knee- and ankle-jerks were normal and equal on the two sides.

The plantar reflexes gave a downward response and the abdominals were certainly obtained with ease on the two halves of the abdomen, both above and below the umbilicus.

Individual movements were executed slowly and imperfectly with the digits of the right hand; approximation of each finger in turn to the tip of the thumb was carried out with effort and was accompanied by an abnormal amount of accessory flexion in other parts of the hand. But he finally succeeded in bringing each finger into contact with the thumb, whether his eyes were open or closed; though in the latter case he frequently brought them together side by side.

His hands could be held out steadily in front of him and the fingers of the right were in fair alinement. Made to separate his fingers and then bring them together again, the movements were somewhat more clumsy in the right hand; but there was no falling away of his fingers when the eyes were closed.

The grasp of the right hand was considerably weaker than that of the left and he complained that it seemed clumsy when he buttoned his clothes. All movements of the right wrist, elbow and shoulder were powerful, but they did not seem to me to exceed those of the left arm to the extent that might have been expected in so strongly right-handed a man.

He walked well and his gait showed no signs of hemiplegia. When driving a motor car he used the right foot for the brake; but with the eyes open he could not stand on his right leg for more than five seconds, although he could balance himself on the left for fifteen seconds.

The movements of the toes of the right foot were more clumsy than those of the left; every action possible on the one side could be carried out on the other, but, when the toes of the right foot were extended, they became abducted, whilst on flexion they came together again. All movements of the right ankle, knee and hip were strongly executed against resistance and there was no sign of incoordination.

I could find no evidence of loss of appreciation of posture or passive movement. He could discriminate the compass points at 1 cm. over the palmar aspect of the fingers of the right hand, and at 3 cm. over the sole of the right foot; there was no obvious difference between the two sides to this test. Localisation was certainly unaffected and he recognised the various tests for shape and form correctly, choosing without fail the duplicate figure from amongst those on the table in front of him. There was no gross loss of sensation to touch, pricking, heat or cold; but the finer tests could not be applied owing to his want of words.

The right hand tended to become blue and cold to a greater extent than the left, especially in the cold weather. Even when warmed it was pinker than the left.

The sphincters were in every way normal.

No. 20

A case of acute and severe Aphasia due to the removal of an extra-cerebral tumour which indented the brain around the meeting point of the inferior frontal and the inferior precentral fissures.

The operation was followed by flaccid right hemiplegia, loss of movement in the same half of the face and tongue, together with the usual changes in the reflexes on the paralysed side. At the expiration of sixteen days all abnormal signs had passed away and there was no difference between the two halves of the body.

The loss of speech was at first profound and she could say "yes" and "no" only. The acts of speaking, reading and writing were all affected at first; even the power of understanding what was said to her was somewhat disturbed. As she regained her capacity to use language, those aptitudes returned first which were least dependent on accurate word-formation. Clinically, within four months of the operation, she had been transformed from a severe example of loss of symbolic formulation and expression into one of Verbal Aphasia so slight that it might have been mistaken for an articulatory disturbance only.

A little more than ten months after the operation, as the result of worry and consequent insomnia, she regressed to a condition in which her defects of speech resembled those found four weeks after removal of the tumour. Speech, reading and writing had grossly deteriorated and many of the serial tests were badly executed. There were no abnormal physical signs.

The causes of her worry were removed and five months later she had recovered to a degree never reached before. She still had obvious difficulty in finding words to express her thoughts, but her powers of reading and writing were greatly improved, problems in arithmetic could be solved correctly and all the serial tests were executed without grave errors. This improvement continued, and has been steadily maintained.

Alice Lucy Esther B., a widow lady of 56, first came under my care on May 29th, 1922, complaining of epileptiform convulsions.

In 1916 she went to bed one night at 10 o'clock apparently in perfect health. As she was falling to sleep she suddenly felt that she could not use her right hand, particularly the thumb and index finger. She sprang up in bed with a sensation of choking and became unconscious, passing urine involuntarily. Two months later she had an exactly similar attack, and in the course of the last six years lost consciousness six times in all. But from time to time she suffered from minor seizures, which began with a "numb feeling" in the thumb; the tip then became flexed towards the palm, the digits "drew up" and she was unable to open them Then the face might become affected; but if the hand was rubbed vigorously the attack would often come to an end without loss of consciousness.

The last seizure, which was a slight one, occurred on May 20th, 1922, and began with the usual symptoms in the thumb and index finger of the right hand. She did not become unconscious, but for six or seven hours afterwards her speech was affected and she was unable freely to express her wishes; by 3 a.m. she had entirely recovered. This loss of speech so greatly alarmed her that she determined to consult a specialist.

When she first came under my care she was an extremely vigorous woman, who not only managed a large household, but carried on with success the business of a decorator and paper manufacturer.

Her pulse was normal, except that the tension was distinctly high (diastolic 120 mm., systolic 190 mm.). The heart was unaffected. Her urine was of a specific gravity of 1020 and contained no albumen or sugar; but in the past she had suffered from glycosuria, which, however, could be completely controlled by a moderate restriction of diet.

A shrewd, capable, North-country woman, her intelligence was much above the average and her mental state had remained unchanged by her illness. Speech had not been affected except during the last attack. She told me: "I knew what I wanted to say, but I could not explain it to anyone; I couldn't seem to put the words together and I couldn't have made a long sentence." When she came under my care, speech, reading and writing were in every way perfect. She carried on her business, kept accounts and made all the arrangements for her stay in London unaided with ease and assurance.

She denied that she ever suffered from headache, but complained of an unpleasant sensation which was "not a pain" behind the eyes and over the vertex. This was increased by stooping or by worry, though not by intellectual efforts or physical fatigue. At no time had her head been sore or tender. She had vomited after the attacks in which she became unconscious, but had not otherwise suffered even from nausea.

Vision was $\frac{6}{6}$ in either eye and the fundi showed no changes of any kind. Hearing, smell and taste were excellent in every way.

The pupils reacted well, ocular movements were perfectly executed and there was no nystagmus. The face moved equally on the two sides: the tongue was protruded straight and withdrawn without deviation.

The right wrist-jerk was somewhat brisker than the left, but the knee- and ankle-jerks were normal and both plantars gave a downward response. In consequence of the laxness of the abdominal wall, the reflexes were obtained with difficulty even to the left of the middle line; on the right side I could not elicit them at any time.

There was no paralysis, paresis, tremor or incoordination. Individual movements were as well executed by the digits of the right as by those of the left hand, and their tone was in no way affected. Her gait was normal and she could stand equally well on either foot with the eyes open or closed.

The most careful sensory examination failed to reveal any disturbance of function. Her power of appreciating the tactile hairs, weight, form, texture, measured movements and the two compass points was equally good on the two sides, and localisation was perfect.

From these signs and symptoms I concluded that she was suffering from the effects of a tumour, probably of extra-cerebral origin, within the left half of the cranial cavity. The absence of sensory defects in the period between the attacks led me to believe that it was situated in front of the fissure of Rolando.

On June 20th, 1922, Mr Wilfred Trotter removed a smooth, lobulated fibrous growth, which measured 5 cm. antero-posteriorly, 4 cm. vertically and 3·5 cm. in depth. Microscopically its structure was that of a fibro-endothelioma. It sprang from the dura mater, which was in turn firmly attached to the bone above it; this was soft and vascular, cutting like cheese. The tumour was so carefully extracted that not even the smallest fragment of cortical tissue adhered to the mass removed. The depression it had produced in the substance of the brain seemed to be centred around the meeting point of the inferior frontal and the inferior precentral fissures.

The wound healed by first intention and the patient showed no evidence of surgical shock or other unpleasant manifestations. But on the day after the operation she was speechless except for the words "yes" and "no"—and even "no" was sometimes wrongly employed when she intended to express assent. This aphasia was accompanied by complete flaccid hemiplegia on the right side of the body with paralysis of the same half of the tongue and lower part of the face. The right plantar reflex gave a definite upward response, and arm- and knee-jerks were brisker than those on the normal side.

From this time onwards she improved steadily day by day both physically and in her powers of speech. As the interest of this case lies more particularly in the order and manner of her recovery, as revealed by systematic examination, I shall divide my report into two portions, the first of which narrates the restoration of her physical powers, whilst the second deals with the much slower return of symbolic formulation and expression.

Physical Examination.

On the *fourth day* after the operation (June 24th) she had recovered considerable strength in the right leg, and could even dorsiflex and plantar extend the right foot. Some power had returned at the shoulder and elbow, and, although individual movements of the digits were impossible, she could close the fingers over mine in a feeble grasp. The lower portion of the right half of the face was completely paralysed, and the tongue deviated grossly to the same side on protrusion. All the deep reflexes on the affected half of the body were brisker than those on the left side; and the right plantar gave a characteristic upward response.

On the *sixth day* (June 26th) power had returned to a remarkable extent; she could make individual movements of the fingers and thumb of the right hand, and the grasp, though weaker than that on the normal side, had greatly increased in strength. All movements were now readily performed by the right leg. Some slight motion had returned to the right half of the face, and the tongue was protruded more nearly in the middle line; she could now lick the right angle of her mouth with ease. The right wrist-jerk was brisker than the left, but the knee- and ankle-jerks were equal on the two sides. On scratching the sole of the right foot, the great toe remained stationary, whilst the others moved downwards and became approximated to one another; similar excitation of the normal foot led to brisk downward movement of all the toes. I could not obtain any reflex from the right half of the abdomen: but even those on the normal side were doubtful, probably owing to the laxity of the abdominal wall.

On the *seventh day* (June 27th) every movement of the right lower extremity was perfect, and crude power had almost completely returned to the right hand. When the arm was held out in front of her, the fingers were in alinement with one another, and they did not fall away on closing the eyes. The lower part of the right half of the face acted voluntarily, though less perfectly than the left, and the tongue was protruded in the middle line. I could discover no sensory loss of any kind. She could appreciate passive movements of 2° in all the digits, and answered "front" or "back" correctly. She had no difficulty in recognising the shape of solid geometrical objects placed in the right hand, and nothing pointed to any "stereognostic" defect.

On the *tenth day* (June 30th) power had greatly increased in the whole of the right upper extremity; individual movements of the fingers and thumb were now possible, and the grasp of the right hand equalled that of the left. The lower portion of the right half of the face was still weaker than the opposite side, but the tongue was protruded in the middle line, and did not deviate on retraction into the mouth. The right wrist-jerk was brisker than the left, whilst the knee- and ankle-jerks were equal on the two sides, and the right plantar gave a completely normal response. Her power of appreciating geometrical shapes was again tested and found to be perfect with either hand.

On the *fourteenth day* (July 4th) the grasp of the right hand was stronger than that of the left, and individual movements of the digits were equally well performed on the two sides. There was no incoordination or ataxy, and the fingers did not fall out of alinement when the eyes were closed. The two wrist-jerks were now equal, and the right plantar exactly resembled that obtained from the normal foot. I was able to elicit a slight reflex from the upper half of the abdomen to the right of the middle line, though not from parts below the umbilicus; but it must be remembered that these reflexes were obtained with great difficulty even on the normal side.

On the *sixteenth day* (July 6th) I could find no definite physical signs pointing to loss of function in any part of the nervous system. The patient was free from headache or discomfort—even the opening in her head did not trouble her. Vision was unaffected, the fields were not restricted, and the fundi normal. The pupils reacted well and movements of the eyes were perfect in all directions. The right half of the face moved well, and I could not observe any difference between the two sides. The tongue was protruded and withdrawn in the middle line. Motor power of both upper and lower limbs, including individual movements of the fingers, was completely restored, and there was no sensory loss of any kind. All the reflexes, except those from the abdomen, were normal and equal on the two sides.

Thus, at the expiration of sixteen days after the removal of an extra-cerebral tumour in the left frontal region, a complete flaccid hemiplegia affecting the face and tongue had cleared up entirely, and no definite difference could be discovered between the reaction of the two halves of the body.

Symbolic Formulation and Expression.

At first she was speechless except for "yes" and "no"—and even "no" was at times wrongly employed. Told to give me her hand or touch her nose, she could do so, but became confused if I specified either the right or the left hand. She seemed to understand simple orders, such as to turn over in bed or move the arm or the leg, but she frequently failed to comprehend the full significance of questions, and was profoundly puzzled by her inability to express her wants.

By the *sixth day* (June 26th) her speech had greatly improved, and she used "yes" and "no" appropriately. She asked spontaneously for an "orange" and for "tea," and employed the following phrases: "I know well enough," "Can't say well enough," "I don't know—no." Asked what she thought of the flowers in her room, she said: "Very pretty, very pretty." She spoke extremely slowly, and evidently formed the words with difficulty; those of more than one syllable tended to be slurred, or were divided by a pause of considerable length into two parts.

She understood simple statements, but was liable to become confused if the words implied a complex order. Told to touch her nose with her right or her left hand, she did so correctly four times in succession; but, when asked to touch her nose or her eye with one or other hand, which introduced a double choice, she failed in four out of eight attempts.

A request to name coins placed before her led to the following result:

A penny	"quinny"
A shilling	"sixpence"
A halfpenny	correct
A two-shilling piece	correct
A sixpence	correct

A penny	correct
A shilling	correct
A halfpenny	"sixpence, halfpenny"
A two-shilling piece	"jew shill-ns"
A sixpence	correct

Asked to name the relative value of two coins laid on the table together, she gave the following answers:

A sixpence and a shilling—"sixpence"
A penny and a shilling—"sixpence, shill-en, two shillings, you know...eleven"
A penny and a sixpence—"fivepence"
A shilling and a two-shilling piece—"one and six"
A sixpence and a two-shilling piece—"sixpence, shill-en"
A halfpenny and a penny—"shill-en"

On the *seventh day* (June 27th) I was able to test her with a set of familiar objects in the usual way.

Table 1.

	Pointing to object shown	Naming an object indicated	Oral commands	Printed commands	Duplicate placed in hand out of sight	Repetition	Writing name of object indicated	Copying from print
Knife	Perfect	Correct	Correct	Correct	Perfect	Correct	rib	Knive
Key	,,	,,	,,	,,	,,	,,	Beeg	Gey
Penny	,,	,,	,,	,,	,,	Punny	penney	Tenny
Matches	,,	"Matcher"	,,	,,	,,	Correct	Mahickes	Mahickes
Scissors	,,	Correct	,,	,,	,,	,,	Secissors	Ssuccoors
Pencil	,,	,,	,,	,,	,,	,,	peicel	Penceil
Key	,,	,,	,,	,,	,,	,,	Bey	Key
Scissors	,,	"Key"; corrected	,,	,,	,,	,,	Sicissors	Scissors
Matches	,,	"Match-ox"	,,	,,	,,	,,	Martchs	Matchers
Knife	,,	Correct	,,	,,	,,	Knive	Bnife	Knife
Penny	,,	"Pea-ny"	,,	Pencil	,,	Correct	peinny	Penny
Matches	,,	"Match ōz"	,,	Correct	,,	,,	Matches	Mahches
Scissors	,,	Correct	,,	,,	,,	,,	Scissars	Ssissors
Pencil	,,	No answer	,,	,,	,,	,,	pencel	Penceil
Penny	,,	"Pence"	,,	Pencil	,,	,,	penny	Penney
Knife	,,	Correct	,,	Correct	,,	,,	Knife	Knife
Key	,,	,,	,,	Knife; corrected	,,	,,	guey	Key
Pencil	,,	"Knife; no, pencil"	,,	Correct	,,	,,	pencel	Pencel

Asked to point to the object on the table which corresponded to the one shown to her or placed in her left hand out of sight, she had not a moment's doubt, but made her choice with great rapidity; the act of matching was evidently performed with ease. She also chose correctly, though more slowly, to oral commands and, when it was given in the form of a printed word, she made two mistakes only. Out of eighteen attempts to name these objects, she was completely successful in ten, and most of her failures were due to defective word-formation; the sounds she uttered bore a definite relation to the word she was seeking. Thus she said "match-er," "match-ox," and "match-oz," for match-box, and "pea-ny" or "pence" for penny. Told to repeat the names after me, her enunciation was better —although she still showed some difficulty in verbal formation. When she attempted to write them down without saying them aloud, most of the words bore some relation to the usual designation of the object before her; but they were extremely poorly written and spelt. The individual letters were badly formed and the structure of the words was defective. This was the case even when she copied them from print in cursive handwriting.

Moreover, a characteristic incident occurred at the beginning of the written portion of these tests. After explaining to her that she was to write down the name of each object as it was shown to her, I handed her a block of paper which I had headed with the word "writing"; this exercised a fatal attraction, and she insisted on copying it instead of recording the name of the object she had just seen. I tore off the sheet, and she began the new one with the same word, but finally after another explanation she started to carry out the task I had set her. This is a good example of the verbal perseveration which is so liable to disturb the records in this class of disorders of speech.

On the same day I tested her with the alphabet. She said the letters spontaneously in due order up to "N," added "V" "P" and then stopped. She made a fresh start and again ran correctly up to "N": after a pause she continued "P Q R S T U V," and with the exclamation "I can't say it," gave up altogether. But, when I said the alphabet, she could repeat it accurately letter by letter. Asked to write the alphabet spontaneously, she produced the following series: *A B C D E F G H I S B J L M M C P* q *B S* t u v w *X Y Y*.

She had great difficulty in copying capitals in cursive script; in fact every letter up to "I" was copied exactly, and she then continued:

(The copy) J K L M N O P Q R S T U V W X Y Z.

(She wrote) 3 4 4 m m o p y T s t U U W X Y *z*.

On the *tenth day* (June 30th) I carried out a complete series of hand, eye, and ear tests with the result given in Table 2.

There was no question that she understood what she was asked to do, although she was occasionally slow in beginning some new form of these tests. Sitting face to face, she succeeded in imitating my movements correctly in eight out of sixteen attempts; in seven her response was an exact reversal, and she made one complete mistake only. But, when they were reflected in the glass, she did not hesitate for a moment. Both oral and printed commands were badly executed, and with the latter she substituted ear for eye on three occasions. Asked to write down my movements, sitting face to face, she simplified the task by naming the right or left hand, omitting any indication of which eye or ear I had touched. This was evidently a severe test, and towards the end her writing became illegible.

She had great difficulty in writing her name and address both spontaneously and to dictation. Not only were the letters badly formed, but some were omitted, whilst others were duplicated, and the whole was illegible except on careful analysis.

On the *fourteenth day* (July 4th) her speech had greatly improved. She gave her name and full address correctly, and with almost perfect enunciation. She talked very slowly and with evident difficulty in finding words; but the nurses insisted that she knew exactly what she wanted. She said to me: "I...been... inkin...improvement" (I've been thinking there has been improvement).

Table 2.

	Imitation of movements made by the observer	Imitation of movements reflected in a mirror	Oral commands	Printed commands	Writing down movements made by the observer
L. hand to L. eye	Correct	Correct	Correct; slow	Correct; slow	right eye
R. hand to R. ear	Reversed	,,	Correct	R. hand to L. ear	right *eye*
R. hand to L. eye	,,	,,	,,	R. hand to L. *ear*	right eye
L. hand to R. eye	,,	,,	R. hand to R. eye	L. hand to R. *ear*	left eye
L. hand to L. ear	,,	,,	Reversed	Correct	left Eay
R. hand to R. eye	L. hand; corrected	,,	Correct	,,	right Eye
L. hand to R. ear	Correct	,,	Reversed	,,	left Esey
R. hand to L. ear	,,	,,	Correct; slow	,,	right ear
L. hand to L. eye	Reversed	,,	Correct	L. hand to R. *ear*	left Eye
R. hand to R. ear	,,	,,	R. hand to L. ear	Correct	left Ear
R. hand to L. eye	Correct	,,	Correct	,,	right eye
L. hand to R. eye	L. hand to L. eye; corrected	,,	R. hand to R. eye	,,	"Can't"
L. hand to L. ear	Reversed	,,	L. hand to L. *eye*	L. hand to R. ear	Illegible
R. hand to R. eye	R. hand to L. eye	,,	Correct	Correct	,,
L. hand to R. ear	Correct	,,	,,	,,	,,
R. hand to L. ear	,,	,,	,,	Reversed	,,

I asked her to repeat three short sentences after me one by one; this she did correctly as follows:

"I have been getting better day after day"; "And I have no sickness or head-ache"; "I was allowed to sit up to have my bed made yes-day af-er-noon" (yesterday afternoon). Told to repeat them as a single sequence, she was unable to do so, saying, "I was allowed to have my bed made yes-day after-noon...No, I can't." I then said all three phrases together, but she failed to repeat them, saying, "I was allowed to...to have my head...Why I ought to say that...I was allowed."

She wrote her name and address spontaneously as follows:

Alicce Lucy Esther B.
16 West Vi er
Bark Pa
Barnsleey.

(Alice Lucy Esther B.
16 West View,
Park Road,
Barnsley).

I printed her name and address and asked her to copy it; but instead of reproducing it letter by letter, she glanced backwards and forwards from the print to the paper and wrote down what she had gathered. The result exhibited exactly the same kind of mistakes as her spontaneous writing; words and letters were so badly formed as to be in places almost illegible. Asked to write anything she wished to tell me, she produced with difficulty and many erasures and corrections, "think have been gettig againg allrthat" (I think I have been getting alright) and "I have been going to have." Asked to interpret these scrawls, she said, "I have been going to say that I have been...I told a sister that...."

I then examined her with the clock tests and obtained the following results:

Table 3.

	Direct imitation	Telling the time	Clock set to oral commands	Clock set to printed commands	
				Ordinary nomenclature	Railway time
5 minutes to 2	Correct	Correct	Correct	Correct	Set 12.40
Half-past 1	,,	,,	,,	,,	Correct
5 minutes past 8	,,	,,	,,	,,	,,
20 minutes to 4	,,	"Quarter to 4; 5 and 20 to; 10 minutes to 4"	,,	,,	Set 2.40
10 minutes past 7	,,	Correct	,,	Set 10.10	Correct
20 minutes to 6	,,	,,	,,	Correct	Whispered "5.40." Set 4.50
10 minutes to 1	,,	,,	Set 10 minutes past, but hour hand before 1	Set 10 to 10	Correct
A quarter to 9	,,	,,	Correct; slow	Correct	,,
20 minutes past 11	,,	"5, 10, 15, 20 past 11"	Correct	,,	Set 10.40
25 minutes to 3	,,	Correct	Set 20 minutes to 3	,,	Correct

She was remarkably bright and cheerful but was puzzled by her failure to express herself and was liable to become confused. When she was right she responded quickly; but if she made a mistake, she said it over under her breath and usually got wrong again. That is to say she made a mistake, appreciated that it was incorrect and then repeated the order in a whisper or aloud, saying it wrong; on this she acted and fell a second time into error. All her actions seemed to be guided by whispered audible or inaudible words, except when she placed the hands of a clock in direct imitation of one set by me; this she carried out rapidly and her lips did not move. She could tell the time slowly, but on the whole correctly, helping herself by counting on her fingers. With oral commands she was certainly dependent on correct repetition of the words said by me, as far as I could interpret her whispers. Given a printed order in the usual nomenclature her lips moved and she then set the clock without looking back at the card; the verbal formulation had fixed the task in her mind and she usually succeeded in placing the hands correctly. But she had great difficulty when the command was printed in railway time; for she tended to set the short hand exactly opposite the hour and then flung the other one into a position corresponding to the number of minutes. Evidently the words "past" or "to," directly preceding the hour, helped her to recognise that the short hand should not be placed exactly opposite the number mentioned in the printed order.

On the *sixteenth day* (July 6th) I again tested her with the alphabet, which she could now say spontaneously without a mistake. Moreover she read it aloud perfectly from print. But, when I gave her the twenty-six block letters and asked her to put them together in order, she said, after much hesitation, "I can't find the right letter." She picked out an "I" and slowly selected A B C F, from this she formed the sequence A B C D E F G L and then gave up, complaining, "I can't do it." Asked to write the alphabet she produced the following series:

A B C D E J G H I J B l m m o p q r s t u

After a pause began again spontaneously:

A B C D E J G H I J B L m m o p q r s t u v w x y ξ.

Each letter was said in a whisper and definitely verbalised. To dictation she wrote the following sequence:

A B C D E E G H I K L m n o *P Q R S J* u v w Y z x,

and she copied the alphabet from print in a very imperfect manner.

On the same day I carried out a series of the man, cat and dog tests.

Table 4.

	Reading aloud	Reading from pictures	Writing from dictation	Writing from pictures	Copying from print
The dog and the cat	"Man and the cat"	"Dog and a cat"	The dog & & Cart	Dog Cat	The Dog & the Cat
The man and the dog	"Man and a dog"	"Man and a dog"	The man and the dog	The man & the dog	The man & the Dog
The cat and the man	"The cat and man"	"Cat and the man"	The cat & the man	The cat & the Man	The Cat & the Man
The cat and the dog	"The cat and dog"	"Cat and dog"	The Cat & the dog	The cal & tthe dog	The Cat & the Dog
The dog and the man	"Dog and the man"	"Dogandtheman"	The dog & the man	The & the man	The dog & the Man
The man and the cat	"A man and a cat"	"Man and a cat"	The man & the cat	The man & the cat	The Man & the Cat
The dog and the man	"A dog and the man"	"Man and..."	The dog & the man	The dog & & Manj	The Dog & the Man
The cat and the man	"The cat and a man"	"Cat and the man"	The cat & the man	The cat & the Man	The Cat & the Man

She read these simple phrases slowly but on the whole correctly and made no essential mistakes when translating pictures into words; once only did she fail to complete the couple shown to her. The content of each sentence, written to dictation, was accurately reproduced, but the structure of the words was defective and the letters were badly formed. These faults were even worse when she wrote from pictures

She found much less difficulty in copying from print; although her writing was poor and the letters imperfect, every word was, however, reproduced in cursive script.

On the *twentieth day* (July 10th) speech was slow and broken by long pauses, but she volunteered many more remarks. Thus she said, "My head is not...quite right...it's...er, numb...otherwise...otherwise...it will do." Asked to explain her difficulty in speaking, she answered, "My difficulty is...I know what I want to say...I don't know how to say it...Sometimes I feel...sometimes I feel...if...if I...if I can't say it...I can't think sometimes...if I could get my thoughts right ...I should be alright."

By this time her speech had so greatly improved that the colour tests were carried out correctly, with the exception that she tended to call red "pink" and orange "red." All were selected without fail to oral and printed commands, and she wrote down their names accurately, excepting that she was puzzled by "helitrope" (heliotrope), her designation for violet.

On the *twenty-sixth day* (July 16th) she wrote her first spontaneous letter; it was coherent and reasonable, but many of the words were badly formed. For instance, she wrote, "I am glod Arthrur won the prize for the windom competion" (I am glad Arthur won the prize for the window competition).

I put her through another series of hand, eye and ear tests, and it is interesting to notice the nature of the improvement in these records.

Table 5.

	Imitation of movements made by the observer	Imitation of movements reflected in a mirror	Oral commands	Printed commands	Writing down movements made by the observer
L. hand to L. eye	Reversed	Correct	Correct	Correct	right to yoo right *ear*
R. hand to R. ear	,,	,,	,,	,,	left to left ear
R. hand to L. eye	Correct	,,	,,	,,	left to right eye
L. hand to R. eye	Reversed	,,	,,	,,	right to left *ear*
L. hand to L. ear	L. hand to R. ear	,,	,,	,,	right to right ear
R. hand to R. eye	R. hand to L. eye	,,	,,	,,	left to right Cay
L. hand to R. ear	Reversed	,,	,,	L. hand to R. *eye*	right to right ear
R. hand to L. ear	Correct	,,	,,	Correct	left to left ear
L. hand to L. eye	Reversed	,,	,,	,,	right to right *ear*
R. hand to R. ear	,,	,,	,,	L. hand to R. ear	left to left ear
R. hand to L. eye	,,	,,	,,	Correct	left to right eye
L. hand to R. eye	,,	,,	,,	,,	right to left eye
L. hand to L. ear	,,	,,	,,	L. hand to R. ear	right to right *eye*
R. hand to R. eye	L. hand to R. eye	,,	,,	Correct	left to left eye
L. hand to R. ear	Reversed	,,	,,	L. hand to R. *eye*	right to left ear
R. hand to L. ear	,,	,,	,,	Correct	left to right ear

When imitating my movements sitting face to face, she made fourteen mistakes, but twelve of these were complete reversals in which she selected right for left and vice versa. When she attempted to write them down all sixteen were erroneously recorded; of these two were reversed, whilst in four she mistook eye and ear.

But oral commands were perfectly executed and, to orders given in print, she made four mistakes only. I then asked her to read them aloud, which she did perfectly, and the errors in their performance were reduced to two. At first she had difficulty in grasping that the printed order read aloud implied an action and was satisfied when the words were uttered; but if they were read silently she at once began to carry out some movement of one or other hand.

On the *twenty-seventh day* (July 17th) she carried out without fail a series of tests with familiar objects, naming them accurately, choosing them to oral or to printed commands and even writing the words correctly. She had now begun to note on paper memoranda of her wants, such as "more diet," "might I have more," "preasure" (pressure) and "tingle," both of which referred to sensations in the head.

On the *thirtieth day* (July 20th) I asked her to write her name and address. She did so correctly, no longer in the form of a signature, but as if it stood on the envelope of a letter sent to her home:

Mrs J. B.
16 West View
Park Rd.
Barnsley.

I then covered this up and requested her to write her name and add the address of the nursing home; but she repeated her previous performance exactly. When I explained to her that I wanted her address in London, where she had daily received letters from her relatives, she replied, "I can't," and made no attempt to write it. I then dictated it to her word by word and she wrote:

Mrs J. B.
The empire nursing hone
Vinsent sq.
Westminster
London S.W.

(i.e. The Empire Nursing Home, Vincent Square, Westminster, London, S.W.)

From print she copied it as follows:

Mrs B.
Ehe empire Nursing Home
Vincent square
Westminsteer E.1111

She was then put through a series of tests with the alphabet. She could now say the letters with ease, both spontaneously and to repetition, and read them perfectly aloud. She wrote them in cursive capitals and her only errors were $\mathscr{T}$ for F, $\mathscr{B}$ for R, $\mathscr{J}$ for T, and the $\mathscr{Z}$ was given several extra turns. They were written more easily to dictation and she copied them perfectly, in both cases employing small cursive script. I then gave her the twenty-six block letters which, after some hesitation, she finally succeeded in placing in their right order to form a perfect alphabet.

On the *thirty-second* and *thirty-third days* (July 22nd–23rd) she was so bright and active that I was able to subject her to a more extensive series of tests.

Her spontaneous speech had still further improved and she attempted sentences of much greater length. For instance: "I went for a drive this morning...I enjoyed it more than in fine weather...It was a bit dull...suited me better...For an hour and a half." She was much troubled that her head had been shaved and had ordered a wig; she inquired, therefore, "Might I...I shall think of it soon... might I...wear hair now?" Intonation was still defective, the pauses were multiplied and tended to fall in the middle of a phrase or at the end of a single word. Speech became syncopated with a repetition of rising and falling accents: e.g. "I seem... to have...a weight... on here" pointing to her head.

She could now name the geometrical shapes placed in her left hand out of sight, calling them respectively "square" (cube), "cork" (cylinder), "marble" (sphere), "nutmeg" (ovoid), "spindle" (cone). With a pyramid she said "oblong ...can't describe it"; then suddenly she exclaimed "pyramid."

She carried out a complete series of clock tests without a mistake, telling the time correctly and setting the hands to oral or to printed commands, whether they were given in ordinary nomenclature or in railway time. She could even write down the time accurately if she was allowed to intermingle at will figures and words.

Table 6.

	Imitation of movements made by the observer	Imitation of movements reflected in a mirror	Oral commands	Printed commands	Writing down movements made by the observer
L. hand to L. eye	Reversed	Correct	Correct	Correct	Correct
R. hand to R. ear	,,	,,	,,	,,	Left hand to left *eye*
R. hand to L. eye	,,	,,	,,	,,	Correct
L. hand to R. eye	,,	,,	,,	,,	,,
L. hand to L. ear	R. hand to L. ear	,,	,,	,,	,,
R. hand to R. eye	Reversed	,,	,,	,,	,,
L. hand to R. ear	,,	,,	,,	,,	Reversed
R. hand to L. ear	,,	,,	,,	,,	Correct
L. hand to L. eye	R. hand to L. eye	,,	,,	,,	Left hand to left *ear*
R. hand to R. ear	Reversed	,,	,,	,,	Correct
R. hand to L. eye	,,	,,	,,	,,	,,
L. hand to R. eye	,,	,,	,,	,,	Reversed
L. hand to L. ear	,,	,,	,,	,,	Right hand to left ear
R. hand to R. eye	,,	,,	,,	,,	Correct
L. hand to R. ear	,,	,,	,,	,,	,,
R. hand to L. ear	R. hand to R. *eye*	,,	,,	,,	,,

The hand, eye and ear tests yielded a much improved set of records. It is true that, when she attempted to copy my movements sitting face to face, she was wrong sixteen times in succession; but of these thirteen were direct reversals and in three attempts only did she mistake the nature of the movement. Oral and printed commands were perfectly executed and she could even write down my actions with five errors only.

Observations made from October 20th to 23rd, 1922
(*four months after the operation*).

She was in excellent physical condition and her urine contained no sugar or other abnormal constituent. The trephine opening was somewhat depressed and pulsated slightly in the sitting posture; this was considerably increased when her head was lowered, but was scarcely perceptible after lying horizontally for a considerable period. She complained of no headache or tenderness, superficial or deep, and had suffered from no fits or seizures of any kind.

Except for her disturbance of speech, I could discover no abnormal signs pointing to any affection of the central nervous system. Movements of the face were carried out equally well on the two sides and the tongue was protruded in the middle line. All the reflexes were normal, including the plantars; I could even obtain them from the right half of the abdomen and there was no longer that difference on the two sides which constituted the earliest and most lasting sign of disease. The grasp of the right hand was stronger than that of the left and individual movements of the fingers were perfectly performed, both the eyes open and shut. The right lower extremity had recovered completely and she could walk three miles without undue fatigue. The most careful sensory examination failed to reveal any abnormality; size, shape, and weight were appreciated equally well with either hand.

Symbolic Formulation and Expression.

She was bright, gay, pleased to come to London and anxious to enjoy its sights. So great was her energy that it was difficult to prevent her from tiring herself unduly and all my observations were made in the morning in the quiet surroundings of my consulting room.

Articulated speech. In spite of profound recovery her speech showed the same defects as before, though to a much slighter degree. She now talked easily, her enunciation was greatly improved and the pauses occurred at longer intervals; yet in principle the defects were of the same kind as before. She was conscious that her speech lacked freedom; she had no difficulty in finding names, but the words were pronounced slowly and the form of the phrase, though it remained essentially grammatical, was frequently altered to obviate verbal difficulties. Thus she said, "Doctor Head...should my head have a big dint in it...if I lie down...for an hour or two...the dint is not there...but if I sit up...any time...a big dint is there...I asked my doctor...he said...it didn't matter...I didn't know...you ...had...cut so much out... until I got home." All her faults depended on inability to discover the exact verbal form she required. If, however, she stumbled over a word, she was loath to leave it uncorrected and had a strong sense of her errors in articulation.

She showed exactly the same defects of speech, when she attempted to repeat a series of phrases said by me, hesitating over such words as "elephants" and "zoological." She did not slavishly follow each individual word, but evidently formulated the meaning to herself and then attempted to express it. This led to the same difficulties as when she talked spontaneously, though every point of importance was correctly seized and she omitted no essential detail.

Understanding of spoken words. She understood everything that was said to her and carried out oral commands perfectly. She could follow and take her part in general conversation, provided she was not hurried.

Reading. Printed commands were correctly executed and she gave a good account of the contents of a paragraph she had read silently. Moreover, she could interest herself in a book, although she no longer read aloud as had been her custom before the operation. Asked to read aloud a selected passage, she succeeded in pronouncing all the words, although she stumbled over many of them and corrected herself in exactly the same way as with spontaneous speech.

Writing. She could write a coherent letter and express herself spontaneously in writing. The only noticeable defects were hesitation and uncertainty over the form of some of the letters or component parts of a word; but she was always able, on reading over what she had written, to detect these errors and to make the necessary corrections. Asked to write down what she had gathered from a selected passage, the contents were given correctly, but the form of the words was defective and the spelling was extremely bad. Throughout her lips moved silently and she was evidently saying the words to herself, although I could detect no sound.

Exactly the same faults appeared when she wrote to dictation, or even when she copied a printed paragraph. She was extremely slow, her lips moved soundlessly as she enunciated each word to herself before writing it down.

All these tests showed that verbal formation and structure were disturbed and she was conscious that, in spite of her great increase in power, she had not regained her normal freedom, when writing spontaneously, to dictation or to copy.

The alphabet. All the letters were said spontaneously in perfect sequence, divided into short groups separated by a pause. She repeated them after me and read them aloud without difficulty. She could write them spontaneously or to dictation with fair accuracy, but translated capitals into cursive handwriting less easily and with several slight corrections in the shape of the letters. Given the twenty-six blocks, the order in which she placed them was correct, except that at first she placed Q for O and omitted U. This she finally discovered, but failed to find its proper place until she had repeated the whole alphabet aloud. Throughout it was evident that any difficulty she might have was with the form or shape of the letters.

A printed paragraph. As a result of what she told me of her visit to the Zoological Gardens, I put in print the following account:

"On Sunday afternoon we went to the Zoological Gardens. We were there from 2 o'clock to 5 and had a cup of tea, when we were tired. It is an immense place and difficult to find, but we took a taxi each way. We saw lions, tigers, elephants, polar bears, a number of large reptiles and many kinds of birds. It was a beautiful afternoon and we enjoyed ourselves greatly."

This she read silently and re-told the story in the following words: "We went to the Zoological Gardens and spent an enjoyable time. We saw there elephants, tigers and various kinds of an-mals. It's a large place and diff-cult to find. We spent an enjoyable afternoon and got home about 5 o'clock in the afternoon."

When she repeated these sentences after me or read them aloud, all her faults were those of enunciation; she stumbled over many of the words, such as elephants and zoological, but finally corrected herself in most instances.

After reading the printed account through again to herself she wrote: "We went to the Zo on Sunday afternoon And spent an enjoyable treat we saw all kind of animals. We had a cup of tea Afterward we came having spent an enjoyable treat."

To dictation she wrote: "On Sunday afternoon we went to the Zo gardens we were there fron two untill five and had a cup of tea when we were tired. It is an immense and difficult to find that we took a taxi each way. We saw lions tigars Elephants and polar baars and a number of large reptiles, and many kinds of birds. It was a beauliful afernoon and we enjoyed ourseilves greatly."

She copied the printed account very slowly; her lips moved and, although she uttered no sound of any kind, it was obvious that she was saying the words to herself before she put them down on paper. She wrote: "On Sunday aflernoon we went to the Zoological Gardens. We were there from 2-0 o'clock to 5-0 And had a cup of tea when we were tired It is an imnense place and difficult to find. But we took a taxi each way we saw lions tigers elephants polar bears a nunber of large reptiles and many kind of birds It was a beautiful aflenmoon we enjoyd ourselves greally."

Numbers and arithmetic. She counted correctly up to a hundred with considerable rapidity and certainty, though some of the numerals were indistinct. The order in which they were given was perfect and she did not hesitate when beginning a new decade.

Addition.			Subtraction.		
325	568	685	864	582	821
432	323	737	432	236	348
757	891	1422	432	346	473

The three simple addition sums were carried out rapidly and without movement of the lips. With the second and third subtraction she said the numbers under her breath incorrectly and, recognising they were wrong, became confused. Finally, however, she succeeded in arriving at the right answer[1].

Coins and their relative value. All the coins were named correctly and she was remarkably accurate in her estimation of the relative value of any two of them placed on the table before her. But she not infrequently found it difficult to arrive at the answer directly without counting up under her breath. Thus, given sixpence and half-a-crown, she whispered "one, two, three, four, five" and then said aloud "five," the correct answer.

She denied she had any difficulty with money and added, "My speech is the worst...you know...if it wasn't for that...I could...go...shopping."

Orientation. She could find her way perfectly and went about alone in her native town. I could not persuade her to produce a ground-plan, because she asserted she had never been able to draw; but she could describe accurately the various pieces of furniture in my room and their relation to one another.

Serial Tests.

(1) *Naming and recognition of common objects.* All these tests were carried out accurately and she could even write down the name of each object as it was shown to her; but her handwriting was poor and some of the letters were malformed, though no word was actually mis-spelt.

(2) *Naming and recognition of colours.* She named all the colours without fail both by word of mouth and in writing, and chose them correctly to oral and printed commands.

(3) *The man, cat and dog tests* were executed perfectly in every respect.

(4) *The clock tests.* She carried out oral and printed commands with considerable rapidity. The time shown on the clock was stated correctly; but, with the higher number of minutes, she tended to count up instead of giving the answer directly. Thus, shown 20 minutes to 4, she said "five, ten, fifteen, twenty to four." She had considerable difficulty in writing down the time and in every instance first enunciated in a whisper the words she ultimately wrote. This preliminary verbalisation, whether right or wrong, determined what she put on to paper and she did not look back repeatedly at the clock face for guidance during the act.

The results of this test were as follows:

Time shown on the clock	She wrote
5 minutes to 2	5 minites to 2
Half-past 1	½ past to 1

[1] At the beginning of our next sitting, when she was fresh, I set her the same sums, which she solved correctly at the first attempt.

Time shown on the clock	She wrote
5 minutes past 8	5 past eigt
20 minutes to 4	5 (erasure) to 4
10 minutes past 7	10 past 7
20 minutes to 6	5.20 to 6
10 minutes to 1	ten minitus to one
A quarter to 9	quarter to nine
20 minutes past 11	twenty past eleven
25 minutes to 3	five & twenty past two

Many of the words were so badly written that it was difficult to be certain of the actual letters employed; thus, minutes was written minitus with no distinction between the up and down strokes belonging to each letter. Verbal structure was inherently faulty and calligraphy suffered.

(5) *The hand, eye and ear tests.* She had completely recovered her power of imitating movements made by me when we sat face to face, and oral and printed commands were executed with remarkable quickness and certainty. The only errors occurred when she was asked to write down silently the movements made by me. Out of sixteen attempts she made three slight mistakes, substituting the *left* for the right ear; in every other case her written statement of the action I had performed was accurate.

Asked if she found these tests difficult, she replied, "No...I seemed to think... or fancy...your right hand was opposite to me...so I put it so."

Observations made on April 29th, 30th and May 1st, 1923
(*a little more than ten months after the operation*).

For a few months following our last sitting she continued to progress favourably and towards the end of the year had almost completely recovered her powers of speech. Then I began to receive increasingly disquieting reports and finally a visit to London was arranged for the end of April 1923.

On her arrival I was shocked at the extent to which she had deteriorated. She complained that she had been greatly troubled by family worries and business affairs. "I have been worried...and I seem as if...as if I can't bear...anything that some people would laugh at...I can't seem to bear anything now...When I'm worried my speech goes bad...Occasionally I've got wrong with my son...and I can't speak a word for the time being."

Her speech had been unaffected until the last fortnight, when she began to be restless and troubled at night.

She had suffered from no fits or epileptiform seizures; but for several months she had occasionally experienced a "numb feeling" on the right side of the mouth and she complained, "It...always comes...when...I'm worried." On April 27th, as she was going to bed, her right hand "came over numb." She was conscious of all her fingers, but they seemed "dead." She felt there was something wrong with her mouth on the right side and "I fancied the leg was a bit affected, but it went off in an instant." There was no convulsion of any kind, she did not lose consciousness and the whole attack passed away in a few moments. After it was over she felt nervous and frightened and "for the next day I hardly knew what I was speaking about."

The trephined area of the skull was in perfect condition; when she was seated, the surface of the tissues which covered it was not above the level of the bone and, although slight bulging occurred on lowering her head, the opening remained soft and pulsated to a slight degree only.

The surface was not sore or tender to the touch. She had suffered from no headache, nausea or vomiting; "but I always have a funny feeling in the head...a fulness...not a pain."

Discs and fundi were in no way abnormal and the pupils reacted well. Movements were equal on the two halves of the face and the tongue was protruded in the middle line. All the reflexes were normal, except those from the abdomen; I was unable to obtain a response from the lower segments on either side or from the right hypochondrium, although a slight contraction could be evoked to the left of the middle line. There was no paralysis or paresis and sensation was entirely unaffected.

Symbolic Formulation and Expression.

She was more anxious and less confident, complaining that she was easily exhausted, especially when she was compelled to talk about subjects that worried her.

Articulated speech. Her power of expression was undoubtedly less than when I examined her in October 1922. She evidently knew what she wanted to say, but could not find the words she required. The groups into which she divided her sentences were shorter and the pauses more frequent and prolonged, but syntax was not otherwise affected. Thus, when explaining her domestic troubles, she said, "You know...he...bothers me...in this way...Well...he...I don't know what to say...but he...wiges (wishes) the business to be...the...well I can't say it... I know what I mean...but I don't know how to say it."

She could find the right names for common objects, but was somewhat slow and not quite perfect with colours. She told the time correctly in spite of some difficulty in finding the requisite words.

She was fully conscious of her mistakes in enunciation and strove to correct them, frequently with success.

She was able to repeat what was said to her and the words were somewhat better formed than when she talked spontaneously.

Understanding of spoken words. She chose a common object or colour and set the hands of a clock without fail to oral commands. With the hand, eye and ear tests, she was somewhat slower and evidently repeated the order under her breath; but she made no actual mistakes.

She understood what was said in ordinary conversation, although comprehension was obviously slower than at the time of the previous examination. Moreover, she again showed the following defective mode of response to directions given by word of mouth. Handed a printed command she was satisfied with reading it aloud and made no choice; it required more than one explanation on my part before she could be persuaded to read the word silently and to indicate the appropriate object on the table. The same difficulty occurred when an object of daily use was placed in her hand out of sight; having named it aloud, she was content and made no attempt to select its duplicate lying in front of her. Once, however, the desired mode of response had been established, all these tests were carried out correctly. Such slowness in comprehending an explanation given by word of mouth showed that she had seriously regressed.

Reading. She could give a fairly good account of what she read silently and chose common objects and colours accurately to printed commands. But she was slow in setting the clock and made several mistakes when the order was given in railway time. In the same way the hand, eye and ear tests were carried out with considerable difficulty although finally, after some hesitation, every action was executed correctly.

When she read aloud, articulation was somewhat defective and the words were ill-formed exactly as if she talked spontaneously.

Writing. Her capacity to express herself in writing had obviously diminished greatly and her written communications from home to me showed how grave had been the regression; they were unusually shortened, words were omitted and the letters badly formed.

She wrote her signature and address accurately, but the script was defective and View was written "Viwe." Asked to relate what she had gathered from a printed account of her visit to the Zoological Gardens, she wrote as follows: "We spent a baoutiful afernoon at the Zootogicol gardens there we saw many kinds of reptile amongst them were lioms tyers polour bears and many other things too mumerous to mention. We had tea there in the ground and arrnved home about 6 oclouck" (i.e. We spent a beautiful afternoon at the Zoological Gardens where we saw many kinds of reptiles, amongst them were lions, tigers, polar bears and many other things too numerous to mention. We had tea there in the grounds and arrived home about 6 o'clock). The same kind of faults appeared, when she wrote these sentences to dictation, and even if the passage was copied directly from print. With every form of test which demanded the act of writing, her lips moved silently and she depended on this non-vocal verbalisation for the words she was about to write. Obviously her power to transform words and letters into their written symbols had deteriorated greatly since my previous examination.

The alphabet. All the letters were said in due order, read aloud perfectly and repeated after me. She could also write them spontaneously, although some of them were badly formed and she replaced n by m. The same faults recurred, when the alphabet was dictated and even if it was copied from print; but it is noticeable that whilst copying she depended on the words she said under her breath rather than on the printed letters before her. Given the twenty-six block letters, she had considerable difficulty in arranging them in order. Finally she produced the following sequence: Λ (V upside down) B C E F G I J K L M N (upside down) O P Q (upside down) R S T U X W Y Z. The V was employed instead of A which with H and D were left on the table and could not be placed in the series. These answers were perceptibly worse than on the previous occasion.

Numbers and arithmetic. She counted correctly up to a hundred, but the words were poorly articulated; fifty became "fivy," sixty "sis-ty."

She was evidently puzzled somewhat by the higher numbers, as shown by her difficulty in setting the clock to printed orders in railway time.

Addition.			Subtraction.		
325	568	685	864	582	821
432	323	737	432	236	348
757	588 (wrong)	1422	432	394 (wrong)	797 altered to 975 (wrong)

These tests show a profound loss of power compared with my previous examination.

Coins and their relative value. She named the various coins one by one with some hesitation and gave their relative value on the whole correctly. For instance, when a sixpence and a half-crown were placed before her she replied on the first occasion "three, er, five" and in the second series of tests "six...no, three and six." With two shillings and a ten-shilling note she exclaimed "eight...oh, six; it isn't right ...five" and on the next occasion she said "don't know...I could work it out."

Serial Tests.

(1) *Naming and recognition of common objects.* All these tests were carried out successfully; but she wrote the names of objects presented to her with much greater difficulty than before. The words were mis-spelt and the letters badly formed; thus she wrote "Bnife, Bniıfe, Knufe" for knife, "penmy, pemny" for penny, "peacil," and then twice correctly, for pencil. On one occasion scissors was written "Scisson" and match-box "Matic box."

(2) *Naming and recognition of colours.* These tests were executed without mistakes; but the words she employed to designate the colours, though always apt, were not infrequently badly written.

(3) *The man, cat and dog tests* were carried out successfully. When reading, either from print or from pictures, these simple phrases, composed of monosyllabic words, her intonation tended to assume a certain rhythmic cadence, e.g. "the... dog and ...the...cat. The...man and...the...dog." If she wrote from pictures, many of the letters were badly formed, although the phrase was correctly composed and its contents accurate; to dictation, her writing greatly improved and when copying it was almost faultless.

(4) *The clock tests.*

Table 7.

	Direct imitation	Telling the time	Clock set to oral commands	Clock set to printed commands		Writing down the time shown on a clock face
				Ordinary nomenclature	Railway time	
5 minutes to 2	Correct	"Two; five minutes to two"	Correct	Correct	Set 1.50	5 minutes to two
Half-past 1	,,	Correct	,,	,,	Correct	½ past one
5 minutes past 8	,,	,,	,,	,,	,,	5 minutes (erased) past eight
20 minutes to 4	,,	"Quarter to four ...er...twenty minutes to four"	,,	20 past 4. "No, *to* four"; corrected	,,	twenty minutes to four
10 minutes past 7	,,	Correct	,,	Correct	,,	tun minmtes past seven
20 minutes to 6	,,	,,	,,	,,	Set 5.35	fine & twenty to six
10 minutes to 1	,,	,,	,,	,,	Correct	tim minites to one
A quarter to 9	,,	,,	,,	,,	Set 8.55	quarter to nine
20 minutes past 11	,,	,,	,,	,,	Correct	twenty minutes to twelve
25 minutes to 3	,,	"Five and twenty minutes to two"	,,	,,	Set 2.45	5 & twenty past tun

She executed oral commands correctly and succeeded in setting the hands, if a printed order was given in the ordinary nomenclature; but, when it was presented in railway time, she made many mistakes, especially with the higher figures. Throughout these tests she moved her lips silently, or occasionally whispered the words.

She told the time slowly and on the whole accurately. She recognised the actual time shown on the clock face; words failed her in which to express what she had correctly appreciated and she had no doubt of the meaning indicated by the hands.

She wrote down the time slowly and laboriously. The formation of the letters and words, together with the spelling, suffered badly and she made a few errors in significance.

(5) *The hand, eye and ear tests.*

Table 8.

	Imitation of movements made by the observer	Imitation of movements reflected in mirror	Oral commands	Printed commands	Writing down movements made by the observer
L. hand to L. eye	Reversed	Correct	Correct	Correct	right to gright eye
R. hand to R. ear	,,	,,	,,	,,	left
R. hand to L. eye	L. hand to R. *ear*	,,	,,	,,	left hand to left ene
L. hand to R. eye	L. hand to L. *ear*	,,	,,	,,	right hand to left eye
L. hand to L. ear	L. hand to R. ear	,,	,,	L. hand to R. ear; corrected	right hand to ryrt *eye*
R. hand to R. eye	R. hand to L. eye	,,	,,	R. hand to R. *ear*; corrected	left hand to luft eye
L. hand to R. ear	Correct	,,	,,	Correct	rigrt hand to left *eye*
R. hand to L. ear	,,	,,	,,	,,	left hand to rigrt *eys*
L. hand to L. eye	L. hand to R. *ear*	,,	,,	,,	right (scrawl) to rigrt eye
R. hand to R. ear	R. hand to L. ear	,,	,,	,,	left hand to laft ear
R. hand to L. eye	Correct	,,	,,	,,	left hand to right *ear*
L. hand to R. eye	,,	,,	,,	L. hand to L. eye; corrected	light e
L. hand to L. ear	,,	,,	,,	Correct	right wand to right (scrawl)
R. hand to R. eye	,,	,,	,,	,,	(Gave up)
L. hand to R. ear	L. hand to L. ear; corrected	,,	,,	,,	,,
R. hand to L. ear	Correct	,,	,,	,,	,,

Oral commands were executed without fault, but those given in print were carried out slowly and with three corrections. Her power of imitating my movements, when we sat face to face, had materially deteriorated and she made eight mistakes in sixteen observations. No wonder, therefore, that she failed grossly when she attempted to write down these movements; in fact, towards the end of this series she gave up, unable to write at all.

Thus four months after the operation this patient had so far recovered that she could carry out most of the serial tests without mistakes. She still showed some lack of freedom in articulated speech and her writing was defective in form rather than content. There were the last remains of the gross verbal aphasia from which she had originally suffered.

But in consequence of much worry she became anxious and her sleep was disturbed. She was easily fatigued and any dispute or domestic trouble would reduce her for a time almost to speechlessness. Then she began to experience abnormal "feelings" in the face and hand of the affected side, which passed away rapidly. Finally, when I saw her in April 1923, she had obviously regressed to a condition akin to that found four weeks after the operation.

CONDITION ON OCTOBER 9TH, 10TH AND 11TH, 1923
(*fifteen and a half months after the operation*).

In consequence of my representations her worries were greatly mitigated and she ceased to take an active part in her business. From this time she improved steadily and, when she again visited London five months later, she was gay and cheerful and her powers of speech had recovered to a remarkable degree.

All "dizzy" attacks and abnormal "feelings" in face and hand had gradually passed away and she suffered from no headache. She slept well and no longer complained of exhaustion.

The opening in the skull was in perfect condition, and did not bulge when she lay flat in bed. It pulsated slightly with any change in position, but this was not grossly exaggerated by stooping.

I could discover no abnormal physical signs on examination of the central nervous system; I was even able to obtain a slight response on scratching the right half of the abdomen, both above and below the level of the umbilicus.

Her arterial tension was still high (systolic 200, diastolic 110), but the heart was not enlarged. The urine was 1015 sp. gravity, and contained no sugar or albumen.

Symbolic Formulation and Expression.

She was an excellent witness and carried out all the tests rapidly and with evident pleasure.

Articulated speech. She still had obvious difficulty in finding words with which to express her thoughts, but the groups were larger and the pauses shorter and less frequent. This was particularly apparent when she narrated her story of her visit to the Zoological Gardens. She could repeat anything I said without fail.

Understanding of spoken words. Oral commands were carried out perfectly and with great rapidity; she obviously comprehended the full meaning of ordinary conversation.

Reading. Printed commands were well executed and there was no longer that hesitation so noticeable at the previous examination. She read the paper daily with interest and complete understanding.

When she read aloud some of the words were poorly pronounced, but her articulation was better than when she spoke spontaneously.

Writing had in every way enormously improved. The simple man, cat and dog phrases were well written in response to pictures and even the movements of the hand, eye and ear tests, when we sat opposite to one another, were accurately described in writing. Moreover, the form of the words and letters was nearly perfect, even when she wrote spontaneously.

The alphabet was said correctly except that she twice omitted H. It was repeated and read aloud perfectly. When written spontaneously, the only faults were that she substituted an m for n and gave the z an extra loop; to dictation she hesitated over h and r, but finally corrected her first attempts and, when copying, she again replaced n by m and bungled the r and w. The block letters, however, were arranged in order successfully.

A printed paragraph. This test in particular showed how profoundly she had improved since our previous meeting. I handed her the printed narrative describing her visit to the Zoological Gardens and she not only told me in great detail what she had read silently, but added, "I might say we went again yesterday. We saw different things that we'd never seen before. It is an immense place and wants a guide really. We went for a couple of hours."

Even the written account was much more nearly perfect and her handwriting was almost normal. She wrote: "When I was last in London We went to the Zoological gardens and enjoyed ourselves immensely. We saw elephants lions and all kind of reptiles, also many kind of birds. When we were tired, we had a cup of tea. We enjoyed ourselves immensely. We had a taxi there and back and all I can say we had an enjoyable time."

When this passage was dictated, the form of some of the words and the character of the writing was still defective, although she put on to paper substantially what I said to her. Asked to copy these sentences from print, she did so with some little difficulty and hesitation, but without omissions or gross mistakes.

Numbers and arithmetic. She counted well up to a hundred and her articulation was perfect until she reached fifty; then she was a little uncertain, whenever the decade number was followed by 6, 7, 8 or 9. Thus she said "fifty-two," but "fif-y eight" and "seven-y nine."

All the six arithmetical exercises were solved correctly, a great improvement on the results of the previous examination.

Coins and their relative value. Coins were named with ease and rapidity and she had no difficulty in stating the relation of any two of them to one another. She could now shop and calculate the change she had to give or receive.

Serial Tests.

(1) *Naming and recognition of common objects* and (2) *of colours.* All these tests were carried out perfectly and, even when she wrote down the names, the words were correctly spelt and rightly formed.

(3) *The man, cat and dog tests* were executed accurately in every respect.

(4) *The clock tests.* She made no mistakes even with the difficult task of writing down the time shown on the clock set by me.

(5) *The hand, eye and ear tests* were carried out with ease, except that, when sitting face to face, she once failed to copy my movements and, on two occasions in sixteen observations was twice forced to correct herself. This is a remarkable change for the better compared with her previous performance. The greatest improvement was shown, however, when she wrote down these movements; every one was accurately recorded and the words were written perfectly.

No. 21

A case of severe Aphasia, due to a vascular lesion in an elderly man. He was first examined a few days after the onset; but a complete series of observations was made eight and a half years later.

There was no disorder of motion or sensation. The reflexes were normal. Vision was in no way affected. The arterial tension was greatly raised and the vessel wall thickened. Otherwise no abnormal physical signs could be discovered.

He was speechless, except for "yes" and "no" and a few automatic expressions. He could not repeat to order anything said to him, even "yes" and "no." He understood most of what he heard, choosing objects and colours correctly to oral commands; yet he failed to execute the more complex tests. He could read nothing aloud and had difficulty in understanding what he read to himself; but he chose familiar objects to printed commands and on several occasions succeeded in selecting a printed card, which bore words corresponding to the colour or to the simple pictures he had just seen. Thus, it is obvious that printed words conveyed some meaning to him. He could write nothing but his surname spontaneously, failed altogether to write to dictation and could not copy print in cursive script. He was unable to say, to repeat, to read or to write the alphabet. He succeeded in writing some of the letters to dictation and copied them with four errors only. He counted with extreme difficulty and failed to reach twenty. Simple problems in arithmetic puzzled him greatly, but he was able to indicate on his fingers with remarkable accuracy the relative value of two coins. He drew a poor representation of a glass from the model and later from memory, but failed completely to draw an elephant.

John B., born in 1855, remained in good health until he reached his fifty-fifth year. He then suffered much financial trouble, his business melted away and he finally gave up work in November 1910. Memory became defective and he found difficulty in recollecting the names of members of his family.

On May 13th, 1911, he rose in the morning well; but at 8 p.m., when he returned from his son's house, where he had been gardening, he seemed strange and was unable to find his words. He went to bed and slept heavily and next morning seemed to be in his usual health; but as the day advanced he became drowsy and strange in his manner. On the 15th, he had obvious difficulty with speech.

On May 17th, 1911, he came to my out-patient department at the London Hospital and was admitted into the wards of Dr Percy Kidd, under whose care he remained until his death nine years later.

Physical Condition in May 1911.

He was a grey-haired well-built man. His pulse was regular, but the arterial wall was thickened and tortuous. The systolic blood-pressure was 190 mm. There were no abnormal signs in the heart. The urine was acid, with a specific gravity of 1014 and contained neither albumen nor sugar.

He was somewhat confused by the difficulty with his speech, but was otherwise intelligent. He complained of no headache and had had no fits or definite seizures. The fundi were clear and the discs normal, but the vessel walls were thickened and had the appearance in places of silver wire; there were no haemorrhages. The pupils were equal and reacted well. Movements of the eyes, face and tongue were well executed. The arm-jerks, knee-jerks and ankle-jerks were brisk and equal on the two sides. The abdominal reflexes were unaffected and the plantars gave a downward response. There was no paralysis, paresis, incoordination or defect of tone. Sensation to pricking and to touch showed no abnormality. The sphincters were unaffected.

Condition of Speech, etc., in May 1911.

He could say nothing but "yes" and "no" together with a few emotional expressions. These he used correctly as, when on breaking the point of a pencil during attempts to write, he exclaimed "I'm sorry." His answers to questions were usually unintelligible. He could not say or repeat his own name; asked, however, if it was "John Beaton" he said "yes."

He understood what was said to him to a remarkable extent provided it did not convey an order; thus on one occasion, when an orange was mentioned over his bed, he searched his locker and brought out a pot of orange marmalade. Even simple orders were sometimes carried out; he put out his tongue, opened or closed his eyes and touched his ear correctly to command. But asked to touch his ear with his left hand he placed it in his mouth and then pulled his moustache.

Given a newspaper with pictures, he looked at it intelligently and pointed out details of interest. He recognised the picture of a cat; shown a kite and asked if it was a balloon he said "no," but replied "yes" when the right name was suggested.

He could not read aloud, but seemed to understand simple words.

He was able to write his name badly after he had been in the hospital for a fortnight and could then copy and write from dictation simple words such as "cat."

Given a key or a penknife he indicated their use in excellent pantomime. He used a comb correctly and tied a reef-knot, when a piece of string was put into his hands. Told to light a cigarette he placed it in his mouth correctly, but spilt the matches; this confused him and he tried to strike one match on the other. Then he recovered himself and carried out the whole act perfectly.

Condition in November 1919 (*eight and a half years after the original seizure*).

The patient remained in fundamentally the same condition; from month to month he attended the clinic of Dr Kidd, through whose kindness I was able to make a complete examination in November 1919.

John B. was then a healthy looking, well-built man of 63. His mental processes were slow, but he was a most willing and interested witness, not infrequently showing remarkable ingenuity in circumventing his disabilities.

The pulse was regular; but the systolic tension was 200 mm., the diastolic 120 mm., and the artery was greatly thickened. The urine had a specific gravity of 1005, was acid, and contained neither albumen nor sugar.

He had suffered from no fits, seizures or other attacks since the initial stroke. He was free from headache and vomiting. The visual fields were unaffected and the fundi normal, except for the degenerated arteries. Pupils, face, tongue, all acted perfectly and there was no disorder of motion or sensation. The abdominal reflexes could be obtained easily from all four segments and the plantars gave a downward response. Arm-jerks, knee-jerks and ankle-jerks were decidedly brisk, but equal on the two halves of the body.

Symbolic Formulation and Expression.

He was now resigned to his condition and spent most of his time in doing little jobs or sitting placidly in his chair. He took evident interest in the tests and, on one occasion only, gave up all attempts to answer in disgust.

Articulated speech. He could use "yes" and "no" correctly in answer to questions, but was otherwise speechless except for a few more or less automatic expressions such as "thank you," "don't know," "I know." He also said "Can't get it," "No, I don't know how to do it," "I know what it is," "I don't know what it says," but the conversation evoked by asking him to draw an elephant (p. 324) was the longest series of coherent words to which he gave utterance.

He was unable to repeat anything said to him. Asked to say "yes," he answered "No, I can't" and told to say "no," shook his head and on one occasion replied "No, I don't know how to do it." He could not repeat any of the phrases he used spontaneously.

Understanding of spoken words. He chose familiar objects and colours correctly to oral commands and understood much that was said in general conversation. But he made many mistakes in setting the hands of the clock; these were due more to misapprehension of the significance of the long and short hands than to failure to comprehend the nature of the order. In the same way he failed repeatedly to carry out the hand, eye and ear tests.

Reading. He could not read aloud even the simple words of the man, cat and dog tests. But this did not prevent him from selecting a card which bore the printed words corresponding exactly to the combination of any two pictures of this series. Moreover, he could choose familiar objects and to a less degree colours in response to printed commands. He even succeeded in ten out of sixteen attempts in selecting a card bearing the name of a colour he had seen.

He was, however, incapable of setting the hands of a clock or carrying out the hand, eye and ear tests in response to printed words, although he occasionally succeeded with the former test if the order was set out in figures.

Writing. Asked to sign his name he wrote "Beadon" but crossed the upward limb of the d, as if it were a t. Apart from this he could write nothing spontaneously.

To dictation he wrote a series of badly formed letters, which bore little or no relation to the words said by me. This also occurred, when he attempted to copy print in cursive handwriting.

The alphabet. He was unable to say, repeat or read the alphabet. Asked to write it he failed entirely even to scrawl upon the paper. He succeeded better in writing to dictation, but the letters were badly formed and he substituted B for D, P for F, G for J, E for Q, K for R, Y for V, M for W, S for Z. Copying was carried out still better and, although the form of each letter was poor, he made fewer substitutions; M stood for N, K for R, V for W, and he could not manage Z at all.

Numbers and arithmetic. Asked to count he said, "One, two, three, four, firth, sixth, seventh, eighth, ninth, tenth, elevenpence"; on a second attempt he said, "One, two, three, four, five, six, seven, eighth, ninth, tenth, eleventh, twelfth." Then he began again exactly as before, but reaching "twelfth" continued "thirteenth, fourteenth, fifteenth, sixteenth, seventeenth, ninth...."

On attempting to repeat the numbers after me he did so correctly up to "ten" and was then unable to go further.

He was given two simple addition and subtraction sums and carried them out as follows:

Addition.		Subtraction.	
325	568	546	613
246	253	132	237
1.6.11.	7.11.11.	416 (wrong)	664 (wrong)

Coins and their relative value. He was unable to utter spontaneously, or to repeat the name of a single coin. But, when I said the words over to him he called out "yes" and nodded his head as I mentioned the correct one.

To test his knowledge of their relative value I asked, "How many of this one go into that one?" and his answers were as follows:

One shilling and a two-shilling piece—He held up two fingers.
A sixpence and a two-shilling piece—Four fingers.
One penny and a sixpence—Six fingers.
A sixpence and half-a-crown—Five fingers.
One penny and one shilling—He held up his right hand with five fingers extended; then he said "nover" (another) and held up his hand again. Next he held up two fingers of the right hand and laid the left index across them horizontally so as to cut them off from the rest of the hand. By this complicated manoeuvre he was able to indicate the high number twelve, which was correct.

One halfpenny and one penny—He said "two."

One penny and a two-shilling piece—He held up both hands with all the fingers extended, twice in succession. Then he exhibited four fingers cut off horizontally by the index of the left hand.

One penny and half-a-crown—He held up the right hand six times in succession to indicate thirty, which was correct.

Thus it was evident that, although he could not utter the names of the coins, he fully appreciated their symbolic significance and relative value.

Drawing. He had never learnt to draw and the result of an attempt to reproduce a glass in outline was very poor. From memory, however, he succeeded somewhat better.

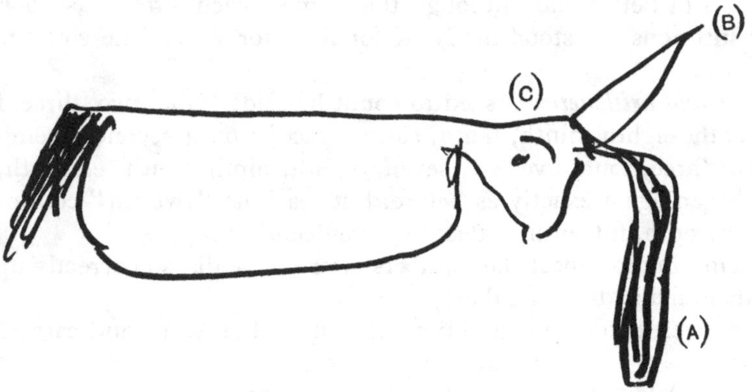

Fig. 28. Attempt by No. 21 to draw an elephant to command.

I then said, "Draw me an elephant. You know an elephant?" and he answered, "Yes, I've been all over, seen lots" (holding up both hands). I enquired, "In India?" "Yes, I've got some on my what you call it." At one time he had been employed as steward on board a boat travelling to India and China and he had brought home some carved figures of elephants, which stood on the mantlepiece of his sitting-room.

The drawing he produced was ridiculous (Fig. 28). Asked "What is this?" (*A*) he said "Er, er, sometimes up that way," indicating that the trunk was sometimes thrown upwards over the back. "What is that?" (*B*) he grasped his own ear, and questioned about (*C*) he said "Don't know," but pointed to his own eye.

Serial Tests.

(1) *Naming and recognition of common objects.*

He had no difficulty in pointing to an object named by me either orally or in print; in each series of eighteen observations he made one error only and his answers were quick and given without hesitation.

But he could not name a single object shown him, although he made me understand in excellent pantomime that he was familiar with their use.

He was unable to write spontaneously or to dictation the names of these common objects, nor could he copy them correctly from a printed card. The letters were badly formed and in most instances what he wrote bore no relation to the word required. Not uncommonly, however, it began with the correct initial.

Table 1.

	Pointing to object shown	Oral commands	Printed commands	Naming an object indicated	Duplicate placed in hand out of sight	Writing name of object indicated	Copied from print	Written to dictation
Knife	Correct	Correct	Correct	"Can't get it" (showed use)	Correct	Baudn	Kolee	Km
Key	"	"	"	"I know what it is"	"	Kinj	Koy	Kest
Match box	"	"	"	Struck a match in dumb-show	"	Meuter	Belddeny	Malndodn
Scissors	"	"	"	"Don't know"; made action of cutting	"	Sangn	Siocolan	Seenlen
Penny	"	"	"	Brought a penny from his pocket	"	Manli	Penny	Pleml
Pencil	"	"	Knife; then penny	Picked up knife and cut the point of the pencil	"	Pleant	Panlod	Pl
Key	"	"	Correct	Made action of turning key in lock	"	Kem	Kny	Kod
Penny	"	"	"	Searched his pockets for a penny	"	Pennl	Ponyl	Pemnli
Match box	"	"	"	Struck a match in dumb-show	"	Manly	Norllondng	Pnondar
Pencil	"	Knife	"	Sharpened pencil with knife	"	Pennl	Pivinl	Pemnt
Scissors	"	Correct	"	Cut with scissors	"	Sannl	Samde	Sinsrssn
Knife	"	"	"	Dumb-show of cutting with a knife	"	Knind	Pannlis	Kmit
Match box	"	"	"	Struck a match	"	Pennel	Pndnchmood	Pandond
Key	"	"	"	Turned the lock	"	Kmnt	Pan	Penml
Pencil	"	"	"	Sharpened point	"	Kmdry	Plenchl	Plannt
Knife	"	"	"	Cut pencil	"	Plant	Plank	Kmsnt
Penny	"	"	"	Searched his pockets for a penny	"	Panck	Pnolon	Pamnt
Scissors	"	"	"	Cut with scissors	"	Samats	Snokerm	Soalsders

(2) *Naming and recognition of colours.* (Table 2.)

He had no trouble in matching a colour shown to him or in picking out the one named by me. But, when it came to indicating the colour named in print he was less certain; he failed five times and had twice to correct his first choice.

He was entirely unable to name a single colour. If, however, cards were laid on the table, each of which bore the name of a colour, he could pick out correctly ten times out of sixteen the one which corresponded to that shown him.

(3) *The man, cat and dog tests.* (Table 3.)

He was totally unable to read any of these combinations either from print or from pictures. But, if the six cards were laid upon the table and he was shown any two of the pictures in combination, he could pick out with accuracy the corresponding printed sentence. So clever was he that, after first choosing "the cat and the man" he corrected the sequence and selected a card bearing the legend "the man and the cat"; the same thing occurred when he was shown pictures of the dog and the cat in this order from left to right. This showed that he not only understood the significance of the printed cards, but recognised the importance of the sequence in which the words occurred.

On attempting to write from dictation he usually produced two words which bore some remote relation to the nouns of the sentence said by me. But when he copied or wrote from pictures, the letters he put together were incomprehensible.

Table 2.

	Pointing to colour shown	Oral commands	Printed commands	Naming	Selecting printed name of colour shown	Copying from print
Black	Correct	Correct	Correct	"No"	Correct	Bdalk
Red	,,	,,	Slow, correct	,,	,,	Kdd
Blue	,,	,,	Green; then correct	,,	Black	Pllu
Green	,,	,,	Yellow	,,	Correct	Kloem
Orange	,,	,,	Yellow	,,	Yellow	Onn
White	,,	,,	Correct, quick	,,	Correct	Wihhode
Violet	,,	,,	,,	,,	Yellow	Vodlet
Yellow	,,	,,	,,	,,	Orange	Ridlms
Black	,,	,,	,,	,,	Correct	
Red	,,	,,	No choice	,,	,,	
Blue	,,	,,	Black; then correct	,,	Yellow	
Green	,,	,,	Yellow	,,	Yellow	
Orange	,,	,,	Yellow	,,	Correct	
White	,,	,,	Correct, quick	,,	,,	
Violet	,,	,,	,,	,,	,,	
Yellow	,,	,,	,,	,,	,,	

Table 3.

	Reading aloud	Reading from pictures	Choosing card with legend corresponding to pictures shown	Writing from dictation	Writing from pictures	Copying from print
The man and the cat	Impossible	Impossible	Chose cat and man; corrected to man and cat	Man Cod	Rmod Ran	loa Man M Bend dang
The dog and the man	,,	,,	Correct	Ben Mon	Mam day	Pamg Bag lan m dann
The cat and the dog	,,	,,	Correct	Cod dag	Cad Mans	Ten dug an Bedg
The man and the dog	,,	,,	,,	Beln M Bag	P man dar	Poa Beanggr
The cat and the man	,,	,,	,,	Cod man	Amd Bnan	Plam c dany
The dog and the cat	,,	,,	,,	C Bog Been	Ram Benary	Plm Bay dandez
The man and the dog	,,	,,	,,	Bundag	Bunny Pay	Ploa man dandez gas
The cat and the man	,,	,,	,,	Codden	Rnan do ag	Plnam dany lmz
The dog and the cat	,,	,,	Chose cat and dog; corrected to dog and cat	Bear Coal	d Bod Buny	Plnamgul Buy
The man and the cat	,,	,,	Correct	Bonard	Man	Plasmdy Buyon

(4) *The clock tests.*

He tended to confuse the two hands, when setting the clock in imitation and to oral command, but in each case was right in six out of ten attempts. But when he was asked to set the hands to printed command expressed in the ordinary nomenclature, e.g. "5 minutes to 8," he failed entirely to understand what was required. If, however, the order was expressed in railway time, e.g. "8.5," he mistook the hands and made several mistakes, but succeeded in carrying it out correctly three times in ten attempts. Asked to tell the time he touched his tongue and shook his head; with the hands at 1.30 he held up one finger cutting it in half horizontally with the opposite index and for "5 minutes to 2" he held up five fingers and then two.

Table 4.

	Direct imitation	Oral commands	Printed commands		Telling the time
			Ordinary nomenclature	Railway time	
5 minutes to 2	Correct	Correct	Impossible	Correct	Impossible
Half-past 1	"	"	"	Set 6.30	"
5 minutes past 8	"	"	"	Set 12.15	"
20 minutes to 4	Set 8.20, confused hands	Short hand at 8, long hand at 4	"	Correct	"
10 minutes past 7	Correct	Correct	"	Short hand at 7, long hand at 10	"
20 minutes to 6	Short hand at 8, long hand at 6	Short hand at 8, long hand at 6	"	Set 5.0	"
10 minutes to 1	Correct	Correct	"	Short hand at 10, long hand at 12	"
A quarter to 9	"	Short hand at 3, long hand correctly	"	Short hand at 12, long hand correctly	"
20 minutes past 11	Short hand at 4, long hand at 11	Correct	"	Correct	"
25 minutes to 3	Correct	Short hand at 11, long hand correctly	"	Short hand at 9, long hand at 2	"

(5) *The coin-bowl tests.*

He failed entirely to carry out any form of this test satisfactorily. To printed command, whether set out in words or in figures, he made no response of any kind. To oral command he was right three times only in fifteen attempts and was usually grossly inaccurate.

(6) *The hand, eye and ear tests.* (Table 5.)

He failed to imitate correctly movements made by me or commands given in the form of pictures. But, when allowed to see them reflected in a mirror, every action was accurately carried out without the slightest hesitation. Both oral and printed commands gave him great trouble and he was totally unable to read or to repeat aloud this series of tests.

Table 5.

	Imitation of movements made by the observer	Imitation of movements reflected in a mirror	Pictorial commands	Pictorial commands reflected in a mirror	Oral commands	Printed commands	Reading aloud printed commands	Repetition of words said by the observer
L. hand to L. eye	Correct	Correct	Reversed	Correct	L. hand to R. eye	"I can't"	Impossible	Impossible
R. hand to R. ear	,,	,,	,,	,,	R. hand to L. ear	"I know what it is; I don't know what it say"	,,	,,
R. hand to L. eye	R. hand to R. eye; then L. hand to L. eye	,,	R. hand to right *ear*	,,	Correct	Shakes his head	,,	,,
L. hand to R. eye	L. hand to L. eye	,,	Reversed	,,	,,	,,	,,	,,
L. hand to L. ear	L. hand to R. ear	,,	,,	,,	L. hand to R. ear	,,	,,	,,
R. hand to R. eye	R. hand to L. *ear*	,,	Reversed; then R. hand to L. eye	,,	R. hand to L. *ear*	,,	,,	,,
L. hand to R. ear	Correct	,,	Reversed	,,	Correct	,,	,,	,,
R. hand to L. ear	Reversed	,,	,,	,,	Reversed	,,	,,	,,
L. hand to R. eye	Reversed; then L. hand to L. eye	,,	,,	,,	R. hand to L. *ear*	,,	,,	,,
R. hand to R. ear	R. hand to L. ear	,,	,,	,,	L. hand to R. ear; then reversed	,,	,,	,,

He died suddenly on the night of January 6th, 1920. No autopsy was permitted.

No. 22

A case of Nominal Aphasia due to a cerebral seizure in an elderly man with raised arterial tension and degenerated arteries. These defects of speech were associated with right hemianopsia, unaccompanied by any other signs of disease in the central nervous system.

Observations made eleven weeks, and again three years after the attack, brought out results which were fundamentally identical in character.

Words were not lacking, but he was perpetually held up for want of the one which exactly expressed his meaning. Articulation and syntax were not otherwise affected and he could repeat what was said to him, if it was not a long and complicated sentence. He had profound difficulty in naming an object shown to him. With colours he was particularly at fault; but, although he could not name them, he could describe how they would be composed from pigments habitually used by a house painter. He understood most of what was said to him and oral commands were performed slowly, though on the whole correctly. The execution of printed commands was grossly defective and he failed to appreciate the meaning of a printed passage read silently. This was even more evident, when he read it to me, and he was not materially aided in understanding what he read by uttering the words aloud. He had never been able to write easily and with freedom and, although he wrote his name and address accurately, he could not compose a short letter. He failed to write down the names of familiar objects and colours, but on several occasions wrote some word of associated meaning or the pigments he would employ to make the colour. It was not the act of writing that was at fault, but the power to discover words of the exact meaning to fit a certain situation and then to transform them into appropriate written symbols. He could copy print exactly, although he could not translate it into cursive script. He counted up to twenty, then became somewhat confused, but ultimately reached a hundred without a mistake. He failed to solve simple problems in arithmetic. Coins were named and their relative value stated correctly. He could draw a jug from a model and from memory, saying "I can see it in my mind"; but he was profoundly puzzled when told to draw an elephant. He failed entirely to construct a ground-plan of the room in which we habitually worked, although he could indicate the position of each salient feature relatively to himself. Orientation was not affected, but he was liable to become confused if he did not see before him the landmarks and guiding points he expected. He had lost the power of reading musical notation and, as he had never played by ear, could no longer use his double-bass.

In the early hours of March 7th, 1920, Alfred B., a man of 65, suffered from a cerebral attack during his sleep. He woke in the morning to find that he could no longer speak easily; there was no paralysis of arm or leg and he was ignorant of the hemianopsia discovered on subsequent examination. On May 12th, 1920, he was admitted to St Mary's Hospital under the care of Dr Wilfred Harris, to whose kindness I am indebted for the opportunity of studying this instructive example of nominal aphasia.

Condition between May 22nd and June 20th, 1920 (*eleven to fifteen weeks after the seizure*).

He was a somewhat worn-looking elderly man, a highly intelligent and skilled artisan. By trade he was a house painter and decorator; but, as he was musical and played both the cornet and double-bass, he was in the habit during the summer of playing in the orchestra at one of the seaside holiday resorts.

His pulse was regular, 68 to the minute, and the systolic arterial tension reached 185 mm., the diastolic 100 mm.; the vessel wall was hard and tortuous. The apex beat of the heart was somewhat forcible and slightly outside the nipple line. Nothing abnormal could be heard beyond an accentuation of the aortic second sound.

He suffered from no headache, giddiness or nausea.

Vision was $\frac{6}{5}$ with either eye, but there was gross right hemianopsia. Form and movement were, however (see Fig. 29), appreciated slightly to the right of the middle line within part of the region of central vision.

The pupils seemed to react to light even from the blind field.

The discs were normal, but the arteries of the fundus were pale in colour and evidently degenerated.

Movements of eyes, face and tongue were perfect. All the reflexes were normal and equal on the two sides. There was no paralysis, paresis, incoordination, tremor, or change in tone in the upper or lower extremities. Sensibility was not in any way disturbed.

The Wassermann reaction was negative both in the serum and cerebro-spinal fluid, and the latter showed no increase in cells or globulin.

Symbolic Formulation and Expression.

Quiet and unemotional, he was neither cast down by failure to answer the tests nor elated by success. If he found much difficulty in executing a task set him, he did not confuse himself by repeated and futile efforts to solve the problem, but simply gave up all attempts to do so. He was most willing to be examined, especially in the quiet surroundings of my consulting room, where he enjoyed talking of his past experiences as a musician. He answered questions readily, but volunteered little information with regard to his disabilities.

He was educated at an elementary school where he learnt to read and spell. He never acquired the art of writing easily; arithmetic on the other hand he always enjoyed.

Articulated speech. Words were not lacking, but he was perpetually held up for want of the one which exactly expressed his meaning. The following remarks, evoked by my enquiry if he had seen many elephants, forms a good example of his defects of speech.

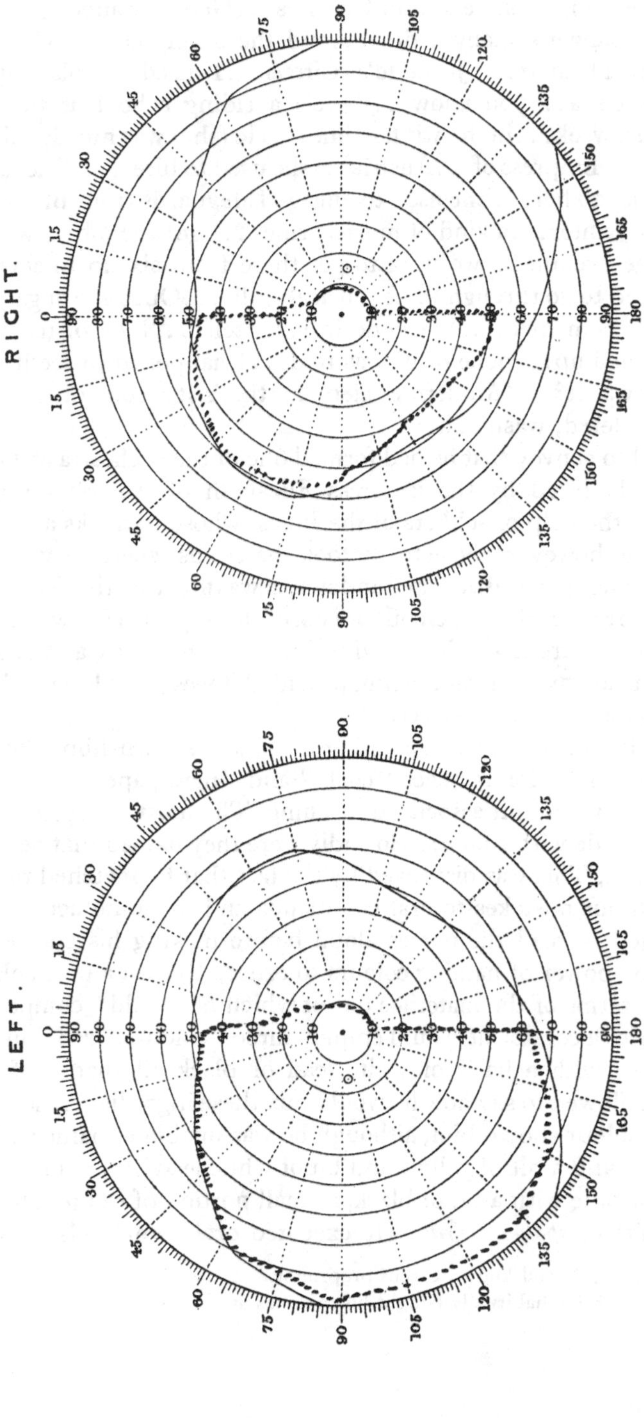

Fig. 29. To show the limitation of the fields of vision in No. 22.

"I've seen 'em in the streets...in Circuses...George Sanger[1], he had a lot... I've played for Sanger's many a time...and the other man...what's his name? ...I've forgot...Jeanette...Jeanette's Circus...I used to play at Gloucester Terrace...There's a...you know...there's a riding school at the back in the mews...Twice a week...in the winter time...He (she) was murdered...what was his (her) name?...Empress of...Austria...she used to hire it...She used to engage seven of us to play to her...She used to engage Lifeguards from Blues...and twice a week...in the winter...a kind of musical ride...I got the job...we used to play for her...in the evening...we used to get there from six up to seven...five up to six...She used to go through these musical drills...Once she engaged Jeanette's Circus and had them there...She rode in it herself...None of us knew who she was till we finished up...none of us was told...I happened to see it in one of the papers...what was it?...'Modern Society'...that's it...one of the papers...yes ...she was murdered, wasn't she?"

He intended to convey that he had formed one of the orchestra at a riding school in Regent's Park, hired by the Empress Elizabeth of Austria for musical drill carried out with the help of soldiers of the Blues, whose barracks are in this neighbourhood. Once, however, she actually took the circus where he was employed.

All the words were well articulated and syntax was not directly disturbed, although his phrases were frequently broken off for lack of the appropriate word. Throughout, he kept firmly to the trend of his narrative, but was frequently at a loss for a name.

He could repeat anything said to him provided it was not a long and complicated sentence; his intonation was perfect.

He had profound difficulty in naming an object shown him. For scissors he substituted "button"; for matches "coals" and "newspaper,"[2] words of fundamentally different form, but associated meaning. The most interesting observations were, however, made with colours. So badly were they named that he was supposed to be colour-blind. This was disproved by the fact that he matched them perfectly, chose them without mistakes to oral commands and made no actual errors, when he was permitted to read the names aloud before making his choice. His defect lay mainly in the power of naming colours to order. Shown a particular colour, he thought of it in terms of the materials out of which he would "compose" a similar paint. As a house decorator he would employ three "colours," red, blue and yellow, and out of these with a basis of white lead or black all shades of pigment are "composed." Allowed to say how he would mix these ingredients, he could indicate the nature of a colour shown him, although he was unable to name it. Thus orange was "a bit of red and a bit of yellow and bit of white lead"; for violet he said "Yes, that's...a bit of blue with a bit of black, a small portion of red just to warm it."

Understanding of spoken words. He executed oral commands slowly and after

[1] A well-known Circus proprietor.

[2] He habitually bought his matches at a newsvendor's.

considerable hesitation, but on the whole correctly. He understood what was said to him in conversation, provided he was not expected to retain an exact memory of a number of detailed statements. For instance, after I had read to him a short account of his musical activities, he could reproduce nothing but "I am a painter and decorator...I can't say it your words...no." Yet, told to tell the story his own way, he neglected no detail, although he employed different words. It was not the significance of the story that troubled him, but the discovery of words with the exact meaning in which to reproduce it.

Reading. The execution of printed commands was grossly defective and he failed to make any choice, when the name of a familiar object was shown to him on a card. The clock was set equally badly whether the order was given in the ordinary nomenclature or in figures (railway time).

He read to himself with extreme slowness passing his finger over one letter after another silently especially in the longer words and he was evidently puzzled even by the simple account of his own musical activities.

This want of comprehension of the meaning of printed words was even more evident, when he attempted to read aloud. He spelt them out letter by letter; this helped him to articulate the words, but did not materially aid him in appreciating their full significance in the narrative.

He was, however, able to reproduce with perfect ease and accuracy the simple phrases of the man, cat and dog tests from pictures, although he had great difficulty in reading them from print. It was not words that were lacking, but the power of recognising the verbal significance of printed symbols.

Writing. He left school young and, although he learnt to read and to spell, he had never been able to write easily or with freedom. This considerably increased the severity of any test which necessitated the act of writing, whether spontaneously or to dictation.

He wrote his name and address correctly, but was completely unable to compose a short letter; after writing "Dear Sir" he ceased to be able to proceed further. He failed to write the names of familiar objects or colours, but on several occasions wrote some word of associated meaning or the ingredients out of which he would compose a pigment of the given colour. The simple phrases of the man, cat and dog series were written correctly from pictures. Thus it was not the act of writing that was affected, but the power to discover words of the exact meaning to fit a certain situation and then to transform them into appropriate written symbols. He copied print in capital letters exactly, which is little more than an act of imitative drawing, but was unable to translate it into cursive script.

Thus, the records obtained with the writing tests varied according to the intellectual severity of the task. He could not write the names of objects shown to him without many mistakes; to dictation the results were somewhat better; copying in cursive script was also defective, but exact reproduction of print was possible.

The alphabet. He said the alphabet spontaneously, read it aloud and repeated it after me perfectly. But he could write no further than H even in printed capitals. When the letters were dictated one by one he wrote $\mathscr{A}$ $\mathscr{B}$ $\mathscr{C}$ $\mathscr{D}$ E F G H I L M N O P R S T U V W X Y Z. Asked to copy the printed alphabet, he produced the following: $\mathscr{A}$ $\mathscr{B}$ c d e f g H i $\mathscr{J}$ K l m n o $\mathscr{P}$ q $\mathscr{R}$ $\mathscr{S}$ t $\mathscr{U}$ $\mathscr{V}$ $\mathscr{W}$ X $\mathscr{Y}$ z.

A printed paragraph. I put together the following sentences taken from the story of his life:

"I was a painter and house decorator. I played the cornet and the double-bass. During the summer I used to take an engagement at the sea. I did six seasons on Deal Pier and one at Hastings. My double-bass was built by Panormo[1], an Italian working in London early in the last century."

This he read to himself silently and was evidently puzzled. After the lapse of five minutes, he said, "I am a painter and house decorator...I was just trying to get the other things underneath...I shall get them directly." I handed the paper back to him and he passed his finger over the words letter by letter, but said nothing, except "I play the cornet and double-bass." He then made no further attempt to convey the meaning of the paragraph he was supposed to have read, saying, "I can't get that somehow."

He read these sentences aloud as follows: "I was a...P A I...painter and ...house decorator...I...P...played...P I played...the cornet...and...the double-bass...During...the...during the...S O...during the summer I... us...ed...I...to...T A K E take...on...E N G A G E M E N T...engagement...at the...S E A...at the sea...I did...P R E no...on...D R E A... D E A L...on Deal pier...and on a...and at...Hast...and at Hastings...B Y, no...B Y, by...D O U R I N G." He then ceased completely puzzled.

After I had read the whole to him aloud and asked him to tell me what he remembered, he said nothing beyond "I am a painter and decorator...I can't say it your words...no." When I replied, "Tell me the story your own way," he at once gave all the details, arranged somewhat differently in his own words. "I'm a painter and decorator. I'm also a musician and I play the cornet and double-bass...and I played on Deal Pier six seasons and Hastings Pier one season. I've a Panormo, double-bass. It's a good instrument...It's an old one...in fact I wouldn't have a new one."

Numbers and arithmetic. He counted slowly and correctly up to a hundred, but failed to solve most of the following simple problems in arithmetic:

Addition.

253	327	586
324	436	254
557 (wrong)	733 (wrong)	740 (wrong)

[1] Vincenzo Panormo, b. 1734 in Sicily, d. 1813 in London where he had long worked.

Subtraction.

856	582	613
432	326	485
424	26 He said "6 from 2, can't do it; 2 from 8 is 6 but I'm greatly mixed now"	98 Here he added forgetting that he was told to subtract

Coins and their relative value. All the coins were named correctly and he stated the relative value of any two of them without mistakes.

Drawing. He made a fairly correct drawing of a jug with the model before him and reproduced it almost exactly from memory. He added, "I can see it in my mind; there's some red on it; there are two figures on it, they are coloured...green I think." All of these details were correct.

Asked to draw an elephant, he was profoundly puzzled and produced nothing, saying, "Yes, quite so, that's the gentleman with the long...yes, quite so, with the long trunk." Finally he exclaimed, "No, I can't think...I can't call (re-call) it, sir." He then proceeded to tell me the story (vide p. 332) of how he played in a circus and formed one of the orchestra for the musical rides of the Empress of Austria.

Drawing a plan. He was told to look round my consulting room and to notice especially the position of windows, doors, tables and fireplace. After moving to another room, I asked him to draw me a ground-plan of the one in which we habitually worked. As a house decorator he was familiar with what I required, calling it a "floor-plan"; but he drew two windows in elevation and, after several ineffectual attempts, gave up, saying, "I know what you mean, but I can't get at it."

I then drew a square in the centre of a sheet of paper to represent the situation of the table at which we sat, indicating also the position of his chair and mine. In response to my questions, he was able to point to the position of the windows, the couch, the cupboards and the door. Asked to state how these objects were situated relatively to the table or to one another, he was unable to do so. He could express their position in space with regard to himself, but not their relation to one another.

Visual images. Throughout these observations he repeatedly said, "I can see it in my mind," when recalling some object he wished to reproduce in words or in a drawing. In the same way, the manner in which he described from memory the coloured figures on the jug he had drawn showed that he possessed visual imagery; but these images could not be evoked at will for the purposes of verbal formulation.

Music had become impossible. For, since he could no longer decipher musical notation, he had ceased to be able to play his double-bass. "I can't read music; I can't tell an *a* from a *b*. It affects me," he said, "the same as reading this," pointing to words in print.

Games. He could not play any card games and had never learnt chess.

Serial Tests.

(1) *Naming and recognition of common objects.*

Table 1.

	Pointing to object shown	Oral commands	Printed commands	Duplicate placed in hand out of sight	Naming object indicated	Writing name of object indicated	Copying from print		Writing to dictation	Repetition
							In printed capitals	In cursive handwriting		
Key	Correct	Correct	No choice	Correct	"Pen...no...I know, but I can't think of it"	Pencil	Correct	Correct	Correct	Correct
Pencil	,,	,,	,,	,,	"That's pencil"	Correct	PENSIL	Paper	,,	,,
Match box	,,	Slow, finally correct	,,	,,	"Er...matches"	Coals	MATCHE BOA	Patch hox	Match pox	,,
Knife	,,	Correct	,,	,,	"Er...knife"	Correct	Correct	Correct	Correct	,,
Penny	,,	,,	,,	,,	"Penny"	,,	,,	Panny	Benny	,,
Scissors	,,	Pencil	,,	,,	"Button...yes, button...a pencil I should say...pen, pen"	"I can't remember"	,,	Eci	Correct	,,
Key	,,	Scissors; "No, that's not it"	,,	,,	"That's er...I know what it is"	"I can't remember"	—	—	,,	,,
Pencil	,,	Correct	,,	,,	"Pencil"	Penicl	—	—	,,	,,
Match box	,,	Slow, correct	,,	,,	"Matches"	Newspaper	—	—	,,	,,
Knife	,,	Correct	"It's K I can see and I. No"	,,	"Knife"	Correct	—	—	,,	,,
Penny	,,	,,	"P...EM...No"	,,	"Penny"	,,	—	—	,,	,,
Scissors	,,	,,	"No, I can only tell I"	,,	"Button"	Scissers	—	—	Sissors	,,

Although most of his answers were finally correct, he found considerable difficulty in executing oral commands, and failed entirely to make a choice to orders given in print. He could not name the various objects shown him without great effort and, in some instances, did not reply at all. It is interesting to notice that by an obvious association of ideas the scissors were called "button." Every word was, however, repeated perfectly after me and he showed no evidence of defective verbal formation.

He could not write down the name of an object with certainty. Sometimes he failed altogether, at others he wrote some word of associated significance, such as "coals" and "newspaper" in place of matches; the latter was explained by the fact that he bought his matches at a newsvendor's shop. To dictation the words though badly spelt were otherwise correct. He copied the printed names laboriously in capitals, but had extreme difficulty in translating them into cursive script. So grossly did this task confuse him that I was compelled to cut short these observations.

(2) *Naming and recognition of colours.*

He was supposed to be colour-blind, because of his defective power of naming colours; but this was shown to be false by the ease with which he matched a colour shown to him and the correctness with which he executed oral commands.

Table 2.

	Pointing to colour shown	Naming	Oral commands	Printed commands	Printed name read aloud and colour chosen		Writing name of colour indicated
					He said	He chose	
Green	Correct	Correct	Correct	Correct	Correctly	Correctly	Wrote nothing
Yellow	,,	"I don't know"	,,	"No, I can't"	Silent	No choice	,,
Red	,,	Correct	,,	Hesitated; chose correctly	Correctly	Correctly	Correct
Blue	,,	"Well, blue, red, blue"	,,	Correct	"Black. No, it's not it's blue"	Black; then correctly	Wrote nothing
White	,,	Correct	,,	Correct	Correctly	Correctly	Correct
Orange	,,	"Well, yellow I suppose... It's on the yellow side"	,,	"Orange I think it is"; chose correctly	,,	,,	Red
Black	,,	Correct	,,	Correct	,,	,,	Correct
Violet	,,	"I'm thinking of what it's made of ...blue"	,,	"No"; no choice	,,	,,	blue and black, small portion of red
Green	,,	Correct	,,	Correct	,,	,,	Correct
Yellow	,,	"That one's yellow, I should think"	,,	"No"; no choice	"No"	No choice	,,
Red	,,	Correct	,,	No choice	Correctly	Correctly	,,
Blue	,,	"Well...blue, really"	,,	,,	,,	,,	,,
White	,,	Correct	,,	Correct	,,	,,	,,
Orange	,,	"There is yellow in both" (placing orange over yellow). "I can't think"	,,	No choice	Correctly; slowly	,,	Red
Black	,,	Correct	,,	No choice	,,	,,	Correct
Violet	,,	"There's red in it and there's blue in it"	,,	"No"; no choice	,,	,,	Wrote nothing

Printed orders were carried out with extreme difficulty and in many instances he failed to make a choice of any kind. But, if he was permitted to read them aloud, the records improved greatly; for in this way he gave himself an oral command.

The most instructive results were obtained when he attempted to name a colour either vocally or in writing. In both cases his answers were grossly defective. Throughout these tests, if he was in doubt about what to call it, he began to consider how a paint of that colour would be composed. A house decorator employs red, blue and yellow with a basis of white lead and by due variation of these ingredients obtains all the tints he requires. Thus, whenever B. failed to recollect the proper name of a colour, he described with remarkable accuracy the materials necessary to produce it. This method of overcoming his defective nomenclature was particularly evident from the following remarks made during his attempts to write down the name of a colour shown to him (cf. Table 2, last column).

Yellow. "It's made with white lead and a bit of...I can't think of it."

Red. "It's made with white lead with a bit of red with it."

Orange. "It's easy enough to make if I'd the stuff; a bit of red and a bit of yellow and a bit of white lead. There are so many tints; there is more red in it than anything." He wrote "red."

Violet. "Yes, that's...a bit of blue with a bit of black, a small portion of red just to warm it." On the second occurrence of this colour in the series, he wrote nothing but said, "I don't know what I called it before...It's made with black, red and a bit of blue; white lead would be the prevailing thing and stain it afterwards."

(3) *The man, cat and dog tests.*

Table 3.

	Reading aloud	Reading from pictures	Writing from pictures	Copying print		Writing to dictation	Reading what he wrote to dictation	Repetition
				In cursive script	In print			
The dog and the cat	"The D O P the dop and H, D O P and T H E C A...Dog and the...dog and the cat"	Perfect	Correct	The cat and the cat	Correct	Correct	"The man and the cat"	Perfect
The man and the dog	"The man and the...H O...the man and the...man and the dog"	,,	,,	Correct	,,	,,	Correct	,,
The cat and the man	"The cat and the...and the man"	,,	,,	,,	,,	,,	,,	,,
The cat and the dog	"The cat and the...dog"	,,	,,	,,	,,	,,	,,	,,
The dog and the man	"The dog and the...cat...That isn't C is it? The dog and the...man"	,,	,,	the man and the cat	,,	,,	"The cat and the...the dog and the man"	,,
The man and the cat	"The man and the...the man and the...cat"	,,	,,	Correct	,,	,,	"The man and the dog"	,,
The dog and the cat	"The man and the cat"	,,	,,	the man and the cat	,,	,,	Correct	,,
The man and the dog	"The man and the...dog"	,,	,,	the man and the cat	,,	,,	,,	,,
The cat and the man	"The cat...and the...man"	,,	,,	Correct	,,	,,	"The dog and the man"	,,
The cat and the dog	"The cat and the...dog"	,,	,,	the cat and the Man	,,	,,	"The man and the...the Cat and the dog"	,,
The dog and the man	"The cat and the man"	,,	,,	the Man and the Man	,,	the god and the man	Correct	,,
The man and the cat	"The man and the...cat"	,,	,,	Correct	,,	Correct	"The man and the...dog"	,,

In response to pictures he could both say these simple phrases and write them down correctly. But he had extreme difficulty in reading them aloud from print. He started by trying to spell out each word letter by letter; becoming confused, he fell back on guessing the words as a whole and in this way succeeded in reading the second half of the series slowly but without mistakes. He succeeded in writing them to my dictation. When, however, he attempted to copy them from print in cursive script, he evidently guessed many of the words and wrote "the man and the cat" for the dog and the man, "the cat and the man" instead of the cat and the dog. If he was allowed to copy the printed words exactly, he did so without mistakes, reproducing each letter stroke by stroke without thinking of them as symbols or words.

(4) *The coin-bowl tests.* He carried out oral commands correctly and explained, "Numbers used to bother me; they don't now." Printed orders, given in figures

(e.g. "1st into 2nd"), were also well executed, if they were read silently. But when he said them aloud before putting them into practice, he was liable to make mistakes, which influenced his subsequent actions adversely.

(5) *The clock tests.*

Table 4.

	Direct imitation	Oral commands	Printed commands		Telling the time	Writing down the time shown on the clock
			Ordinary nomenclature	Railway time		
5 minutes to 2	Perfect	Correct	Correct	Correct	Correct	5 minutes to twelve
Half-past 1	"	"	Set 2.30	Set 1.20	"	Correct
5 minutes past 8	"	"	Hour hand at 1; long hand at 20 past	Correct	"	"
20 minutes to 4	"	"	Correct	Set 3.30	"	"
10 minutes past 7	"	"	Set 10 minutes *to* 7	Set 7.0	"	"
20 minutes to 6	"	Confused hands	Correct	Correct	"	twenty minets past six
10 minutes to 1	"	Correct	Set 20 minutes to 1	Set 12.15	"	Correct
A quarter to 9	"	"	Set 9.45; "Oh! that's ten"; then correct	Correct	"Quarter to twelve"	"
20 minutes past 11	"	"	Hour hand at 11; long hand at half past	"	"Quarter past eleven"; then correct	twenty minetus past eleven
25 minutes to 3	"	"	Set 25 minutes to 9	Said "Two twenty three" and set 2.23	Correct	twenty five minetus to three

Oral commands were executed slowly with one mistake only in ten observations; this depended on confusion between the significance of the two hands. Throughout the whole of this series, he tended to set the short hand directly opposite the figure indicating the hour and not in proportion to the number of minutes shown by the long hand. With "20 minutes to 4," "10 minutes to 1" and "5 minutes to 2" he failed to recognise that it should have been placed somewhere short of the hour named.

Printed commands, whether given in the ordinary nomenclature or in railway time, were badly executed and, even if the clock was set correctly, the answer was given after much hesitation.

He told the time on the whole accurately but with some difficulty. In the same way he wrote down the time with two mistakes only, although both writing and spelling were very defective.

(6) *The hand, eye and ear tests.* (Table 5.)

He imitated slowly and inaccurately my movements sitting face to face, or pictorial commands held in his hand; but, as soon as they were reflected in a mirror, his answers were given rapidly and with perfect ease.

Oral commands were performed without mistakes; on the other hand, printed orders were carried out badly and he frequently confused eye and ear. His power of reading them aloud was so defective that he was thereby puzzled rather than aided in carrying them into execution.

He wrote down my movements with fair accuracy and three out of the four mistakes consisted in confusing eye and ear.

Table 5.

	Imitation of movements made by the observer	Imitation of movements reflected in a mirror	Pictorial commands	Pictorial commands reflected in a mirror	Oral commands	Printed commands	Printed commands read aloud and executed: He said	Printed commands read aloud and executed: Movement executed	Writing down movements made by the observer
L. hand to L. eye	Correct	Correct	Correct	Correct	Correct	R. hand to L. *ear*	"L. hand to L. *ear*"	L. hand to L. *ear*	Correct
R. hand to R. ear	”	”	”	”	”	Correct; slow	Correctly	Reversed	”
R. hand to L. eye	Reversed	”	R. hand to R. eye	”	”	R. hand to L. *ear*	"R. hand to L. *ear*"	R. hand to L. *ear*	R. hand to L. *ear*
L. hand to R. eye	”	”	Reversed	”	”	R. hand to R. *ear*	"L. hand to R. *ear*. E A R... yes, *ear*"	L. hand to R. *ear*	L. hand to L. *ear*
L. hand to L. ear	Reversed. "Oh! that was the wrong hand"	”	Correct	”	”	Reversed; "No"; then correct	Correctly	Correct	Correct
R. hand to R. eye	Correct	”	L. hand to L. *ear*	”	”	R. hand to R. *ear*	"R. hand to R. *ear*. No, it isn't. Oh! R. eye"	First to ear; then correct	R. hand to R. *ear*
L. hand to R. ear	Reversed	”	Reversed	”	”	Correct	"L. hand to R. hand...head ...H A R... No"	Did nothing	Correct
R. hand to L. ear	”	”	”	”	”	”	Correctly	Correct	”
L. hand to L. eye	Correct	”	"I done the wrong hand, I think"	”	”	L. hand to L. *ear*	"L. hand to L. *ear*"	L. hand to L. *ear*	”
R. hand to R. ear	”	”	L. hand to L. *eye*	”	”	Correct	Correctly	Correct	”
R. hand to L. eye	”	”	Reversed	”	”	R. hand to L. *ear*	"R. hand to L. *ear*"	R. hand to L. *ear*	”
L. hand to R. eye	”	”	”	”	”	R. hand to R. *ear*	"L. hand to R. *ear*"	L. hand to R. *ear*	”
L. hand to L. ear	”	”	”	”	”	Correct	Correctly	Correct	”
R. hand to R. eye	”	”	”	”	”	R. hand to R. *ear*	"R. hand to R. *ear*"	R. hand to R. *ear*	R. hand to L. eye
L. hand to R. ear	”	”	Correct	”	”	Correct	"L. hand to L. ear, to R. ear"	L. hand to L. ear; then correct	Correct
R. hand to L. ear	R. hand to R. ear	”	Reversed	”	”	”	Correctly	Correct	”

Condition between March 17th and April 5th, 1923 (*three years after the stroke*).

Three years after the attack he was physically in much the same state, although his powers of speech had somewhat improved.

His pulse was regular, 68 to the minute; the systolic tension was 175 mm., the diastolic 85 mm. There were no abnormal signs in the heart, beyond slight displacement outwards of the apex beat and accentuation of the aortic second sound.

Gross right hemianopsia was the only sign pointing to a lesion of the central nervous system.

Symbolic Formulation and Expression.

Though slightly less severe, his defects of speech were essentially identical with those discovered on my first series of observations. He still complained that he had difficulty in finding names, especially for colours. But he described accurately how he would compose each tint from the pigments at his disposal as a house painter. Moreover, when shown blue and yellow, he failed to name them directly and yet he employed both words in attempting to describe how he would make these colours. With the former he said, "I don't know what colour it is; there is blue in it" and with yellow "It's got yellow in it; I can't tell what colour you'd call it." It was not words that were lacking, but the power to fit an appropriate verbal symbol to an object or conception.

He read to himself with considerable difficulty and hesitated greatly when reading aloud (vide infra, p. 342).

He could write his name and address correctly; but, asked to compose a letter to me, he produced the following very slowly and with much effort: "Dear Doctor Head May I. offer my services to you as painter and decorator. I see the Outside of your." He then ceased, saying, "I'm afraid I hardly know what I'm doing; I seem to get mixed, I'm afraid it's badly done." When he attempted to write down what he had been told or had read to himself his handwriting was bad and he was unable to communicate his thoughts spontaneously in writing (vide p. 342). To dictation he succeeded somewhat better and he could now copy a printed paragraph in cursive script, although he failed to do so consistently with the printed letters of the alphabet.

The alphabet. He said the letters in due order spontaneously, repeated them after me and read them aloud perfectly. Given the twenty-six block letters, he had extreme difficulty in arranging them in sequence, because, even if he knew which one he required, he could not always recognise it amongst those scattered on the table. Thus he chose X for K, saying, "That's a K isn't it; I want K, I can't tell it when I see it." When in doubt, he would try various letters to see if they fitted the gap he had left; for instance, after P he said, "It's Q I want," but tried and rejected V. He succeeded ultimately in putting together the alphabet, leaving a space between J and L. Seeing the K alone on the table, he exclaimed, "Oh I've found the K at last" and placed it in its proper position. Throughout he was hampered by want of immediate recognition of the significance of the letters as they lay in disorder before him.

He wrote the alphabet spontaneously with much effort and several corrections. To dictation he succeeded somewhat better, employing capitals and small letters indiscriminately. He could not translate print into small cursive letters, and yet, when the alphabet was placed before him in this script, he reproduced every one of them correctly. It was not the power of writing these signs that was at fault, but the capacity readily to convert one form of letter into another.

A printed paragraph. I handed him the same sentences containing details from his life given on p. 334. He read them to himself with great effort and finally said, "I'm a bass player...Now I've forgotten...I remember, but I can't say it...It's most peculiar...I did six months at Deal Pier and one at Hastings...I play the cornet and double-bass...That's not exactly as that's written...I can't remember it...It's very peculiar."

He read it aloud as follows: "I was a painter and...and house decorator...I play the cornet...and the...double-bass...During the summer...I used to take an engagement...at the sea...engagement at the sea...at the sea...I did...six seasons at Deal...Pier...and one at Hastings...My...double-bass...was built by Panormo...and I...played...morning and evening...an Italian...an Italian working in...London...early in...in...early in...last century."

When I asked him to tell me how much he remembered of what he had just read aloud, he said, "I played on Deal Pier six seasons...Hastings one season... I've got it in my head, but I can't say it."

He was given the printed page and, after reading it silently again, was told to write down what he remembered. He replied "I'm lost," but wrote "I was a painter and decorator by trade I used to play the double-bass and cornet."

To my dictation he wrote: "I was a painter and house decorator. I played the cornet and the doable Bass. during the summer I used to take an engagement at the sea. I did six seasons on Deal Pier and one at Hastings. My double Bass was built by Pernormo an Ettellian working in London early in the last Centuray."

He copied the printed paragraph perfectly in cursive script and his handwriting, which had been previously scarcely legible, greatly improved in character.

Numbers and arithmetic. He counted perfectly up to twenty, but then became confused between the numbers of this and of the succeeding decade. Allowed to go back and to begin again at twenty, he counted without a single mistake up to a hundred.

He still had profound difficulty with simple addition, but solved two out of the three problems. He could not subtract at all and gave up all attempt to do so, saying, "For the life of me I don't know what to do there."

Coins and their relative value. He named all the coins correctly and stated their relation to one another; in each case, however, it was necessary to repeat the question formally.

Drawing. He drew the outline of a jug fairly well from a model and reproduced it almost exactly ten minutes later from memory. Asked if he could see what he had drawn, he said, "Yes I can see the jug...just an ordinary jug...no colour except the drawing on it...and there's a tree there...green isn't it...there's a little colour on the handle...I can see it quite well." All these details were correct.

Told to draw an elephant, he failed completely, saying, "I know quite well what it is but I don't...I'm just trying to call it to mind." When I asked him what an elephant was like, he replied, "It has the... (moving his hand down from his nose to his waist) the what you call it...the trunk...comes down here (repeating the movement)."

Drawing a plan. He was completely unable to draw a ground-plan of the room in which we worked; but, if I mentioned its various salient features, he could indicate the position which they would bear to the place where he habitually sat.

Orientation. He had no difficulty in finding his way in the neighbourhood of his home, but he could not be trusted in the streets of London alone. He was liable to become confused, if he did not see before him exactly the landmarks and guiding points he expected.

Music. He was still unable to read musical notation and had sold his double-bass, as he could no longer play it.

Serial Tests.

(1) *Naming and recognition of common objects.* (Table 6.)

He still showed considerable hesitation in choosing familiar objects to oral and printed commands and in naming them to order.

When he attempted to write down the names, he made two definite mistakes and twice failed to reproduce the difficult word "scissors." But he wrote them correctly to dictation and was able to copy them from print in cursive handwriting.

(2) *Naming and recognition of colours.* (Table 7.)

He named the colours badly and tended as before to describe the materials out of which they could be composed; for instance, with violet he said, "It's got a lot of blue in it, it wants a bit of red and blue." Shown blue, he explained, "I don't know what colour it is, there is blue in it," and yellow, "It's got yellow in it, I can't tell what colour you'd call it." This showed that the defect did not lie in verbal formation; for both "blue" and "yellow" could be evoked for descriptive purposes, but not as names indicative directly of a colour shown. He remarked, "It's most peculiar, I can't ask for them; but if I sat down I could match it. I'm a good colourman, I could make it. I know if it's the same, but I can't ask for it."

Oral and printed commands were executed slowly and with the former he tended to become confused between blue and violet, orange and yellow.

Shown a colour, he could sometimes choose the printed card which bore its name, although in three instances he failed entirely. On one occasion, after selecting with considerable hesitation the card which bore the word "violet," he laid the coloured silk across the card, as if he were matching two colours, and said, "Yes, that's right isn't it?"

He still had much difficulty in writing down the names of colours shown to him, but he could write them fairly well to dictation and copied them from print in cursive script.

Table 6.

	Pointing to object shown	Oral commands	Printed commands	Naming	Duplicate placed in hand out of sight	Writing name of object indicated	Writing to dictation	Copying print in cursive script	Repetition
Knife	Correct	Scissors. "The knife you said"; corrected	Correct	Correct	Correct	Correct	Correct	Correct	Correct
Key	,,	Scissors	Correct; very slow	,,	,,	,,	,,	,,	,,
Penny	,,	Correct	Correct	,,	,,	,,	,,	,,	,,
Matches	,,	,,	,,	,,	,,	,,	,,	,,	,,
Scissors	,,	,,	,,	"I can't think of the name of it"	,,	"I can't; it's scissors isn't it?"	,,	,,	,,
Pencil	,,	,,	Correct; slow	Correct	,,	Correct	,,	,,	,,
Key	,,	Scissors	Correct	,,	,,	"Knife"	,,	,,	,,
Scissors	,,	Correct	Hesitated; then correct	,,	,,	"I don't know how to make S"	,,	,,	,,
Matches	,,	Correct; slow	Correct	,,	,,	Correct	,,	,,	,,
Knife	,,	Correct	Hesitated; correct	,,	,,	,,	,,	,,	,,
Penny	,,	,,	Correct	,,	,,	,,	,,	,,	,,
Matches	,,	Correct; slow	,,	,,	,,	,,	,,	,,	,,
Scissors	,,	,,	,,	Correct; slow	,,	"Scissers"	,,	,,	,,
Pencil	,,	,,	Hesitated; correct	"Knife"	,,	Correct	,,	,,	,,
Penny	,,	,,	Correct	Correct	,,	,,	,,	,,	,,
Knife	,,	Correct; slow	,,	,,	,,	,,	,,	,,	,,
Key	,,	Scissors	Pencil	,,	,,	,,	,,	,,	,,
Pencil	,,	Correct	"No, that's it"; correct	,,	,,	,,	,,	,,	,,

(3) *The man, cat and dog tests*. (Table 8.)

He now read these simple phrases aloud correctly though very slowly from print, but was able to produce them with ease and rapidity in response to a combination of any two pictures. He could write accurately from pictures or to dictation and copied the words from print in cursive handwriting without mistakes. It is interesting to notice that these simple phrases could be evoked most easily from pictures both for articulated speech and written reproduction.

(4) *The coin-bowl tests*. Oral commands were perfectly executed and he made no mistakes to printed orders, provided he did not read them aloud. If, however, he attempted to utter the words, he spelt them out letter by letter, often incorrectly, and so confused himself. These observations were almost exactly similar to those made nearly three years before.

Table 7.

	Pointing to colour shown	Naming colour shown	Oral commands	Printed commands	Printed name read aloud and colour chosen: He said	Printed name read aloud and colour chosen: He chose	Writing name of colour shown	Writing name to dictation	Copying name from print in cursive script	Choosing card bearing name of colour shown
Black	Correct	Correct	Correct	Correct	Correctly	Correctly	Correct	Correct	Correct	Correct
Red	”	”	”	”	”	”	”	”	”	”
Blue	”	“I don’t know what colour it is; there is blue in it”	Violet	Correct; slow	”	No choice	“I can’t think of it”	”	”	Violet
Green	”	Correct; very slow	Correct	Correct	”	Blue; then correctly	Black	”	”	No choice
Orange	”	“Red...No, it’s yellow”	Yellow	”	”	Yellow	Yellow bit of red	”	”	”
White	”	Correct	Correct	”	”	Correctly	Correct	”	”	Correct
Violet	”	“It’s got a lot of blue in it. It wants a bit of red and blue”	Blue	”	”	Blue, doubtful	Blue	Violate	”	No choice
Yellow	”	“It’s got yellow in it. I can’t tell what colour you’d call it”	Orange	Correct; very slow	”	Correctly	Correct	Correct	”	Correct; very slow
Red	”	Correct	Correct	”	”	”	“I can’t”	”	”	”
White	”	”	”	”	”	”	Correct	”	”	”
Yellow	”	“I’ve forgotten...a warm tint...yellow”	Red; then white; then orange	”	”	”	”	”	”	”
Blue	”	“It’s got blue in it”	Violet	”	”	Correctly; slow	Violet	”	”	Correct; slow
Green	”	Correct	Correct	”	”	”	Correct	”	”	”
Black	”	”	”	”	”	”	”	”	”	”
Orange	”	Red	Yellow	Yellow	”	”	Red	”	”	Yellow. “It’s too red to be yellow”
Violet	”	“It’s got blue and a little red”	Correct	Blue	”	”	Violate	Violate	”	Correct; very slow

Table 8.

	Reading aloud	Reading from pictures	Writing from pictures	Writing to dictation	Copying from print	Reading what he wrote to dictation	Repetition
The dog and the cat	Correct; slow	Correct	Correct	Correct	Correct	Correct	Perfect
The man and the dog	,,	,,	,,	,,	,,	,,	,,
The cat and the man	,,	,,	,,	,,	,,	"The cat and the dog...man"	,,
The cat and the dog	Correct	,,	,,	,,	,,	Correct	,,
The dog and the man	"The dog and the cat. No"; corrected	,,	,,	,,	,,	"The dog and the cat...man"	,,
The man and the cat	Correct	,,	,,	,,	,,	Correct	,,
The dog and the man	,,	,,	,,	,,	,,	,,	,,
The cat and the man	,,	"Dog and the man"	,,	,,	,,	,,	,,
The dog and the cat	,,	Correct	,,	,,	,,	,,	,,
The man and the dog	,,	,,	,,	,,	,,	,,	,,
The cat and the dog	,,	,,	,,	,,	,,	,,	,,
The man and the cat	,,	,,	,,	,,	,,	,,	,,

(5) *The clock tests.*

Table 9.

	Direct imitation	Oral commands	Printed commands		Telling the time	Writing down the time
			Ordinary nomenclature	Railway time		
5 minutes to 2	Correct	Correct	Correct	Correct	Correct	Correct
Half-past 1	,,	,,	Correct; very slow	,,	,,	,,
5 minutes past 8	,,	,,	Confused hands; short hand at 1, long hand at 8	Set 5, and 8 minutes to the hour	Correct; slow	five munites past four
20 minutes to 4	,,	,,	Correct	"It's 40 minutes past 3"; finally correct	,,	twenty minutes past 8
10 minutes past 7	,,	,,	,,	Correct	Correct	Correct
20 minutes to 6	,,	,,	Confused hands	Set 8.10	,,	,,
10 minutes to 1	,,	,,	Correct	Set 12.20	,,	ten minutes to eleven
A quarter to 9	,,	,,	Set 9	Correct	,,	quater to eight
20 minutes past 11	,,	,,	Correct	Correct; slow	,,	Correct
25 minutes to 3	,,	,,	Set 20 minutes to 3; then 25 minutes *past*	Set 2.25	"Ten minutes past seven"	,,

Oral commands were correctly though slowly executed. But he tended to set the short hand of the clock opposite the number of the hour mentioned; for "twenty minutes to six" he placed it so that it pointed to the figure 6 and "a quarter to nine" was set in the same ambiguous manner.

Printed commands were carried out equally badly, whether they were given in the ordinary nomenclature or in railway time. He confused the significance of the two hands and made all possible mistakes arising from want of appreciation of symbolic meaning.

He told the time on the whole correctly, though after considerable hesitation, and made several errors, when attempting to write it down.

(6) *The hand, eye and ear tests.*

Table 10.

	Imitation of movements made by the observer	Imitation of movements reflected in a mirror	Pictorial commands	Pictorial commands reflected in a mirror	Oral commands	Printed commands (silently)	Printed commands read aloud and executed		Writing down movements made by the observer
							He said	Movement executed	
L. hand to L. eye	Correct	Correct	Correct	Correct	Correct	L. hand to R. eye	Correctly	Correct	Reversed
R. hand to R. ear	,,	,,	,,	,,	,,	R. hand to R. *eye*, corrected	,,	,,	Correct
R. hand to L. eye	,,	,,	Correct; slow	,,	,,	R. hand to L. *ear*, corrected	,,	,,	,,
L. hand to R. eye	R. hand, corrected	,,	Reversed, corrected	,,	,,	Correct	,,	,,	,,
L. hand to L. ear	Correct	,,	Correct	,,	,,	,,	,,	,,	,,
R. hand to R. eye	,,	,,	,,	,,	,,	,,	,,	,,	,,
L. hand to R. ear	,,	,,	Reversed	,,	,,	,,	,,	,,	,,
R. hand to L. ear	,,	,,	Corrected	,,	,,	Correct; very slow	,,	,,	,,
L. hand to L. eye	,,	,,	Correct	,,	,,	Correct	,,	,,	,,
R. hand to R. ear	,,	,,	,,	,,	,,	Correct; very slow	,,	,,	,,
R. hand to L. eye	R. hand to L. *ear*	,,	,,	,,	,,	Correct	,,	,,	Right hand to left *ear*
L. hand to R. eye	Correct	,,	L. hand to L. eye, corrected	,,	,,	,,	,,	,,	Correct
L. hand to L. ear	,,	,,	Corrected	,,	,,	,,	,,	,,	,,
R. hand to R. eye	,,	,,	Correct	,,	,,	Correct; very slow	,,	,,	,,
L. hand to R. ear	,,	,,	,,	,,	,,	,,	,,	,,	,,
R. hand to L. ear	,,	,,	,,	,,	,,	,,	,,	,,	,,

He imitated my movements slowly, when we sat face to face, but with rapidity and certainty if they were reflected in a mirror. Pictorial commands were also badly executed, except when shown as a reflection.

Printed orders were performed with considerable hesitation and he showed a tendency to confuse eye and ear. But if he was permitted to read them aloud, he executed them without mistakes.

He wrote down the movements made by me, when we sat face to face, with two errors only, a distinct improvement on his previous record.

No. 23

A case of congenital disorder of speech in an otherwise intelligent young man. He was first examined by me at the age of twenty-two and again two and a quarter years later with almost identical results. He had never been able to learn to read and write with ease and found difficulty with simple arithmetic.

His defects of symbolic formulation and expression were akin to those in certain cases of Nominal Aphasia. He did not lack words, but insisted that he could not find those which aptly expressed his meaning. He named common objects correctly after some hesitation and was slower and less accurate with colours. He could carry out oral commands and understood what was said in ordinary conversation. Printed orders were less readily executed and he failed to comprehend exactly all he read to himself silently. He was unable to write down the name of an object or colour shown him; nor could he reproduce in writing the contents of a printed paragraph he had read. His writing was equally defective when the words were dictated by me. He could, however, copy print in cursive script showing that the fundamental fault lay in the power to translate speech into written symbols rather than in the mechanical act of writing. He failed to say or to write the alphabet spontaneously, to write it correctly to dictation, or even to put together the block letters in due sequence. He could count, but was unable to solve simple problems in arithmetic. Coins were named correctly and with some effort he was able to state their relative value. Orientation was unaffected, but he failed to draw an accurate ground-plan of the room in which we worked. He could sing, provided he did not attempt to find the words, and had a keen ear for faults in music played by others.

Carlos C. was sent to me in 1920 at the age of 22 because, although he was highly intelligent, he had never been able to find words in which to express his thoughts. He could not learn like other boys at school, and had reached the second standard only at thirteen years of age, when he left.

He was a twin, the seventh and last child of a healthy family; the other twin was a sister, who was in every way normal and strong. There was no collateral nervous disease of any kind and his relatives belonged to a sound farmer stock.

He was a broad, sturdy young man of middle height and splendid physical development, strongly right-handed, throwing, bowling and batting in the normal manner.

He had never been ill in his life and loved his work on the farm. His master spoke very highly of his ability and the patient said there was nothing he could not do if he was not compelled to talk about it.

Physically, he showed no abnormal signs of any kind. He had not suffered from fits or seizures and was entirely free from headache. The visual fields were not restricted; he was myopic, but could be corrected to $\frac{6}{6}$ with glasses, and the fundi were in every way normal. Hearing was extremely acute; smell and taste were poorly developed, but the deficiency lay within the limits of health. All reflexes, superficial and deep, were normal. There was no paralysis, paresis, incoordination or tremor and all forms of sensation were perfect.

Condition between November 13th and 27th, 1920.

Symbolic Formulation and Expression.

He was bright and cheerful, a little shy until his confidence was gained, but an excellent witness. If he was badly puzzled he tended to flush and become vexed and disturbed; otherwise he carried out all the tests quietly and persistently up to his capacity. He complained, "I get cross sometimes and seem to make myself worse." Whenever he could execute a task easily, for instance, if he was asked to match an object or colour he had seen, his replies were given with great rapidity and certainty. On one occasion I held up the blue silk and he at once called out "It isn't here"; the duplicate had fallen unseen to the floor, but he recognised that this colour was not amongst those on the table before him.

He said, "I can see it all myself, but I can't explain it to other people." "When I think of anything everything seems to be rolling along; I can't hold it. I think of one thing and, when I'm talking to anybody, a number of things keep rolling in my head all of a moment. I can see what it is. I seem to see it myself, but I can't put it properly into words. My mind won't stop at one thing; they keep on rolling. Myself, I imagine you're only thinking of what you are talking about; when I'm talking to anybody it seems a lot of things keep going by."

"When I want to put my mind to do anything, there is something won't let me. If I go to feed sheep, things keep passing in my mind. I do it, but whilst I'm doing it, things keep coming in my head; I can't hold it whilst I'm talking about it."

Introspectively he was slow, because he had difficulty in formulating his thoughts in words. Thus, the most valuable observations are those where he volunteered some explanation during a series of tests without any question from me.

It was difficult to record these remarks exactly; for, if I did not succeed in writing them down immediately, he was unable to recall what he had said. Suppose he had made some statement with regard to a test he was executing and I asked "What did you say?" he probably would reply, "I can't keep it in my mind, not more than half." But, if I remained silent and continued the same series of observations, he would probably repeat his previous remark, often in different words, but with the same significance. The most certain method of stopping introspection was to ask, "What did you say?"

He was naturally gay and cheerful and his general capacity, as judged by his actions, was above the average. He came of a race of farmers, but was working as a labourer, because he could not take a position of command owing to his difficulty in expressing himself. But he carried out his work splendidly. "If my master tells me to do anything I know what I've got to do, but I can't explain if there are any hard words in it." He was particularly good at mechanical jobs and, after taking a bicycle to pieces, could put the parts together again perfectly.

Articulated speech. No fault could be found with his spontaneous speech except that he had difficulty in discovering names and words in which to express his thoughts. He would make a statement, and, finding it inadequate, try again. This gave his phrases a clumsy turn, but the words were correctly pronounced and the rhythm otherwise perfect. When he was struggling to find the name for an object, he occasionally employed some word approximate in sound, as "night" for knife; but this rarely occurred in ordinary conversation.

He had considerable difficulty in giving names to familiar objects or to colours, even after he had heard them or read them during a full series of observations with oral and printed commands.

He could, however, tell the time correctly. This aptitude seems to have been due to special education; his school-mistress, finding that it was difficult to teach him like other children, concentrated on the clock. "I learnt to tell the time quick at school," he said; "the governess had a large one, a large one, same as this," holding up my test-clock, "I learnt to say 'em quite quick."

He could repeat what was said to him accurately, provided the content of the phrase had a simple meaning, as in the man, cat and dog tests; but if it was complex he was liable to forget exactly what he was asked to repeat.

Understanding of spoken words. In ordinary conversation he understood what was said to him and carried out simple orders without fail. Thus he chose the various familiar objects perfectly to oral commands, but made several errors with the colours, a more abstract choice. He set the clock accurately and ultimately succeeded, after considerable hesitation, in executing the hand, eye and ear tests when I gave the order by word of mouth.

Reading. He complained, "When I read the paper, I can read the words, not all of 'em; I can see the word on the paper, but I can't seem to put it together in my head." Given a printed passage and asked to read it to himself, he was unable to describe what it contained. He said, "I should have fairly to learn that before I could get hold of it."

To printed commands even familiar objects were badly chosen and he made many mistakes with colours. He set the clock imperfectly when the printed order was given in the ordinary nomenclature, and his answers were not materially improved by transposing it into railway time. Although he ultimately set "Five minutes past eight" correctly, he complained, "Minutes, that's a hard word, and eight I couldn't see at first. When I see a hard word first, like that, I can't sift it out; then it seems to come." With "A quarter to nine" he failed, and said in explanation, "I can't see that; I can't seem to get the sound."

The hand, eye and ear tests were carried out slowly and imperfectly; on several occasions he ultimately succeeded after correcting his previous errors. Moreover, throughout these responses to printed commands, read to himself, his lips moved although no sound was audible.

Asked to read aloud the monosyllabic words of the man, cat and dog tests, he started by spelling them letter by letter and was puzzled. But after saying "D O T dot; no G O T, no," he suddenly exclaimed, "the dog and the cat," which was correct. From this time he read the words accurately and did not attempt to decipher them letter by letter.

The following observations showed how completely he depended on a general impression of the words and not on their integral structure. I asked him to read aloud the phrases of the man, cat and dog tests from the manuscript he had just produced in response to pictures. This contained many faults; dog was frequently spelt "god" and in most instances the two nouns stood alone coupled by "and"; but he read them aloud exactly as if the whole phrase had been set out perfectly, blind to the manifest defects of the copy.

When he attempted to read a longer passage aloud, he failed so badly that its meaning was incomprehensible both to the auditor and to himself; many words were missed altogether and he could not understand those which he spelt out letter by letter.

For the most part he read aloud correctly the printed orders of the hand, eye and ear tests and carried them out perfectly; but, if he said them wrong, he was liable to be misled, although there was no doubt that he was helped in their execution by reading them aloud.

Writing. He wrote his name and address, but was unable to compose a letter, and complained, "I can't see the words: I'm fond of writing, but this stops me; I'd like to write all day; same as when I want to put my mind to do anything there is something won't let me."

His power of writing the names of familiar objects or colours shown to him was very defective. He said, "I've got to thoroughly learn a word before I can write it; like 'country,' I can see the c and the y at the end; yet I can't seem to put it together." Asked what he saw, when I said the word "Horse," he replied, "I see H O R S E; I don't see a picture of a horse. I fancy I can see a picture if I want to."

Shown the time on a clock face, he transcribed it extremely badly; letters were defective, even simple words were poorly spelt and many of the verbal expressions were not completed. After attempting to write twenty minutes to four, he said, "I can't seem to get hold of that. I can imagine I can see how long a word it is ...twenty; but I can't see all the letters to it." Shown ten minutes past seven, he replied, "I got that, but I can't seem to put 'em together, not the letters"; and yet he had no difficulty in telling the time correctly.

He wrote down the movements made by me during the hand, eye and ear tests much better than might have been expected from the gross defects in reading the names of familiar objects or the position of the hands of a clock. Holding up his pencil, he would make a movement towards the right or the left corresponding to the hand employed by me and wrote it down correctly. He then looked up at my face to determine which eye or ear I had touched. No word was said and usually he did not move his lips. Throughout the whole of these tests I kept my hand in position until he had completed his record.

In spite of this capacity to transcribe movements made by me, he wrote the names of the man, the cat and the dog extremely badly when they were presented in the form of pictures; not only was dog frequently written "god," but the whole test was poorly executed in spite of its apparent simplicity.

He was completely incapable of taking down a consecutive paragraph to dictation, although the monosyllabic phrases of the man, cat and dog series were reproduced correctly. Whilst writing them, he frequently repeated the words in a whisper or by means of soundless lip-movements, and in this way retained the names in his memory until the time came to put each one upon paper. Thus, when I dictated "the cat and the dog," he immediately wrote "cat," whispering "the dog" in order to remind himself of what was to follow.

Repetition of the words actually said by me undoubtedly aided him to write a simple group of nouns correctly. But self-dictation was of little help, if he had first to formulate the suitable expression unaided. Thus, although he could tell the time correctly, he wrote down what he said in a grossly defective manner. Similarly, he named the colours aloud with fair accuracy, but transcribed the words he had uttered extremely badly.

On the other hand, he copied printed words in cursive script with great ease and his handwriting at once improved noticeably. Even the long and complicated paragraph was on the whole remarkably well transcribed, although at the end he could not retail the meaning of what he had written.

The alphabet. He said the letters in the following sequence: "A B C D E F G H A...A I J...K N M O B...No, not B...V X Y Z."

Asked to write the alphabet he produced A B C D e m... and then ceased altogether.

When the letters were dictated, he wrote A B C D E F G H I J K L M N O P Q R S T U V W x y z.

He copied them correctly, in most instances transcribing the printed letter into its cursive equivalent, a b c D e f g h I j K l m n o p Q r s t u v w x y z.

He could read the alphabet aloud perfectly without the slightest hesitation or mispronunciation.

A printed paragraph. He chose the following passage from *David Copperfield*: "The gentleman spoken of was a gentleman with a very unpromising squint and a prominent chin, who had a tall white hat on with a narrow brim and whose close fitting drab trowsers seemed to button all the way up outside his legs from his boots to his hips."

He read this silently to himself and then said, "I can't get it at all; like same as that word 'brim,' I seem to have got that and yet I haven't." He began again, "The gentleman, spoke; no that's wrong, I forget. Same as that piece there, I should have fairly to learn that before I could get hold of it."

He read it through again to himself, but could not put down in writing a word of what it contained.

He then read it aloud as follows: "The gentleman, spoke of the...of was... that seems funny...P U I N T...can't get that word; and I can't get that word C H I N chattin, who had a...with a W H I T E white hat on...with a, can't get that...two words...and those cross...can't get that. I can see what they are, but I can't seem to explain them." After he had read the passage in this fashion, he was asked what it conveyed to him and he replied, "I can't get it at all."

To dictation he could write nothing; but he copied the paragraph as follows in cursive handwriting: "The gentleman spoken of was a gentleman with a very unpromising spuint and a prominent chin. Who had a tall white hat on with a narrow flat brim and whose cloefitting drab trousers seemed to button all the way up outside his legs from his boots to his hips."

Asked to tell me the sense of what he had written he replied, "I seem to have got it, but I can't seem to say it. I can see some of the words."

Pictures. When he was shown any two pictures of the man, cat and dog series he had no difficulty in finding the appropriate words. But, if he attempted to write them down, he tended to employ "god" for dog and once replaced cat by "dog."

As soon as pictures were made to carry commands, as in the hand, eye and ear tests, they were badly carried out; but, if the same diagrams were reflected in a mirror, his responses were perfect in every particular.

Moreover, pictures embodying a joke or a story were appreciated to the full provided it was not necessary for complete comprehension to include the printed legend.

Numbers and arithmetic. He could count correctly, but somewhat slowly. When set simple arithmetical exercises, he said, "I learnt more since I've been away from school"; for he was fully aware of the drawbacks of his defective powers of formulation.

The six sums were carried out as follows:

Addition.			Subtraction.			
462	228	345	654	852	713	
235	734	868	432	427	325	
697	962	1213	222	425	588	(wrong)

After completing the third addition sum, he said, "That's wrong, I made a mistake." Allowed to see it again, he went over it figure by figure aloud and said, "No, that's right." He realised that the answer to the last subtraction was wrong, but wanted to change the 8 in the second column and to replace 5 by 4, which would have been wrong. Here he had a sense of error, although his attempted corrections would have made the matter worse.

Names and relative value of coins. Coins were named with comparative ease; their relative value, though ultimately given in correct terms, was arrived at slowly and with obvious labour. In many instances he carried out the calculation on his fingers or by counting instead of expressing the relation immediately. He had no difficulty with change during the transactions of daily life.

Drawing. He drew a spirit-lamp and a mug fairly well from the model, reproducing them poorly from memory. But, when I asked him to describe the coloured pattern on the mug, he said, "Blue and white, all black lines. Then there was...I can see that colour, but I can't seem to draw it." He then took the drawing he had made from memory and added a series of marks between the lines intended to represent the tree-like pattern, saying, "There were leaves round there." It was obvious that his visual image contained more than he was able to translate into a formal drawing.

Asked to draw an elephant, he said, "I can see what it is, same as I can see a horse, what that is," and at once drew a fairly accurate picture of a horse followed by a poor representation of an elephant. When I enquired, "Is there anything you have left out?" he answered, "The horns, I think they've got a horn there," pointing to the mouth. He then added, "I've left out his ear, I forgot," and, when told to add the lacking parts to his drawing, he said, "I forget where they go."

During his attempt to draw an elephant he remarked, "I can't see him quite clear. I think I recognise everything. I can see the elephant, I seem to see the two horns down from each side of that...what you call it...trunk. I can't seem to draw it. If I sit and look at it, it seems as if in a few minutes I can do some more."

Orientation and plan drawing. He had no difficulty in finding his way and was able to guide his sister from the station to my house. But he was completely unable to describe to her or to me how he came. Any attempt to express the way he would travel or the route along which he had passed led to confusion, and he was unable to express what he wanted to say.

After we had worked together for several days in the same room, he was asked to draw a plan, indicating its main features. He marked out an oblong, but filled it in with drawings of windows, door and fireplace in elevation.

When, on the other hand, I drew a quadrilateral to represent the shape of the room he indicated the relative position of the various objects with remarkable accuracy, provided he was not asked to draw them. In fact, a plan drawn by me to his dictation contained more detail than I could have remembered had I been asked to construct it myself.

Music. He complained that when singing he had no difficulty with the tune, but could not get the words. In the same way, "when they are playing the violin or piano, I can tell them if they go wrong; I hear the sounds alright, how they ought to go."

Games. He was able to amuse himself with card games so long as they did not demand complex acts of formulated memory and expression. Thus he took part in family whist, but could not play it seriously. He complained, "I can't seem to keep them in my head, Hearts, Kings, Queens,...what's gone. I can remember them, yet I don't seem to come to the sound of it. I *can* play, only I can't seem to keep in my head what's gone."

He had never learnt to play chess or draughts.

Serial Tests.

(1) *Naming and recognition of common objects.*

Table 1.

	Pointing to object shown	Oral commands	Printed commands	Naming an object indicated	Duplicate placed in hand out of sight	Writing name of object indicated	Copying the printed names in cursive hand-writing
Knife	Correct	Correct	Correct	Correct	Correct	Ken	Correct
Key	,,	,,	,,	,,	,,	Kent	,,
Penny	,,	,,	,,	,,	,,	Correct	,,
Matches	,,	,,	,,	,,	,,	Mams	,,
Scissors	,,	,,	,,	,,	,,	Senaser	,,
Pencil	,,	,,	,,	,,	,,	pener	,,
Key	,,	,,	Knife; then correct	,,	,,	Kert	,,
Scissors	,,	,,	Correct	,,	,,	Senlis	,,
Matches	,,	,,	,,	,,	,,	Males	,,
Knife	,,	,,	,,	,,	,,	Kent	,,
Penny	,,	,,	,,	,,	,,	penney	,,
Pencil	,,	,,	Penny	,,	,,	penler	,,
Scissors	,,	,,	Correct	"Key"; then correct	,,	Scaers	,,
Pencil	,,	,,	Key	Correct	,,	pener	,,
Penny	,,	,,	Correct	,,	,,	Correct	,,
Knife	,,	,,	Key	"Night"	,,	Kenl	,,
Key	,,	,,	Correct	"I can't say just the word." "Oh! key"	,,	Correct	,,
Matches	,,	,,	,,	"Mat; no matches"	,,	Mates	,,

He selected quickly and without hesitation the duplicate of an object seen or placed in his hand. He had no difficulty in making a correct choice to oral commands, but was slower and less certain when the order was given in print. He said, "That's where I go wrong; sometimes I know just as well, but they don't come quick enough.

At school, the easy words I could pick out, the hard words I used to make a blunder." Asked to name each object in turn as it was indicated to him, he was ultimately successful after considerable hesitation.

He wrote the names with extreme difficulty in letters that were hesitating and badly formed. He would begin correctly, but gave up, saying, "That's wrong, I can't"; "I've got to thoroughly learn the word before I can write it."

Asked to copy them, he did so with perfect accuracy and his handwriting was excellent. He said, "That's easy; at school I used to have a book and copy it off on a slate, what they call it, trans-cription."

(2) *Naming and recognition of colours.*

Table 2.

	Pointing to colour shown	Oral commands	Printed commands	Naming colour shown	Writing down name of colour shown	Name of colour said aloud and then written		Printed name read aloud
						He said	He wrote	
Black	Correct	Correct	Correct	Correct	Brack	Correctly	Brack	Correct
Red	,,	,,	,,	,,	Correct	,,	Correctly	,,
Blue	,,	,,	"Is it mauve, purple?" No choice	,,	Buo	,,	Bures	,,
Green	,,	,,	Correct	,,	gr	,,	grn	,,
Orange	,,	Yellow; "that's lemon"	Violet	"Light red; not mauve. Don't know"	Ouer	,,	"I can't get the sound of the first letter"	"I think that's mauve"
White	,,	Correct	Correct	Correct	Write	,,	Write	Correct
Violet	,,	,,	,,	"Purple, I think"	Poe	"Purple"	per	"Vi-let"
Yellow	,,	,,	"Don't know what it is." No choice	"Lilla"	Cream	"Lilla"	le	"I can't get that"
Red	,,	Orange	Correct	Correct	Correct	Correctly	Reed	Correct
White	,,	Correct	,,	,,	,,	,,	Wrid	,,
Yellow	,,	,,	Green	"Lilla, lella. I can't say it properly"	loe	"Lilla"	li	"I can't get that"
Blue	,,	,,	Correct	Correct	Bues	Correctly	Bul	Correct
Green	,,	,,	,,	,,	Grrens	,,	gnre	,,
Black	,,	,,	,,	,,	Back	,,	Brack	,,
Orange	,,	Violet; "that's mauve"	Yellow	,,	Oeni	,,	"I can't get first letter"	"Mauve"
Violet	,,	Correct	"I can't see that"	"Purple"	Bl	"Purple"	pur	"Vi-let"

He named the colours uncertainly and was slow and hesitating in his choice, both to oral and printed commands. He wrote the names extremely badly and his handwriting was not improved by allowing him to utter the words aloud before transferring them to paper.

When he attempted to read the printed names aloud, he not only failed with orange and yellow, but substituted "mauve" for the former, showing how little he depended on the actual form of the word that stood on the card he held in his hand.

(3) *The man, cat and dog tests.*

Table 3.

	Reading aloud	Reading from pictures	Writing from pictures	Writing from dictation	Repetition	Reading what he had written	Copying
The dog and the cat	"The D O T dot; no, G O T; no the dog and the cat"	Correct	The dog and cat	Dog and the Cat	"Dog and the Cat"	Perfect	Correct
The man and the dog	Correct	,,	Man and God	Man and the Dog	"Man and the dog"	,,	,,
The cat and the man	,,	,,	Cat and man	Cat and the Man	Correct	,,	,,
The cat and the dog	,,	,,	Cat and God	Cat and the Dog	,,	,,	,,
The dog and the man	,,	,,	God and mon	Dog and the Man	"The man...the man and the cat..." Corrected on repetition of words by observer	,,	,,
The man and the cat	,,	,,	Man and Cat	Man and the Cat	Correct	,,	,,
The dog and the man	,,	,,	God and Man	the Dog the Man	,,	,,	,,
The cat and the man	Correct. "No, that's wrong; no, it's right"	,,	Cat and man	the Cat the Man	,,	,,	,,
The dog and the cat	Correct	,,	Dog and Cat	the Dog the Cat	,,	,,	,,
The man and the dog	,,	,,	Man and Dog	the Man the Dog	,,	,,	,,
The cat and the dog	,,	,,	Cat and Dog	the Cat the Dog	,,	,,	,,
The man and the cat	,,	,,	Man and Dog	the Man the Cat	,,	,,	,,

Asked to read aloud these simple phrases, he began by spelling out each noun incorrectly; then he suddenly said, "the dog and the cat," which was accurate. From this time onwards he did not think of the composition of the words, but read them as a whole; he remembered how the phrases were built up and gave to each one in turn the couple of nouns set out on the printed card. Once only did he hesitate, saying, "No, that's wrong; no, it's right, I thought it was a different letter at the end."

He could translate pictures into words correctly, but wrote them down extremely badly; dog was frequently written "god" and was substituted for cat in the last phrase of the series. And yet when he was given this faulty copy and was asked to read it aloud, he produced a set of perfect phrases just as if they had been written without mistakes; he paid no attention to "god" and "mon," but read them as if they were "dog" and "man" respectively.

The content of each phrase was correctly written to dictation although he tended to omit either the conjunction or one of the articles. He frequently repeated one of the nouns in a whisper or by means of silent lip-movements; thus, when I dictated "the cat and the dog," he wrote "cat," saying in a whisper "the dog" in order to remind himself of what was to follow. He reinforced his memory by silent or whispered repetition.

When he was asked to copy the printed cards, he exclaimed, "That's a lot easier," his handwriting improved greatly and he produced a faultless copy.

(4) *The clock tests.*

Table 4.

	Direct imitation	Oral commands	Printed commands		Telling the time	Writing down the time	Telling the time aloud and writing it down	
			Ordinary nomenclature	Railway time			He said	He wrote
5 minutes to 2	Correct	Correct	Set 2.55	Set 1.25. "That's not right"	Correct	five too two	"Five minutes to two" (correct)	five to two
Half-past 1	„	„	"I can't get that word." Set 12.30	Correct	„	hl past one	"half past one" (correct)	haft past one
5 minutes past 8	„	„	Correct; very slow	„	„	five past eight	"Five minutes past eight" (correct)	five min past eight
20 minutes to 4	„	„	Correct	„	„	twenty fast for	"Twenty to four" (correct)	tw to for
10 minutes past 7	„	„	Correct; great hesitation	Set 6.50 (ten minutes *to* 7)	„	ten past sis	"Ten past seven" (correct)	ten past sem
20 minutes to 6	„	„	Correct	Set 5.45	„	too six	"Twenty to six" (correct)	lwe two six
10 minutes to 1	„	„	„	Set 12.25. "No." Set 12.55. "That's right"	„	ten to one	"Ten to one" (correct)	ten two one
A quarter to 9	„	„	"I can't see that; I don't seem to get the sound." No response	Correct	„	Qeag to E	"Quarter to nine" (correct)	quer two nines
20 minutes past 11	„	„	Set 7.20	„	„	lw past E	"Twenty past eleven" (correct)	lw past E
25 minutes to 3	„	„	Finally correct	„	„	five tw	Five and twenty	five twe to three

He could tell the time, carry out oral commands and set one clock in direct imitation of another with great accuracy. He said, "I learnt to tell the time quick at school. The governess had a large one...a clock...same as this," pointing to the one he held in his hand, "I learnt to say 'em quick." Finding the difficulty in teaching him like other boys, she had concentrated her efforts on such practical acquirements as telling the time and the names and value of coins.

If I set the time on a clock face and asked him to write it down silently, he did so extremely badly; the simplest words were mis-spelt, many of the expressions were not completed and some were wrong. With the hands at twenty minutes to four he said, "I can't seem to get hold of that. I can imagine I can see how long a word it is...twenty...but I can't see all the letters in it." In the same way, when the clock showed 7.10, he wrote "ten past sis" (six), saying, "I got that, but I can't seem to put 'em together, not the letters like."

Even when permitted to say the time aloud, which he did perfectly, he was unable to transfer it to paper; he explained his difficulties by saying, "I can't get twenty" or "seven" or "eleven."

He had great difficulty in executing printed commands given either in ordinary nomenclature or in railway time. He pondered over the clock like a chess-player contemplating some position of the game and his lips moved silently. He could not translate the verbal and numerical symbols into the corresponding position of the hands of the clock and complained, "I can't get that word," "I don't see that, I don't seem to get the sound." Given "5 minutes past 8" he said, "Minutes, that a hard word and eight I couldn't see at first, like that, I can't sift it out; then it seems to come." He missed "A quarter to 9" saying, "I can't see that, I can't seem to get the sound."

(5) *The coin-bowl tests.*

He had no difficulty in executing oral commands or those given in printed figures; but he was somewhat slower and made two mistakes when the order was set out in full on the card, as for instance "second penny into third bowl." Permitted, however, to read it aloud, he shortened the phrase to "second into third" and carried out the manœuvre without hesitation.

(6) *The hand, eye and ear tests.* (Table 5.)

Throughout all forms of these tests which necessitated formulation, the movement was carried out in two stages; first he selected and held up the hand he was about to employ and then he carried it to that eye or ear which seemed to him to fulfil the command. He was equally bad at carrying out pictorial commands; even if the act was performed correctly he was slow and hesitated in his choice. On the contrary, he imitated my movements seen in a mirror or executed an order given in the form of a reflected picture in one stage, bringing the correct hand at once to the part indicated.

In the same way, when translating the movements made by me into written words, he first held up his pencil to the right or to the left according to the hand I had employed, wrote this down correctly, and then looked up in my face to determine which eye or ear I had touched. No word was said and usually he did not move his lips. Throughout the whole of these tests I kept my hand in position until he had completed his record.

To oral commands he produced an almost perfect series of responses, but the movements were made in two stages and were wanting in promptness. Printed orders were executed somewhat less easily and his lips usually moved, although no sound could be heard. When he was permitted to read them aloud, they were carried out somewhat more easily; but he tended to become the victim of his errors in nomenclature.

Condition in February 1923 (*two years and three months later*).

Owing to the kindness of Dr Riddoch I was able to make another complete series of observations after an interval of two years and a quarter.

With the exception of his defects of speech, I could find no signs pointing to any abnormal condition of the central nervous system. The visual fields were not

Table 5.

	Imitation of movements made by the observer	Imitation of movements reflected in a mirror	Pictorial commands	Pictorial commands reflected in a mirror	Oral commands	Printed commands	Printed commands read aloud and executed: He read	Printed commands read aloud and executed: Movement executed	Writing down movements made by the observer
L. hand to L. eye	Correct	Correct	L. hand to R. eye	Correct	Correct	Correct	Correctly	Correct	Correct
R. hand to R. ear	R. hand to R. *eye*; corrected	,,	Correct	,,	,,	,,	,,	,,	,,
R. hand to L. eye	Correct	,,	Reversed; corrected	,,	,,	,,	,,	,,	,,
L. hand to R. eye	,,	,,	Correct	,,	L. hand to R. *ear*. "No," corrected	L. hand to R. *ear*. "No," corrected	,,	,,	,,
L. hand to L. ear	R. hand, corrected	,,	,,	,,	Correct	Correct	,,	,,	,,
R. hand to R. eye	R. hand to L. eye	,,	R. hand to L. eye	,,	,,	,,	,,	,,	,,
L. hand to R. ear	Correct	,,	Correct; then L. hand to L. ear	,,	,,	L. hand to R. *eye*	,,	,,	,,
R. hand to L. ear	,,	,,	Reversed	,,	,,	Correct	,,	,,	,,
L. hand to L. eye	,,	,,	,,	,,	,,	L. hand to L. *ear*; corrected	,,	,,	L. hand to R. eye
R. hand to R. ear	,,	,,	,,	,,	,,	Correct	,,	,,	R. hand to R. *eye*; corrected
R. hand to L. eye	,,	,,	,,	,,	,,	,,	"R. hand to L. *ear*"	R. hand to L. *ear*	Correct
L. hand to R. eye	Reversed; corrected	,,	R. hand. "No," L. hand; then corrected	,,	,,	,,	Correctly	Correct	,,
L. hand to L. ear	L. hand to R. ear	,,	Correct	,,	R. hand to L. ear; corrected	,,	"L. hand to R. ear"	L. hand to R. ear	,,
R. hand to R. eye	R. hand to L. eye	,,	Correct; slow	,,	Correct	R. hand to R. *ear*; corrected	"R. hand to R. *ear*"; then correctly	Correct	,,
L. hand to R. ear	Correct	,,	Correct. "No"; then reversed	,,	,,	Correct	Correctly	,,	,,
R. hand to L. ear	,,	,,	Reversed	,,	,,	,,	,,	,,	,,

restricted, there was no loss of motion or sensation and the reflexes were unaffected. His general health was excellent.

Symbolic Formulation and Expression.

The serial tests and other methods of examination yielded results which were almost identical with those obtained more than two years previously. The records revealed no new features, but they were accompanied by many remarks on the part of the patient which threw light on the nature of his disabilities. These I shall attempt to summarise before entering into a detailed description of the various affections of speech.

He complained, "I seem to have got the idea of everything, yet it comes and goes. Same in reading, singing, anything. I seem to have got the frame, I can't get the name." He frequently recognised that he had made a mistake, even when he was unable to correct it. He said, "I can see how to do a thing, but I can't explain it. Same as carpentering or anything like that; I seem to have got the frame of it, I know how to do it, but I always get mixed up. I can't always explain it." "The words seem to go faint, seem to come and go; I lose it again." Evidently repeating a word or an order fixed it; for he insisted, "If I keep saying it, it comes plain to me, I know it."

"I can't find my words; if I could find my words I'd be clever in life. I seem to have the frame of everything, but I don't seem able to hold it, it's gone. And yet I can tell you how long a word is, how long it is this way," drawing a pencil horizontally across the paper, "and yet I couldn't count how many letters it has. I can count the beginning if it is easy, but I can't count any more, if it is a hard word." "It's finding the words that's my difficulty," and he gave as an example that copying was easy, but writing to dictation troubled him; he added, "It's the same with sums; I can get the easy ones, but when I come to the hard ones I am done."

He insisted that his main difficulty lay in finding names or appropriate words in which to express his thoughts. One day, for instance, after leaving me he did not return to the hospital at once, but went to a restaurant in the neighbourhood of my house for dinner. At our next sitting he described to me exactly where it was situated without once using the words right and left, which confused him. He said that he first turned "to this side," holding up his right hand; then "to this side," holding up the left, "where they have the road up and round by the station to a restaurant near opposite the Marble Arch." Every detail was accurate. As he retraced his steps in imagination, he knew how he turned and what he saw, but he was quite incapable of formulating this as "I took the first to the right, then the first to the left, turning to the right by the station."

Any act which required verbal formulation he called "thinking." Thus, after imitating my movements reflected in a mirror with quickness and accuracy, he said, "It is easy; there is no thinking. Same as with counting; when I count I don't think.

Throughout, he explained the fleeting character of his ideas and images. When attempting to reproduce an experience, he repeatedly said, "I see it, then it goes; I can't see it always, not clear enough to put down." "Same with card playing. I play quite well, but I guess. I can't remember what has gone out. If anyone asked me what's gone, I couldn't tell them; but I get it right." "It always goes faint and I can't seem to get it when I want to" was a comment he made whilst attempting to draw an object from memory.

The defects of *articulated speech* were identical with those observed more than two years before. Words were correctly pronounced and rhythm was disturbed solely in consequence of the difficulty he experienced in finding the right word to express his meaning. He named common objects correctly, but was slower and less accurate with colours; he could still tell the time with astonishing accuracy. Repetition was not materially affected.

Understanding of spoken words. He carried out oral commands on the whole accurately, although with some hesitation and several rapid corrections.

Reading. He was slow in executing printed commands and, although he set the clock correctly when the order was given in the ordinary nomenclature, he failed badly with railway time. This was evidently due to the care with which he had been taught the time at school, whereas he was not equally familiar with the method of stating it in figures.

He had obvious difficulty in understanding what he read to himself, as shown by the results obtained with a selected paragraph (vide infra, p. 363). Failure to appreciate the details of the descriptive passage led to want of comprehension of its meaning.

He read aloud badly, failing to enunciate many of the words, even though he spelt them letter by letter correctly. Moreover, to read a command aloud did not materially add to its correct execution.

Writing. He wrote his name and address and composed the following letter after extreme deliberation and with many erasures and corrections:

"Dear Sir[1]

I thanking you so much for treat me at your House. It is a lot better to give me a full treat at your house and what it would at the Hospital I thanking you so much for paying my fine From the Hospital to your House. It is quite nice to get out of the Hospital for a few hours

from

Carlos C."

[1] This was intended to signify: "Dear sir, I thank you so much for treating me at your house. It is a lot better to give me a full treatment at your house than what it would be at the Hospital. I thank you so much for paying my fare from the hospital to your house. It is quite nice to get out of the Hospital for a few hours."

After reading a test paragraph (vide infra) silently, he wrote down what he had gathered from it extremely badly; many of the words were incomplete and the whole would have been incomprehensible without a knowledge of the printed text.

His writing was not materially improved when I dictated the words; yet he could copy print in cursive script without error. It was not the act of writing that was at fault, but the power of transforming the names of objects he had seen or words he had heard into written symbols. Once they were given to him, he could make the movements necessary to reproduce them correctly. He said, "We used to have copybooks and my writing was good. It's finding the words that's my difficulty; same as dictation, I used to get bothered in that."

The alphabet. Asked to say the letters of the alphabet spontaneously he did so correctly up to G. Then he began again, finally producing the following series: "A B C D E F G H I K N O P Q W X Y Z." But he repeated them after me without a mistake and enunciated them perfectly.

When he attempted to put down the alphabet on paper spontaneously, he wrote: A B C d e f g H I j k m n o P w.

He succeeded somewhat better to dictation, although he became confused towards the end of the alphabet: *A* b c d e f g h I j k l m n o p Q M S l u v w x y.

On the other hand, he copied the printed alphabet correctly in cursive script, except that he tended to employ capitals and small letters indiscriminately.

Given the twenty-six block letters he put together the following imperfect sequence: Λ (V upside down) B C D E ſ (J upside down) G H I K M N O Q S T. He then gave up, saying, "I don't know which comes next." But as soon as I dictated the order in which the letters should follow one another he had no difficulty in constructing the alphabet.

A printed paragraph. I laid before him the following passage, asking him to read it silently and to tell me what it conveyed to him. "The gentleman spoken of had a very ugly squint and a prominent chin. He was wearing a tall white hat with a narrow flat brim and riding breeches with yellow leather gaiters. He carried in his hand a switch, with which he tapped his boots, as he talked in a hoarse voice."

He evidently experienced great difficulty in appreciating its meaning and complained, "I can't seem to get everything." He began, "The gentleman they were speaking of...had a cheerful speech," but came to a stop and asked to be allowed to read the passage again. After he had done so he said, "He carried in his hand a swim..." and, unable to continue further, gave the following explanation: "I've got thoroughly to get hold of it...I've got to read it many times...It would come to me later in the day...It would come to me in rotation...That's the same with anything...It may come to me this afternoon, or to-night, or any time."

He then read the passage aloud as follows: "The gentleman spoke of had a very general speech and a C H I N...He was waiting a tall white hat with a... that's where I can't...F L A T...B R...bringing...and...I can see but I can't see the front word...B R E E C H E S. He carried in his hand a...S W I T C H ...swiz." He suddenly said, "Leather...whilst I was thinking of that (switch) leather came" and then continued, "with which he...tapp-ed...his boots as he walked in a H O A R S E...I can see the next word, but I can't say it."

I read these sentences through to him and asked him not to try to remember the words, but to tell me what they called up in his mind. He replied, "I can see the man...I can see him with his leather gaiters and riding breeches and hat and a swish...squint eyed and a funny chin...There was something else...did you say he had a beard on his chin? No, not that; there was something else...I see someone with a black hat, black coat and waistcoat and yellow riding breeches and gaiters with boots and a switch...looking down he is with his squint eyes. I should see that for an hour or more. He'll keep coming on my mind."

After he had read the passage again to himself silently, he wrote down what he remembered as follows: "the gentl spoken of had a very he had a sw in his hand sw eye leather ga on as he wh a a long sguing b on he got a p C. to his Boots with." He then said, "I can see him...but I can't seem to put him into words as I ought to...It seems to go too quick in rotation. I can see his head and his squint...then I see his breeches and his leather gaiters...carrying a swish in his hand...There's another word I can't get...then about his boots...let me see that was H A P P E D wasn't it?"

To my dictation he wrote: "th gentt spon of had a very ley sw and a po cgih he was w a tall white hat with a falt pun and rying br with lolare g er he carried in his hand a ws with he lop his boots as he told in a horses v."

But when he copied these sentences from print in cursive script he made no mistake of any kind and the character of his handwriting enormously improved.

Numbers and arithmetic. He counted up to a hundred without difficulty and explained that he was able to do so because "when I count I don't think."

Addition.			Subtraction.		
462	228	345	654	852	713
235	734	868	432	427	325
897 (wrong)	962	1213	222	435 (wrong)	5 7 (unfinished)

Names and relative value of coins. All the coins were named and the relative value of any two of them stated without mistakes; but throughout his lips moved silently and the answer, though finally correct, was obviously arrived at with effort. He had no difficulty with money in the transactions of daily life.

Drawing. I asked him to draw anything he chose and he produced a remarkably detailed representation of his home. One of the windows was blackened over with shading and he explained, "That was a window, but they've closed it up; it's all blank." This I found on enquiry to be correct. Asked if he could see the house, he said "Oh! yes...yes, if I put my mind on it, I can see it clearly."

He drew a jug from a model, reproducing it somewhat feebly from memory. He said, "It's not clear enough to put it down; I only guess it, then it goes. I can't see it always; I saw it all full and then it went. It always goes faint and I can't seem to get it when I want to."

He produced a poor drawing of an elephant to order, and becoming confused made many corrections. He explained, "I can see it, but it keeps coming and going. It's more of a guess."

Orientation and plan drawing. He was able to find his way about the streets unaided. Once he had been over the ground, he remembered whether he had to turn to the right or to the left, although he became confused directly he attempted to express it in words. He described exactly how he went from my house to a restaurant in the following words: "To this side (holding up the right hand), then to this side (holding up the left), where they have the road up and round by the station to a restaurant near opposite the Marble Arch."

I took him into another part of my house and asked him to draw a plan of the room in which we usually worked. He drew a quadrilateral, marked in the table, but indicated our positions at it wrongly. In spite of this primary error, the mirror, cupboards, fireplace and door into the laboratory were indicated with accuracy, but the main doorway and windows were omitted entirely.

I then drew an outline figure of the room with a square in proper position to represent the table. I asked "Where do you sit?" and then "Where do I sit?" and in both instances he answered correctly. I then told him to point to the place of each salient object in turn; this he did with remarkable accuracy, so long as I did not require him to formulate the relation of any two of them to one another. Thus, it was obvious that it was his power of formulation, rather than his perceptual aptitude, which was at fault.

Images. After he had drawn a jug placed before him, it was removed from his sight, and he then described its shape and coloured pattern in the following terms: "I can see it; it's white with a blue edging and crinkly all round the handle. There's a boy on one side and a woman on the other, green I think." All these details were correct.

I then showed him the wooden figure of a Venetian guitar player in a white mask, dark cloak and three-cornered hat. Five minutes afterwards he said, "I see it. He's playing...I've been trying to think what they call those things. He's standing on a board. He's got a sluch (slouch) hat on. I can see the statue and then it's gone; it flies over, it comes up and then goes faint and then comes again." Here again he emphasised the fluctuating nature of his visual images and the difficulty he found in describing them to order.

Serial Tests.

(1) *Naming and recognition of common objects.*

Table 6.

	Pointing to object shown	Oral commands	Printed commands	Naming an object indicated	Duplicate placed in hand out of sight	Writing name of object indicated	Writing name to dictation	Copying the printed names in cursive handwriting
Knife	Correct	Correct	Key	Correct	Correct	Kinee	K	Correct
Key	,,	,,	Correct. "I missed the first...knife"	,,	,,	Correct	Correct	,,
Penny	,,	,,	Correct	,,	,,	,,	,,	,,
Match Box	,,	,,	,,	,,	,,	Box M	match	,,
Scissors	,,	,,	,,	,,	,,	S le	s l	,,
Pencil	,,	,,	Correct; slow	,,	,,	pen l	p l	,,
Key	,,	,,	Correct	,,	,,	Kye	Correct	,,
Scissors	,,	,,	,,	,,	,,	s l	s l	,,
Match Box	,,	,,	,,	,,	,,	Match	match	,,
Knife	,,	,,	Correct; slow	,,	,,	Ken	knfe	,,
Penny	,,	,,	Correct	,,	,,	Correct	penney	,,
Match Box	,,	,,	,,	,,	,,	match	match	,,
Scissors	,,	,,	,,	,,	,,	s l	s l	,,
Pencil	,,	,,	Correct; slow	,,	,,	p l	pennle	,,
Penny	,,	,,	Correct	,,	,,	peneny	penney	,,
Knife	,,	,,	,,	,,	,,	kife	kinfe	,,
Key	,,	,,	,,	,,	,,	Correct	Correct	,,
Pencil	,,	,,	,,	,,	,,	p l	p l	,,

The main interest of these records lies in the difficulty he experienced in writing down, either spontaneously or to dictation, the names of familiar objects; in many instances he wrote the first letter, but could not complete the word. Yet every word could be copied correctly from print in cursive characters.

(2) *Naming and recognition of colours.*

He showed considerable uncertainty and hesitation in naming colours, such as orange, violet and yellow, and in making an accurate choice to printed commands. Occasionally he failed even when permitted to read the names aloud before selecting the colour.

He wrote the names of colours shown to him very imperfectly and was equally at fault when the words were dictated; but he copied them perfectly from print in cursive script. He then said, "That's easy. If I could find my words I'd be clever in life. I seem to have the frame of everything, but I don't seem able to hold it, it's gone."

(3) *The man, cat and dog tests.* There was a slight tendency throughout to reverse the order or to substitute one name for the other, e.g. the cat and the man in place of the cat and the dog; but in every case he ultimately corrected his mistakes. All these simple phrases were written correctly in response to pictures or to dictation and he copied them perfectly from print in cursive characters.

Table 7.

	Pointing to colour shown	Naming colour shown	Oral commands	Printed commands	Name read aloud and colour chosen		Writing down name of colour shown	Writing names to dictation	Copying names from print in handwriting	Colours named aloud and written down	
					He read	He chose				He said	He wrote
Black	Correct	Correct	Correct	Correct	Correctly	Correctly	Correct	Correct	Correct	Correctly	Correctly
Red	”	”	”	”	”	”	”	”	”	”	”
Blue	”	Correct; slow	”	Correct; very slow	”	”	Bu	Bu	”	”	Blure
Green	”	Correct	”	Correct	”	”	Correct	Correct	”	”	Correctly
Orange	”	“Something like red, a sort of purple”	”	Violet	”	”	Onllo	O en	”	”	O en
White	”	Correct	”	Correct	”	”	Correct	Correct	”	”	Correctly
Violet	”	“Purple”	”	”	”	”	g Vi	Villet	”	“Orange; that’s wrong, violet”	Vi it
Yellow	”	“Lellow”	”	No reply	“Violet”	Violet	lollow	O ow	”	“Lellow”	lollowe
Red	”	Correct	”	Correct	Correctly	Correctly	Correct	Correct	”	Correctly	Correctly
White	”	”	”	”	”	”	”	”	”	”	”
Yellow	”	“Lellow”	”	Violet	“Violet”	Violet	lollow	lollow	”	”	low
Blue	”	Correct	”	Correct	Correctly	Correctly	Bure	Bur	”	“Ber-lew”	Brlu
Green	”	”	”	”	”	”	Correct	Correct	”	Correctly	Correctly
Black	”	”	”	”	”	”	”	”	”	”	”
Orange	”	“I can see that, but I can’t. . .”	”	”	”	”	Ou	O eu	”	“Or-age”	O eu
Violet	”	“Orange; no, purple”	”	”	“I can’t get it”	No choice	Vi	Villit	”	Correctly	V. it.

(4) *The clock tests.*

Table 8.

	Direct imitation	Oral commands	Printed commands: Ordinary nomenclature	Printed commands: Railway time	Telling the time	Writing down the time
5 minutes to 2	Correct	Correct	Set 5.55	Correct	Correct	5 minnts to two (correct)
Half-past 1	,,	,,	Correct	,,	,,	Haft past one (correct)
5 minutes past 8	,,	,,	,,	,,	,,	5 past 8 (correct)
20 minutes to 4	,,	,,	,,	,,	,,	20 muntes to 4 (correct)
10 minutes past 7	,,	,,	,,	Set 10.7; then 7 and 10 minutes to the hour	,,	10 past 7 (correct)
20 minutes to 6	,,	,,	,,	Set 4.40; then correct	,,	20 muntes to 6 (correct)
10 minutes to 1	,,	,,	,,	Set 12.55	,,	10 muntes to one (correct)
A quarter to 9	,,	,,	,,	Correct	,,	Our to 9 (correct)
20 minutes past 11	,,	,,	,,	Set 12.20	,,	20 past 11 (correct)
25 minutes to 3	,,	,,	,,	Correct	,,	25 to 3 (correct)

These records were almost identical with those obtained two years previously. He told the time well and executed printed commands correctly, though somewhat slowly if given in the ordinary nomenclature. He was less familiar with railway time and made several mistakes to orders in this form, which he tended to translate into the ordinary nomenclature, saying, e.g. "2.35 is five and twenty to three, isn't it?" When writing down the time he employed figures instead of words, and his answers were consequently somewhat better expressed than on the previous occasion.

(5) *The hand, eye and ear tests.* (Table 9.)

Here again the records almost exactly corresponded to those obtained two years before. When imitating my movements as we sat face to face he responded slowly and made several mistakes; but, as soon as they were reflected in a mirror, he said, "It's easy; there's no thinking. Same as counting; when I count I don't think."

Oral commands were executed slowly; he made no actual mistakes, but was uncertain between eye and ear, especially if he had to cross the face. This difficulty was accentuated when the order was given in print, and he complained, "I get bothered eye and ear."

When writing down the movements made by me, he hesitated and made several corrections, although he finally completed this task without error. First, however, he wrote which hand I had employed; then, after looking at me again, he decided on the eye or the ear that I was touching. The act was carried out in two separate parts and thus made easier of execution.

Table 9.

	Imitation of movements made by the observer	Imitation of movements reflected in a mirror	Pictorial commands	Pictorial commands reflected in a mirror	Oral commands	Printed commands	Printed commands read aloud and executed		Writing down movements made by the observer
							He read	Movement executed	
L. hand to L. eye	Correct	Correct	Correct	Correct	Correct	*Ear*; corrected	Correctly	Correct	Correct
R. hand to R. ear	,,	,,	,,	,,	,,	Correct	,,	,,	,,
R. hand to L. eye	Reversed	,,	Reversed	,,	,,	,,	"R. hand to L. *ear*"	R. hand to L. *ear*	,,
L. hand to R. eye	Correct	,,	Correct	,,	,,	,,	Correctly	Correct	,,
L. hand to L. ear	L. hand to R. ear	,,	,,	,,	,,	,,	,,	,,	,,
R. hand to R. eye	Correct	,,	,,	,,	,,	,,	"*Ear*"; corrected "eye"	,,	,,
L. hand to R. ear	,,	,,	L. hand to L. ear	,,	,,	,,	Correctly	,,	Corrected
R. hand to L. ear	,,	,,	R. hand to R. ear	,,	,,	,,	,,	,,	Correct
L. hand to L. eye	R. hand; corrected	,,	Correct	,,	,,	,,	,,	,,	Corrected
R. hand to R. ear	Correct	,,	,,	,,	,,	,,	,,	,,	Correct
R. hand to L. eye	,,	,,	,,	,,	*Ear*; corrected	*Ear*; corrected	"L. *ear*, L. eye; I always say it wrong"	L. *ear*; corrected	Corrected
L. hand to R. eye	,,	,,	,,	,,	Correct	Correct	Correctly	Correct	Correct
L. hand to L. ear	,,	,,	,,	,,	,,	Corrected	,,	,,	,,
R. hand to R. eye	,,	,,	,,	,,	,,	Correct	,,	,,	,,
L. hand to R. ear	,,	,,	,,	,,	,,	,,	,,	,,	Corrected
R. hand to L. ear	,,	,,	Reversed	,,	,,	,,	,,	,,	Correct

At first sight it might seem as if this patient was a pure example of agraphia; but closer examination showed that much more than writing was affected. He constantly insisted that he was unable to discover appropriate words or names to express the contents of his mind. He possessed plenty of words, but found difficulty in applying them. As these defects of speech had existed all his life, he had been compelled to learn to read and write under the most unfavourable conditions. Consequently both these aptitudes suffered severely, more particularly the power of translating names into written symbols. The act of writing was possible, as shown by the way in which he copied print in cursive script and wrote down the simple phrases of the man, cat and dog tests in response to pictures. His main defect lay in want of power to find words with a meaning that exactly fitted a certain situation.

No. 24

A case of Semantic Aphasia, due to a vascular lesion in an elderly man. There were no abnormal physical signs beyond the affection of speech.

His principal defects of symbolic formulation and expression consisted in want of capacity to appreciate the general significance of details, however presented, and inability to deduce from them their logical consequences. He also failed to recognise, or was unable to retain in his mind, the full intention of an act he was about to perform spontaneously or to order. Thus, he frequently misunderstood the ultimate significance of pictures, especially in conjunction with a printed legend. During any series of tests he repeatedly forgot what he was expected to do and reflection of my movements in a mirror confused, rather than aided him, in imitating them correctly.

He talked rapidly in somewhat short and jerky sentences, as if afraid of forgetting what he wanted to say. He named objects slowly but correctly and did not lack words, although in ordinary conversation he occasionally used a wrong expression. He could repeat anything said to him provided it did not consist of a long and involved sentence. Single words and short phrases were perfectly understood and he executed even complex oral commands. If, however, he developed a false general conception of what he had heard, he was unable to correct it and became confused. Although he could carry out printed commands, he had great difficulty in understanding what he read to himself or aloud. Given a series of sentences which led by consecutive steps to some general impression, he was unable to reproduce what he had read. He wrote his name and address perfectly, but could not place on paper without the grossest mistakes his own ideas or the gist of something he had heard or read. To dictation he wrote well, except that he was confused by his errors in spelling. He copied slowly but perfectly. He counted with accuracy and wrote the numbers without difficulty; arithmetical problems puzzled him and were solved with effort. Coins were named correctly, but he expressed their relation to one another clumsily and was confused by the monetary transactions of daily life. Drawing was very defective, even with a model before him. Orientation was gravely affected and he failed entirely to construct a ground-plan of the room in which we habitually worked.

J. H. P., aged 65, a Doctor of Medicine, consulted me on January 26th, 1921, because he was unable to understand what he read. There had been no stroke or seizure of any kind to account for this condition; but, two weeks before I saw him, he had begun to notice some difficulty in reading, which had increased considerably a couple of days before his first visit to me.

He was an elderly man who did not look unduly old for his age. His pulse was 72 to the minute and regular, but the arterial wall was somewhat hard; the systolic tension was 220 mm., the diastolic 120 mm. The apex beat of the heart extended 1·5 cm. to the left of the nipple line and this was confirmed by percussion. No murmurs were audible, although the second sound at the aortic area was loud and booming. The specific gravity of the urine was 1030; it was acid and contained neither albumen nor sugar.

He suffered from no headache, nausea or vomiting. Vision in the right eye was $\frac{6}{6}$ and the field was perfect; but the left eye was nearly blind from an injury in childhood. The right disc was normal; the left fundus showed profound choroidal changes and detachment of the retina. Hearing, smell and taste were unaffected. The pupils reacted normally, and all movements of the eyes, the face and the tongue were well carried out. The reflexes, including the plantars and abdominals, were normal and equal on the two halves of the body. There was no paralysis, paresis or incoordination, nor could I discover any changes in sensibility even to measured tests.

He was a right-handed man, who had always thrown and played lawn-tennis in the usual manner. He could not cut with the loose-jointed scissors held in the left hand.

There was no evidence of apraxia. He could extract a match from the box, strike it, light a cigarette and blow out the match again with perfect ease. He tied a common knot and converted it into a reef knot without difficulty. He used a knife, spoon, towel, hair and nail-brush correctly. He was able to carry out rapidly in pantomime the act of striking a match and lighting from it an imaginary cigarette; he showed how he would brush his hair without a brush and wash his face with a supposititious sponge.

Condition of Symbolic Formulation and Expression between January 26th and February 18th, 1921.

For the last three or four years his daughter had noticed some lack of mental energy and initiative, especially since he gave up medical practice some eighteen months before I first saw him. But he was a man of wide interests, keenly occupied with politics and sociological questions. Most of his time had been spent in reading and his disability thus deprived him of his greatest amusement and solace.

The following remarks, made during one of the pauses in my examination, give a good idea of his general intellectual powers: "Now on this Irish question, I like, even now that I am ill, the irrationality of their arguments...not necessarily criminal, but irrationality of numbers...why they go for the destruction of the English nation, though they themselves have been conquered. The same thing applies to the Indian question. Why are the crown colonies so dissatisfied, while the free colonies are perfectly satisfied? These are the subjects that interest me and I think I can rationally reason upon."

"I was talking to an Egyptian the other day, a Doctor, and he said, 'We hate you. I am educated, but I am treated as a black nigger. We hate you and we teach the tradition.' Even the Cyprus (the inhabitants of Cyprus) are trying to get under the...get under the Greek. The Egyptians would like to be under the Turk. We have to find the cause of this trouble; we have a large Empire."

Articulated speech. He talked rapidly in somewhat short and jerky sentences, as if he was afraid of forgetting what he wanted to say. He did not lack words, although in ordinary conversation he occasionally used a wrong expression. Thus, he said "My son is just home from Ireland. He is a flying man. Takes the ship (aeroplane or machine) about to carry the police, to give information, to carry the letters of the police. He is not allowed to fire; for some reason the Government stopped that. Ready to be murdered any day, the young man. For instance, young F., son of an old friend of mine, served for four years in the Artillery and got the C.M. or something (M.C., i.e. Military Cross). He was the only one of fourteen not killed. Lay twenty-four hours, his head knocked in by a bucket (musket), no by a rifle. He is recovering."

Intonation was perfect and syntax was not affected apart from the errors in phrasing due to faulty composition.

He could repeat perfectly anything said to him, provided it did not consist of long and involved sentences.

Understanding of spoken words. Single words and short phrases were perfectly understood and he could even carry out the complex hand, eye and ear tests to oral command. Moreover, he was able to take in the contents of a newspaper, when it was read aloud. But, if he once became puzzled, he floundered along unable to recover himself unless he started afresh; for once he had developed a false general conception of the significance of something he had heard he was unable to correct it.

Reading. His most serious complaint was of his inability to read. "For reading I can only see...understand one verse, a line or so and then I lose it." Yet he could carry out even the complex printed commands of the hand, eye and ear tests with two minor errors only. He was, however, puzzled when asked to set the clock to orders given in print. It was not so much the detail that confused him as the general significance of the act he was asked to perform. Given a series of sentences, which led on by consecutive steps to some general impression (vide infra), he was unable to reproduce what he had read.

Even if he was permitted to read the words aloud, which he did without serious mistakes, they conveyed little to his mind. Sentences correctly pronounced seemed to him questionable and he failed to give a coherent representation of their meaning.

Writing. He wrote his name and address perfectly. When I asked him to place on paper spontaneously the gist of the political conceptions he had just laid before me, he produced the following sentences. "Why are National Colonies dissastified (dissatisfied)? India Eagptian (Egyptian) Crpress (Cyprus) all dissatified and hating the English. Where as the free Colonies are loial (loyal). the natives of Egypt say the (they) know the govt is good but they admit they hate us. and would rather be under a bad govt such as the Turk. This appears to be due to gealousey (jealousy) and due to the educated man he as he believes looked down upon and the contempt of olor" (due to the educated man, who, as he believes, is looked down upon and the contempt of colour).

This is a good example of the difficulty he found in composing his thoughts, so that they could be transferred to paper; and such want of ability was even more evident, when he was asked to write down the sense of what he had read.

The faults of spelling, obvious in spontaneous expression on paper, were also present, when he attempted to write down the names of common objects. With colours he was more successful, and in the man, cat and dog tests the words were correctly written in response to pictures.

To dictation he wrote well except that he became confused by his errors in spelling.

He could copy slowly but perfectly, following each word as he did so with his finger.

A printed paragraph. I handed him the following sentences in print and told him to read them silently. "But my country now is Italy where I have a residence for life and literally may sit under my own vine and my own fig tree. I have some thousands of the one and some scores of the other with myrtles, pomegranates, oranges, lemons and mimosas in great quantity. I intend to make a garden not very unlike yours. In a few days, whenever the weather will allow it, I have four mimosas ready to place in front of my house and a friend who is coming to plant them."

Asked to put down on paper what he had gathered he wrote "I have Italy as my country and mimosa, 4 bushes" and then ceased.

The printed paragraph was again placed in his hands and he read it through silently and deliberately. He then said "I know Italy. I have an interest in Italy. You know it...and mimosas and pomegranates. I forget the rest."

He read it aloud as follows: "But my country now is Italy where I have a residence for life and literally may sit under my own vine and fig tree. I have thousands of the one and some scores of the other with myrtles...That's not good sense is it?...with pomegranates, oranges, lemons and mimosas in great quantity. I intend to make a garden not very unlikely yours...unlikely...unlike yours and in a few days, whenever the weather will allow it, I have four mimosas in place in front of my house and a friend who is coming to plant them."

I then demanded "What is it about?" and he replied "Well, the country is Italy. You have this mimosa and these shrubs. You intend to make a garden not very unlike...You have four mimosa and a friend...I have to take the ideas as they come. I think it is a difficult subject; it is involved. It wants concentration of thought. That's what I can't do."

To my dictation he wrote "But my country now is Italy where I have a residence for life and literaly six under my own vine and own vigtree. I have some 1000 of the one and scores of the other with Myrtles, Ponegranates, Oranges, Lemons and Mimosas in great quantity. I intend to make a garden not very unlike yours. In a few days when even the weather will allow it I have 4 mimosas ready to place in front of my house and a friend who is coming to plant them."

He then copied the whole paragraph without a mistake looking back perpetually to the printed sheet and following the words with the index finger of his left hand.

But, when I asked him to recapitulate what he had learnt from the sentences he had so often read and written, he answered, "I've a general idea of it. It's Italy. You have there mimosas, pomegranates and so on...and, er, you make a home in Italy for life. I don't remember anything else."

Finally he added, "I'm wonderfully clear minded in some respects. I know, but I can't keep it in my mind. I've no constraint of thought and if I attempt it I get worried. I've no sequence of ideas; involved sentences are inapplicable."

Numbers and arithmetic. He could count perfectly and wrote the numbers without difficulty.

But he complained that he was "very stupid" over arithmetic and he was slow over even simple exercises in addition and subtraction.

Addition.			Subtraction.		
586	675	956	865	953	814
413	318	467	423	627	286
1019 (wrong)	993	1423	442	326	528

Coins and their relative value. All coins were named correctly. But, when any two were placed on the table before him and he was asked how many of the one went to the other, his answers, even if correct, assumed a curious form. He tended to build them up by successive statements rather than by direct apprehension.

Thus:

A halfpenny and two and sixpence—"Two and six...twice twenty...one five and two pence."

A penny and two shillings—"One and twenty-four."

A sixpence and a shilling—"One in twelve...one in two."

A sixpence and two shillings—"One in two...two shillings...one in four."

Occasionally as with sixpence and two and six he would give a prompt and correct answer "five."

In ordinary life he found considerable difficulty with change.

Drawing. He made a poor drawing of a spirit-lamp on the table in front of him and failed altogether when the model was removed. He was entirely unable to draw an elephant to command, saying of the scrawl he produced, "No, I can't; it's more like a bird anyway."

Orientation and plan drawing. He could not be trusted out of the house alone since his illness; for, although he might be able to find his way he was liable to curious mistakes. Thus, after he had visited me many times on foot, one day he made his daughter ring the bell at No. 4, Montagu Street, a house which in aspect and surroundings bore no relation to No. 4, Montagu Square. He was misled by the name and failed to recognise the absence of my brass plate on the door and the fundamentally different appearance of the house.

The number and indications on an omnibus conveyed nothing to him; he had to be told on each occasion which one to take.

Asked to draw a ground-plan of my room, he failed entirely; the various objects were marked down in false relation to one another and in impossible positions. The fireplace and windows were omitted and the diagram had no outlines, although he strove to indicate the shape of each individual object, such as my rotating chair and the table at which we worked.

General significance of pictures. I asked his daughter to choose a picture that would have amused her father before his illness. As he was profoundly interested in politics she chose a cartoon of Mr Lloyd George playing the harp from the same score as M. Briand, who held in his hand a French horn. This he was shown and he said, "It's the Welsh Prime Minister with the Celtic instrument and the other man has a musical instrument, a blowing instrument. He's a foreigner probably; whether he's a French editor I don't know." I then uncovered the legend beneath the picture, "The world's premier duettists," and he replied, "I don't understand it; it doesn't help me."

He had no difficulty in recognising the details of a picture, but he could not appreciate its composite meaning. As he was a Doctor I thought a humorous drawing of the man who liked the sulphur waters of Harrogate would appeal to him; but he failed completely to see the point either of the drawing or of the legend. He said, "No, I don't see it. The man who liked it. The pump room. He's been to the beer house because he liked it." I asked, "Is it a beer house?" and he replied, "He's a man who goes into the public bars and drinks the pump...like Bath and these places." I said, "Suppose it was Harrogate?" He answered, "He's been drinking the Pump-room waters; they're mostly sulphur. I suppose the other man is laughing because he likes it. There, you see what difficulty I have."

Images. He undoubtedly possessed some power of visual imagery. Thus when I said to him "rose," he assured me that he saw a red rose projected in space before him. He added, "I can see your hall-door and your dining-room. I see your furniture, which is very pretty. I thought you had a taste, an appreciation of furniture. I saw the gentleman (my father's portrait in the waiting-room), I saw his bearded face and I wondered was it your father or yourself. I noticed the antique mirror there. I can still see them all in my mind."

But as soon as he was commanded to describe some object, such as my front door, which he had seen many times, he was liable to make absurd mistakes. He said the door was brown instead of green and thought the front of the house was grey instead of white; and yet he described the three bells on the door-post and placed my brass plate correctly. But he was obliged to reconstruct the name it bore, saying, "I see the name in front of me now. I confused it first with Heath, then with an old friend of mine Heard, and now I have corrected it."

Thus visual images could be evoked spontaneously or in response to a word; but he did not possess the power of employing them with certainty as symbolic formulae.

Comprehension of the general aim or significance of an act. He understood what he was required to do during the estimation of his field of vision; but he suddenly seemed to forget my instructions altogether. When corrected, he said, "Now that's the peculiarity of my memory I can't remember what I've got to do now. It's gone."

In the same way, when I was testing his power of appreciating form, the solid objects of different shapes were placed on the table in front of him and he was asked to point to the one which corresponded to the object he held in his hand. He asked "Where am I to find it?" and to my reply "On the table," he said "Oh yes, now I see, yes," and every subsequent response was perfect. This slowness in recognising the full intention of an act he was asked to perform tended to appear more or less with all the tests.

Thus, he was able to use the loose-jointed scissors perfectly with his right hand and failed to cut properly when they were held between the opposite thumb and index finger; this is the normal result for a right-handed person. The test interested him greatly as a medical man; but he completely failed to understand the cause of the phenomenon or the significance and effect of the loosened joint, even when it was explained to him as he held the scissors alternately in the right and left hand.

Serial Tests.

(1) *Naming and recognition of common objects.* He had no difficulty in choosing objects shown to him or named orally and in print. He gave their names somewhat slowly but correctly. The only errors in this series of tests occurred when he attempted to write down the names. Thus he wrote "knife, key, car (for penny), match, sessors, pencil, key, cissors, match, knife, penny, piencil."

(2) *Naming and recognition of colours.* All these tests were carried out accurately. He chose the right colours to oral and printed commands, named them correctly and wrote down for each one an appropriate designation.

(3) *The man, cat and dog tests.* Here again he carried out the various tasks set him perfectly. He read the phrases aloud from print and pictures, repeated them, wrote them from pictures and to dictation, and copied them without difficulty.

(4) *The clock tests.* (Table 1.)

This series of tests gave him the greatest trouble and led to many errors. He could set one clock in direct imitation of another, but failed both to oral and printed commands. There was evidently gross misunderstanding of "to" and "past"; and yet he was pleased with his performance and said "I seem alright there." When the printed command was given in the ordinary nomenclature, he set the hour hand opposite to the figure on the clock face, oblivious of the number of minutes; thus for "10 minutes to 1" he set 1.10. But when the order was given in railway time, e.g. "12.50," he set the hour hand at 12 and placed the other one at the correct number of minutes. He told the time accurately, though his nomenclature varied considerably; thus "a quarter to 9" became "45 minutes past 8" and "25 minutes to 3," "35 minutes past 2." This was also evident when he wrote down the time shown on the clock, although his answers were less correct.

(5) *The coin-bowl tests.* These were carried out perfectly to oral or printed commands and he read the words aloud, executing each order without fail.

Table 1.

	Direct imitation	Oral commands	Printed commands		Telling the time	Writing down the time shown on a clock face
			Ordinary nomenclature	Railway time		
5 minutes to 2	Correct	Correct	Set 2.5	Correct	Correct	55 min past 1
Half-past 1	,,	,,	Correct	,,	,,	thirty min past 1
5 minutes past 8	,,	,,	Set 8.55	Set 8.55	,,	Correct
20 minutes to 4	,,	Set 4.20	Set 4.20	Set 3.20	,,	Forty min past 3
10 minutes past 7	,,	Correct	Correct	Correct	,,	Correct
20 minutes to 6	,,	,,	Set 6.20	,,	,,	40 min past 5
10 minutes to 1	,,	,,	Set 1.10	,,	,,	Fifty mins past 1
A quarter to 9	,,	Set 9.15	Correct	,,	,,	45 mins past 9
20 minutes past 11	,,	Correct	,,	,,	,,	40 min past 11
25 minutes to 3	,,	Set 3.25	Set 3.25	,,	,,	Thirty five min past 2

(6) *The hand, eye and ear tests.* (Table 2.)

Commands given orally were well executed and he made two errors only, when they took the form of printed words read silently to himself. But he imitated my movements extremely badly, sitting face to face, and failed to an equal degree when the orders were given in the form of pictures. Moreover, reflection in the mirror puzzled instead of helping him; before the test began, he was shown what he was expected to do, but did not grasp the general significance of what he saw. He had an idea that he must make a movement opposed to that which seemed to him the natural one and said, "It's more puzzling in the mirror; I see it's a left-hand mirror; I don't think there is anything abnormal about that; I have to remember that it's the opposite to what I see in the glass." Seeing one of the picture cards on the table, he said, "I see that's the right (correct), but it would be left in the mirror." After all these tests were completed, he added, "I think I must have been wrong about the mirror. I was conscious of something wrong, I was conscious that it was left. You had two mirrors; no, you had one mirror and two reflections, that made it left." This is a characteristic example of the way in which he became confused over the general principles underlying some particular act.

Asked to write down the movements made by me without formulating them aloud, he fell into numerous errors; these were mainly mistakes between eye and ear and, with one exception, right and left were indicated correctly.

Table 2.

	Imitation of movements made by the observer	Imitation of movements reflected in a mirror	Pictorial commands	Pictorial commands reflected in a mirror	Oral commands	Printed commands	Writing down movements made by the observer	Reading aloud and executing printed commands
L. hand to L. eye	Correct	Reversed	Correct	Reversed	Correct	Correct	Correct	Correct
R. hand to R. ear	R. hand to R. *eye*	,,	,,	,,	,,	,,	R. hand to R. *eye*	,,
R. hand to L. eye	R. hand to R. eye; corrected	R. hand to R. eye	R. hand to R. eye	,,	,,	,,	Correct	,,
L. hand to R. eye	L. hand to L. eye	Reversed	L. hand to L. eye	R. hand to R. eye	,,	L. hand to R. *ear*	L. hand to L. eye	,,
L. hand to L. ear	Correct	R. hand to R. *eye*	Correct	L. hand to R. ear	,,	Correct	Correct	,,
R. hand to R. eye	,,	Reversed	,,	Reversed	,,	R. hand to R. *ear*	R. hand to R. *ear*	,,
L. hand to R. ear	L. hand to L. ear; corrected	,,	L. hand to L. *eye*	Correct	,,	Correct	Correct	,,
R. hand to L. ear	Correct	L. hand to R. *eye*	R. hand to L. *eye*	Reversed	,,	,,	,,	,,
L. hand to L. eye	,,	Reversed	Correct	,,	,,	,,	L. hand to L. *ear*	,,
R. hand to R. ear	,,	,,	R. hand to R. *eye*	,,	,,	,,	Correct	,,
R. hand to L. eye	R. hand to R. eye; corrected	R. hand to R. eye	Correct	,,	,,	,,	R. hand to L. *ear*	,,
L. hand to R. eye	R. hand to L. eye; corrected	R. hand to R. eye	L. hand to L. eye	L. hand to L. eye	,,	,,	L. hand to R. *ear*	,,

He improved considerably under treatment and his blood pressure was reduced to 180 mm. systolic and 120 diastolic.

His speech showed signs of recovery and he went to India where he died suddenly on January 24th, 1922.

No. 25

A case where the Semantic defects were of congenital origin. They were associated with no abnormal physical signs of any kind. From childhood this patient had recognised that she was unlike other persons. She had extreme difficulty in learning to read, to write and to carry out even simple arithmetical calculations. But, in spite of her disabilities, she was unusually intelligent and originated the idea of open-air schools, which she actually carried into execution. Her introspective notes formed a valuable addition to the results of my examination.

Miss A. C. S., born in March, 1867, was a professional gardener. She first consulted me in 1910, because no one had been able to explain the peculiar mental clumsiness from which she had suffered all her life. At that time I had not invented any of my serial tests and ordinary methods of examination failed to reveal the nature of her disability. But I promised her that, if at any time I should obtain the key to the condition, I would let her know; she, therefore, gave me an extended series of sittings between February 14th and April 5th, 1920. To her I owe a most valuable criticism of my methods; for she would think over them, ponder their aim and bring me a written account of her opinion with regard to their value in elucidating her condition.

History. She always knew she was not like other people. She was extraordinarily alive to all matters of experience and speculative questioning, but she did not learn to read until she was thirteen years of age. She attended no school, being taught at home by governesses; she had no regular lessons after twelve, for it seemed a hopeless task to teach her reading, writing and arithmetic. Her father, a school inspector, who took endless trouble with her education, always said, "The way to your mind is by all sorts of roundabout paths, through hedges and over ditches."

After all organised lessons had ceased, she learnt to read "with a rush"; but she first read intelligently some years later, when she stopped in a house where there was a copy of the *Encyclopaedia Britannica*. She read one article after another and this awakened her desire for theoretical knowledge.

From fifteen to twenty her life was spent in the practical details of nursing her mother and drudging over household affairs. At about twenty she began to appreciate how different she was from others and became unhappy and shy.

She determined to have a profession and joined the Horticultural Department of a provincial university without matriculation; for she could never pass an examination. She left with much knowledge, which she put to practical use, but without a diploma.

Finally, in 1907, she originated the idea of open-air schools and, after reading several papers on the subject, was made secretary of the association. On the practical side she succeeded in establishing and running life on open-air lines in several schools, but her organising work was greatly hampered by her difficulty in writing and in expressing her thoughts in a coherent manner. Moreover, the efforts she made to transmute thought into words led to chronic fatigue, and she was ultimately compelled to relinquish her post.

Condition between February 14th and April 5th, 1920.

Physical Examination.

She was a well-built, somewhat thin and worn looking woman of 53. There were no abnormal signs of any kind beyond the defects of speech, reading and writing.

She was definitely right-handed; she habitually threw and cut with the right and could not use the loose-jointed scissors with the left hand (Gordon's test).

Vision was R. $\frac{6}{5}$ and L. $\frac{6}{9}$ poorly. The right eye was a little hypermetropic, the left slightly myopic. The fields of vision were not restricted and no scotomata could be discovered, even when the plotting was carried out on a large screen. The discs were normal.

Symbolic Formulation and Expression.

She was an unusually intelligent woman, whose mental processes were continually hampered and checked by a congenital defect in symbolic expression. In many instances she was fully conscious of the nature of her disability and from long experience had learnt how to circumvent it; but some of her difficulties were insuperable. These had ruined her administrative efficiency, especially the impossibility of expressing her thoughts easily in writing.

She was a most willing subject for examination; in fact throughout she adopted a critical attitude to the tests I applied and at the end of each series dictated notes, which were often of the greatest value.

Articulated speech. She was able to find all the words and names she required in ordinary conversation and the syntax and balance of her phrases were unaltered. Articulation was usually perfect; but if she was tired, confused or vexed she developed a true stammer. This defect first appeared during the period of her life from about fifteen to twenty, when she realised that she was not as others are; she became shy, and with this want of self-confidence developed a slight but distinct stammer.

During our sittings this articulatory fault was rarely present, unless she arrived at my house tired; but on one occasion (February 29th), after she had stammered to an unusual extent, the following passage occurred amongst the written notes she presented to me at our next meeting: "I am stamming badly over this sitting. Is the reason because my mind was full of another aspect of the case—the causes at the back of it? I have had to put all these thoughts completely out of my mind, and find difficulty in adjusting myself to what has to be done."

She could say the alphabet perfectly but added, "I can say it full tilt, but I can't go slow. If I am looking up a word in a dictionary or card catalogue, I forget how the letters come and have to say the alphabet through. If my word begins with Le, I may look at Lt, and then go on for ever so many pages before remembering that E comes before T."

The days of the week and months of the year were given without a mistake, and she found no difficulty in repeating words or short phrases said to her.

Understanding of spoken words. At first sight she seemed to have no difficulty in understanding what was said to her. She chose common objects and colours to oral commands and could even set the clock correctly, if the order was worded in the common nomenclature; but if it was given in railway time, with which she was relatively unfamiliar, she was much slower and less accurate. She executed the hand, eye and ear tests to oral commands with hesitation and obvious effort, although her answers were ultimately correct; this was mainly due to the confusion between right and left, which she attempted to resolve by the following complicated reasoning: "I said, when he said 'right,' it was this hand; therefore, if he says 'right' this time, it is the same, if he says 'left' it is the other."

Her difficulty in comprehending the full significance of spoken words came out perpetually in daily intercourse. She complained that she was unable to "hold in her mind" a task explained to her in the course of conversation. "I must have the conditions, which will enable me to take it by degrees in such small parts that it makes me useless for life." This want of understanding was not in any way confined to spoken words, but was a feature of all attempts at symbolic comprehension.

Reading. She could read aloud without a mistake and with perfect enunciation. Moreover, to utter the words seemed to add greatly to her power of understanding them and she had little difficulty in executing a printed command, provided she was permitted to say it aloud.

When she read a passage silently she was liable to miss its general significance; she would fail to appreciate some essential point and this would lead to confusion (cf. Jokes, p. 386). But printed commands were on the whole well executed, even if they demanded choice between relatively similar acts.

Writing. She wrote the alphabet on the whole correctly; but at D she paused and after a while continued from F, omitting E altogether. She stopped again at Q but continued correctly to the end. The letters were written some of them in printed capitals, others in cursive script, and she added in explanation, "I never can do the same thing; I must have variation."

The character of her handwriting depended on the ease or difficulty of the task; thus, she copied printed matter in excellent cursive script, but any attempt to express general ideas led to profound deterioration. "So long as I take in the sense at a glance, I can put it down from sheer habit."

Her spelling suffered in the same way; the harder the task the worse it became, until the faults reached a degree unknown in an educated person. The names of a set of common objects were spelt on the whole correctly, with the exception of scissors. As soon as she had finished this test, she wrote for me the following explanation, illustrating the confusion into which her writing fell when she attempted to convey some general idea: "Cissors and penny difficult because one must choose between alternatives and there is knothing (nothing) to guid. K in knife is quite striking and easy to remember. With the other things they couldn't be different." To this she appended the further note, suggested by the word "knothing." "This is excellent for showy (showing) up what goes on. My mind is always a little in advance of what I say or write. Hence constant confusion, see 'knothing'! It must be because the conection of the k and n which is coming is vividly present and connected up between hand and memory and visual picture of kn."

The days of the week were written without mistake, but as soon as I asked her to write the months in sequence she said, "This is going to be a bother because of the spelling," although the only mistake she made was "Feburary." Finally she added, "This does not get hold of my real difficulty. When I think we are different to what we were in last week (the month had changed from March to April), I have to learn to write April and begin M, which I cross out or change into April. I never know what I shall write in consequence."

Selected printed passage. She was given the following passage from Landor's letters and told to read it to herself silently: "To his sisters. But my country now is Italy, where I have a residence for life and literally may sit under my own vine and my own fig-tree. I have some thousands of the one and some scores of the other with myrtles, pomegranates, oranges, lemons, gagias and mimosas in great quantity. I intend to make a garden not very unlike yours at Warwick; but, alas, time is wanting. I may live another ten years, but do not expect it. In a few days, whenever the weather will allow it, I have four mimosas ready to place round my intended tomb, and a friend who is coming to plant them."

As a professional gardener this passage was of peculiar interest to her and, asked to tell what she had understood, she said, "Well our man is evidently living in a pleasant warm climate in which he wants to have things the only one of which is mimosa. He is writing to a friend and says he wishes his garden to be like one at Warwick. He has four plants for his tomb, which I think are mimosas and a friend is going to look after them...Oh! and he may live another ten years but did not expect to do so."

I then dictated this passage to her and she wrote it correctly except for "litterally" and "toombe." As soon as she had finished she said, "This is an excellent test. I might never have seen the beginning of it. I did not think I had ever read anything about Italy; I had entirely missed that he was living in Italy. I inferred a warm climate because he was growing mimosas."

She was next asked to write down what she remembered of the dictated passage. She wrote:

"To his sisters.

The writer is in italy and tels of his garden in which he has fig trees and vines pomgranates and many other things. He wishes to make a garden resembling the one at Warwick, but time is short and he fears it will not be done. When the weather is good he has for transplanting 4 mimosa bushes and those a friend is to plan round his intended toumb."

She added, "I don't think I missed out anything except the many things he grew in his garden"; but it is noticeable that she changed the passage into oblique narration.

She read the passage aloud without a mistake and with perfect enunciation. Now, asked to write what she remembered of its contents, she enormously improved and gave an almost perfect account. "Italy is now my home and I literally sit under my own vine and fig trees of which I have some thousands of the one and many hundreds of the other. I have also in the garden memosas gagias and numerous other things. I had hoped to make a garden something like yours at Warwick, but fear time may be lacking! I may live another ten years but do not expect to do so. I have 4 memosa bushes to go round my intended toumb and when the weather is fitting a friend is coming to plant them."

She added, "I wasn't at all sure if it was thousands of vines or of fig trees. The form of the sentence stuck in my mind, it was so picturesque, but I did not know what applied to which. When I read it I was able to appreciate the literary beauty of it, but now I have to write it myself I am nowhere."

Arithmetic. She was given the following simple sums:

Addition.				Subtraction.			
586	675	956		865	953	814	
413	318	467		423	627	286	
999	993	1443	(wrong)	442	326	728	(corrected to 528)

She passed the mistake in the third addition unnoticed, but said, "These little things give me no difficulty. It is when sustained effort is required that I fail. I can't add up a column of figures."

Coins and their relative value. She had no difficulty in naming any coin placed before her; but, when she attempted to state their relative value she was slow, hesitated and made several mistakes. Her answers were as follows:

One penny and one shilling—Correct.

One halfpenny and two shillings and sixpence—"How stupid; I shall want a piece of paper to do it. I put it into shillings; I do it in bits. Thirty-six."

Sixpence and two shillings and sixpence—Correct; very slow.

One penny and two shillings—Correct. "This is done in two operations; twelve pennies into a shilling. Then twice twelve."
One halfpenny and sixpence—"Twenty-four."
One penny and two shillings and sixpence—"It's quite a bother to add 24 and 6 together. That is what I am trying to do. I try to do it by remembering that five sixes is 30." She gave no final answer.
One halfpenny and one shilling—Correct and quick.
One penny and two shillings and sixpence—Correct. "I said a penny into a shilling goes twelve and multiplied by two."
One halfpenny and sixpence—Correct and quick.
Sixpence and two and sixpence—Correct but slow.
One penny and two and sixpence—Correct but slow.
One penny and one shilling—Correct. "That's the easiest of all."
One halfpenny and one penny—Correct.
One penny and two shillings—Correct and quick.
One halfpenny and two shillings and sixpence—Correct but slow.
Sixpence and one shilling—Correct.
One halfpenny and one shilling—Correct and quick.
One halfpenny and one penny—Correct and quick.
Sixpence and two shillings—Twice.
One halfpenny and two shillings—Correct.

She added, "You can easily stump me with the matter of change. If somebody counts out change to me I become absolutely confused and really don't know. For instance, I had a pound and owed my friend eight shillings and twopence. We neither of us had any pennies and I was lost, for I could not see what my change was. I would have taken anything in change unless I could work it out on paper with a pencil. I make all sorts of mistakes in this way."

Drawing. She had been taught to draw and had learnt to block out the object on paper; but the result of her attempt to draw a candlestick from a model was not up to her preparation or knowledge. She could not bring it within the limits of the sheet of paper nor did she place it directly in the centre.

Asked to draw it from memory she made a bad reproduction of her previous drawing. "I can see the brass candlestick and I know it wasn't fat in the middle like this (pointing to her sketch). If you ask me where the largest part was, I cannot tell you. I can see the square base. I can see the mass, but I can't remember the detail to draw it."

On another occasion she made a good sketch of a spirit-lamp from a model; but, when asked to reproduce it from memory, the result was not a replica, but was built up by argument with herself. "I said to myself, there was the wick, then there was a disc out of which the wick came. I remembered the general form and the top and the wick inside."

When I requested her to draw an elephant, she produced a picture distinctly resembling this animal, except that she gave it a bushy tail and forgot the tusks.

After she had finished she exclaimed, "I haven't put the tusks in. I can't remember where they come. They come from just below the eye I think; but I don't know, I believe they are teeth and should come out of the top of the jaw really."

After making several attempts to argue the question out to herself she requested, "May I do a diagrammatic picture according to what I know about tusks and teeth and noses and all that, on the assumption that the elephant is like every animal is?"

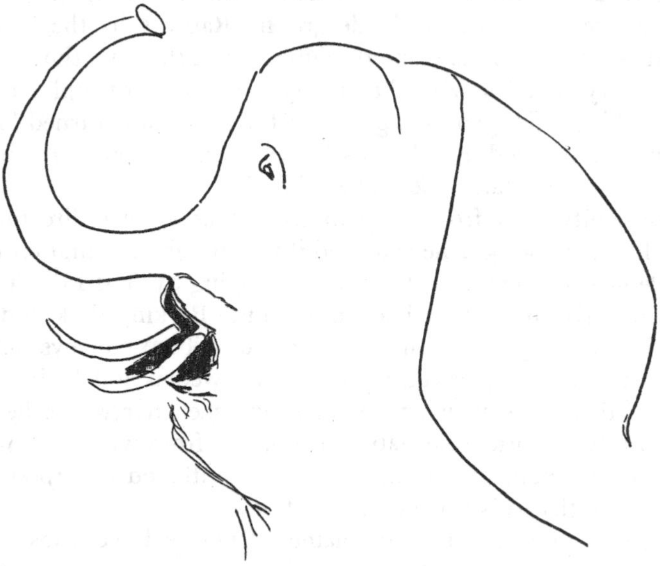

Fig. 30. Successful attempt by No. 25 to draw the head of an elephant.

She then produced the above drawing, carrying on a running commentary as each part was filled in. "This is my diagrammatic picture. It is made up of what I know about tusks and teeth and noses. I think what all animals have and then make it up. I made an open mouth; then I put in the teeth. I got rid of the nose by putting it like that (elevated). That's all I can do."

She drew an excellent plan of the room in which we worked, marking the position of the various pieces of furniture correctly. "I put myself and then I went round the room putting in the fireplace and then the couch and so on. The way I got it was by putting in each thing as I remembered it. I made no general plan. Those were all the things I could remember in the room. I was not sure of the alcoves on either side of the fireplace. I knew there were other chairs, but could only remember the two chairs and the round chair at your table. I could see the things I put in quite clearly."

Orientation. She had great difficulty in finding her way for the following reasons. So long as she could pass automatically from place to place she reached her destination with ease; but, as soon as she was compelled to think, she was liable to become confused. Thus, she had firmly associated the Marble Arch with Montagu Square, and this again with my house. But one day she got out of the Tube at the Bond Street station in error; then she was lost. For she expected to see the Marble Arch in front of her as if she had alighted at that station; not seeing it, she was confused until a messenger boy showed her the way. On another occasion she wanted to reach the Underground Railway by the British Museum station, but went in error to the Holborn Tube, across the way, though she travelled on these lines every day. She waited patiently in the row of people, until she slowly reached the booking office; on asking for her ticket she was turned back, and then for the first time recognised that she was in the wrong station. "It's because of this sort of thing that I can't take a permanent job."

Another difficulty arose from her inability to follow given directions; right and left bothered her and she became confused if told to take the first on the right, etc.

Again, "People say to me, what 'bus are you going by, and I don't know. When I see a 'bus with 'Barking' on it, I see in my mind Barking Park and then I know that's where I want to go. A number (on the omnibus) conveys nothing at all." In the same way she had planned a journey to Sweden and had in her pocket a complete set of tickets. But, when the cabman asked her where he should drive to, she had entirely forgotten the station in London from which she was to set out. She talked round the subject with him until he mentioned Liverpool Street, when it flashed upon her that this was her destination.

Jokes. "It may be ages," she complained, "before I see a joke. It makes no difference if it is in words or pictures."

On one occasion I showed her a picture from "Punch" in which a tramp is being taken to task by a country gentleman, who says, "It's about time you chaps started to do something; hard work never killed anybody." The mendicant replies, "You are mistaken, Sir, I lost three wives through it."

She said, "There's no joke in it; he lost three wives through the war. I suppose he lost three wives, but I don't know what by." About ten minutes later she exclaimed, "Oh! now I see it. It was the wives who were killed by work." She laughed heartily and added, "That's very characteristic; when once I have seen it, I wonder how I have been so silly not to have seen it at once."

When she left me she was in the habit of writing down her impressions and handing them to me at our next meeting. Amongst these notes occurred the following suggestive thoughts on this experiment, which I transcribe exactly. "It was not so much that I did not see the joke, but that I did not see anything. This is *most characteristic*; I make my remarks upon it before I have read all the words, before I have really looked at the picture. The one word 'kill' calls up war associtus (associations). I jump to the conclusin (conclusion) that it is a war joke. As I do not see where the joke is, I think it is a bad one and put the thing down. When Dr Head jogs my attention to it again *then* I see I have missed something; *then* I see what the picture stands for. Then I put it altogether and see the joke! But the interesting part in this test is that Dr Head's jogging of the attention was equivalent to *interest* in subject matter when alone. Just as the one word 'kill' in this case turned me off the whole thing, so one word or sentence beary (bearing) upon sonethy (something) of interest will jog my attention in the same way and cause me to read a passage or a page over and over again untile (until) I get its full meaning. But this *has* to be done; and if the interest is not there to 'jog,' the effort is not made because one is unconscious that an effort is needed."

Other intellectual aptitudes. "I must have the conditions which will enable me to take it (the task) by degrees, in such small parts that it makes me useless for life."

Thus, she could not boil an egg without writing down the time she put it into the water. "When I want to write 1920, I begin with 20 and build up round it. The new thing in the dates is the 2; I therefore begin with this and then build up the rest. To-morrow (March 1st) I shall be faced with March. I shall therefore begin with an F and turn this into an M. It helps me to start. I put something onto the paper and then change it into what I want."

She had to make a model of an open-air school for exhibition at one of the museums, and was told the space that would be placed at her disposal. She knew she could not work to a general scale and so got a carpenter to cut for her blocks of wood 10 inches by 5 inches. She then built up her model on a scale of one inch to a foot, putting together the pieces in detail. "I planned it to cover 12 feet square; it wasn't until I got to the exhibition that I discovered it covered a space of 24 feet each way. I knew I was working an inch to a foot, but I could not work it out so as to get the total space."

She complained of the extraordinary variations in her powers. "There is a saturation point with regard to learning. You improve fairly quickly and then you come to a deadlock. If I am tired my trouble is to remember the most ordinary things at will, such as my own name, the number of my house, or any ordinary thing that ordinary people learn automatically."

"A long thing like a prayer is quite impossible. If I thought about the Lord's prayer, I should certainly fail. When I had to read it aloud at family prayers, the only way was to fix my mind on something else, like one chimneypot being higher than another, and then fire away. If I fixed my mind on the book I should be certain to get stuck."

The significance of summer-time bothered her greatly. "With summer-time you put the clock on or back, I don't know which. In the middle of the day I stop and think; the clock says eleven. Before we altered, it would have said ten or eleven. I get at it by thinking how we should be when it was dark. Then

I remember that at seven o'clock last night it was light, but that before it used to be dark at seven o'clock. I get at it round about."

Images. She could see the outlines, colour and lighting of visual images that recurred spontaneously or in answer to command. "But I cannot see letters like I see you or the Tube station, when I am away from you."

She could not reproduce voices, the sound of church bells, scents, tastes or touches, as is so commonly the case with normal persons, whose memory is strongly visual in everyday operations.

Movements could be well imagined; she could think of herself as closing the door, turning a key or carrying out similar actions. But such complex orders as those of the hand, eye and ear tests confused her badly.

Thus, her images, which seemed to belong mainly to the visual type, were intact; but she had difficulty in evoking them in response to a direct command, unless it was of a simple nature.

Games, etc. She knew how to play whist, but her game was spoilt by her tendency to become confused. "I am interested in the problem of which card to play, but I forget what has been played and so cannot play with other people."

She could not put together any form of puzzle, "It's that kind of thing that distracts me."

In billiards she was unable to make any stroke off the cushion, and ceased to try to learn.

Serial Tests.

(1) *Naming and recognition of common objects.* All these forms of examination were carried out with ease except writing the name of the object indicated. The nomenclature was correct but the spelling of scissors ("sisors" and twice "cisors") was faulty. She added the following explanation: "Some difficulties I can argue out; scissors and penny are difficult because you could spell them differently; but if I stop to ask whether there are two or one 'n' in penny there is nothing to help me." As a matter of fact, in all these examples the word "penny" was spelt correctly.

Later she wrote, "Cissors and penny difficult because one must choose between alternatives and there is knothing (nothing) to guid. K in knife is quite striking and easy to remember. With the other things they couldn't be different." She read over what she had written and added the following note: "This is *excellent* for showy (showing) up what goes on. My mind is always a little in advance of what I say or write. Hence constant confusin (confusion), see 'knothing.' It must be because the connection of the k and n which is coming is vividly present and connected up between hand and memory and visual picture of kn[1]."

[1] This is a frequent form of mistake in typewriting.

(2) *Naming and recognition of colours*. All forms of this test were carried out perfectly. "There is no difficulty," she said. "It's because it's the direct think. There's no translation." After writing the names of the colours correctly, she added, "There is nothing to think about here. The writing is therefore much better than where there are other things to be thought about." This was in fact true; her handwriting was excellent.

(3) *The man, cat and dog tests*. She wrote these simple phrases well to dictation or from pictures, copied them accurately and read them aloud with perfect intonation.

She found this test easy, "but there is great difficulty in reading matter that has to be thought about. Suppose there had been any detail to remember. Suppose I had had to put dog with a big D and cat with a little c, my difficulty would have come out. I should not have been able to hold in my mind the task you wanted me to carry out. If I can get the sense into a spell of attention so long ——— I can do it; but if the spell of attention required is so long ——————— I am lost before I come to the end. In the Bible, Proverbs was the only part I could read to myself understandingly, because I could grasp the whole idea at a go without getting tired."

(4) *The clock tests*. (Table 1.)

This was a splendid method of revealing her disabilities. She could set one clock in direct imitation of the other and found no difficulty in executing oral commands, provided I employed the ordinary nomenclature; but, if I gave them in railway time, they were carried out imperfectly. She tended to set the hour hand directly opposite the figure on the clock face, and on one occasion pushed it back instead of forward in her attempts to give it a position proportionate to the number of minutes. (10 minutes to 1.) "If you say twenty minutes to three, that is quite easy and I see it; I visualise it and there is no problem. But if you say 2.45 I have to go to the clock and have to tot up two forty-five."

Asked to set the clock to a command in ordinary nomenclature, printed as on Table 1, partly in numerals and partly in words, she was slow and made three errors, mistaking "to" for "past" the hour. "I say to myself 'to' or 'past' and I look at it many times before I get it right. You see what a labour life is, can't you?"

Yet, so soon as the printed order was expressed in railway time, she not only carried it out more quickly, but set the two hands exactly. For, as the card lay always before her, she did not have to remember both the hour and the minutes, as with oral commands, but could see the one and refer back to the card for the other. "It is very much easier. If I have one card in front of me, as in this test, I see it in a moment. I put one hand to 2 and then work the other round to 35." When, however, the ordinary nomenclature was employed she became confused as to the contrasted significance of "to" and "past."

Table 1.

	Direct imitation	Oral commands		Printed commands		Telling the time	
		Ordinary nomenclature	Railway time	Ordinary nomenclature	Railway time	In words	In numbers
5 minutes to 2	Correct	Correct	Correct; slow	Correct	Correct	Correct	"Two fifty-five"
Half-past 1	,,	,,	,, ; quick	,,	,,	,,	Correct
5 minutes past 8	,,	,,	Correct	Set 5 minutes *to* 8	,,	,,	,,
20 minutes to 4	,,	,,	3.20; then correct	Correct	,,	,,	Correct; very slow
10 minutes past 7	,,	,,	Correct	Set 10 minutes *to* 7	,,	,,	Correct
20 minutes to 6	,,	,,	,,	Correct	,,	,,	Correct; very slow
10 minutes to 1	,,	,,	Short hand at 12, long hand at 50. Thus pushed hour hand *back*	,,	,,	,,	Correct
A quarter to 9	,,	,,	Correct	,,	,,	,,	,,
20 minutes past 11	,,	,,	,,	Set 20 minutes *to* 11	,,	,,	"Eleven forty. No, eleven twenty"
25 minutes to 3	,,	,,	,,	Correct	,,	,,	Correct

When it came to telling the time verbally, she again found it easier to use the ordinary nomenclature, which was more familiar to her than railway time. "Three forty," she explained, "that's quite a long business. I first look at the small hand to know what the hour is. I see it is nearer four than three. But I know that I have to begin by talking about three...Then I look at the big hand and I add ten minutes to the half-hour. It is easy to remember that the half-hour is thirty, so I add ten to make forty. Then I tend to forget the hour, whilst I'm doing this. Some things seem to stick without the slightest effort, and 2.30 and 2.15 as being the half-past and quarter-past have always stuck." Then she added, "It isn't that you can't do it, but it takes time. If anyone hurries you, that comes to the same thing as not being able to do it at all."

But, as soon as she was asked to tell the time without the use of spoken words by picking out a card, it mattered little whether the legend was in the ordinary nomenclature or in railway time.

If she was allowed to say the time aloud before she wrote it down, she was the victim of what she said. Thus, for "five minutes to two" she both said and wrote "eight five," and she made several similar errors. Throughout, her manner of writing the time varied and sometimes she adopted one form sometimes the other. She said, finally, "You see, I must always obtain variation."

(5) *The coin-bowl tests*. These gave her no difficulty; she executed oral and printed commands rapidly and without error. She was equally quick whether the order was given in the form of "1st into 3rd" or "first penny into third bowl," for in both instances she reduced it in her own mind to "first into third," etc.

Table 1 (*continued*).

Choosing a card corresponding to the time shown on a clock		Writing down the time shown on a clock		Telling the time aloud and then writing it down	
Ordinary nomenclature	Railway time	Ordinary nomenclature	Railway time	She said	She wrote
Correct	No choice	5 to 2 (correct)	1.55 (correct)	"Eight five"	8.5
,,	Correct	½ past 1 (correct)	1.30 (,,)	"One thirty" (correct)	1.30 (correct)
,,	,,	5 past 8 (correct)	8.5 (,,)	"Five past 8" (correct)	5.8
,,	Correct ; slow	20 to 4 (correct)	3.40 (,,)	"Ten to 4"	10 to 4
,,	Correct	10 past 7 (correct)	7.10 (,,)	"Ten past 2"	Ten past 2
,,	,,	20 to 6 (correct)	5.20	"Twenty to six" (correct)	20 to 6 (correct)
,,	Correct; very slow	10 to 1 (correct)	12.50 (correct)	"Ten to one" (correct)	10 to 1 (correct)
,,	Correct; slow	quarter to 9 (correct)	8.45 (,,)	"Quarter to 9" (correct)	¼ to 9
,,	Correct	20 past 11 (correct)	11.20 (,,)	"Twenty past 11" (correct)	20 past 11 (correct)
,,	,,	25 to 3 (correct)	2.35 (,,)	"Twenty five to 3" (correct)	25 to 3 (correct)

But on one occasion, when starting this test, she made a curious and characteristic mistake; she called the penny lying to her extreme left the "first," although the "first bowl" was the one to the extreme right. I pulled her up and she said, "That is most characteristic; if I can make a change of this kind I always do."

(6) *The hand, eye and ear tests.* (Table 2.)

This method of examination threw much light on her difficulties. She was puzzled, when she attempted to imitate my movements, and after the fourth observation of his series, she said, "I am going to dismiss from my mind all right and left and simply say to myself 'you use the opposite of what he does.' I shall be safe if I use the opposite hand." Then she added, "If it were important exactly what part of the eye or ear I touched, it would make me much slower." She was also slow, hesitating and fell into error when carrying out pictorial commands.

But she imitated correctly both my movements and pictorial commands when reflected in the glass. "Here there isn't anything to think about at all. I think the picture was easier than the actual movement because of the line down the centre, which gave me the idea if it was the same side or crossed. When *you* made the movement, I had to think harder."

Oral and printed commands were carried out slowly, but on the whole correctly. "They seem to me about the same. I said to myself 'when he said right it was this hand'; therefore if he says right this time it is the same, if he says left it is the other.' I am not quite certain if I take in all the command at a go. I take in right hand; then I look again and if I have not moved my hand I am liable to forget the

Table 2.

	Imitation of movements made by the observer	Imitation of movements reflected in a mirror	Pictorial commands	Pictorial commands reflected in a mirror	Oral commands	Printed commands	Printed commands read aloud and executed		Writing down movements made by the observer
							She read	Movement executed	
L. hand to R. ear	Reversed	Correct	Reversed	Correct	Correct	Correct	"L. hand to R. *eye*"	L. hand to R. *eye*	Left hand towright ear (correct)
R. hand to L. eye	,,	,,	Correct	,,	,,	,,	Correctly	Correct	righ hand to left eye (correct)
R. hand to L. ear	Correct	,,	,,	,,	,,	,,	,,	,,	right hand
L. hand to L. eye	L. hand to R. eye	,,	,,	,,	,,	,,	,,	,,	left hand to left eye (correct)
R. hand to R. ear	Correct	,,	,,	,,	,,	,,	,,	,,	right hand to right ear (correct)
L. hand to R. eye	Correct; very slow	,,	,,	,,	,,	,,	,,	,,	Left hand to
L. hand to L. ear	Correct	,,	,,	,,	,,	,,	,,	,,	left hand to left ear (correct)
R. hand to R. eye	,,	,,	,,	,,	Correct; slow	,,	,,	,,	right hand to right eye (correct)
L. hand to R. ear	L. hand to R. *eye*; corrected	,,	R. hand; corrected	,,	L. hand to L. ear: corrected	L. hand to R. *eye*; corrected	,,	,,	Left hand to right ear (correct)
R. hand to L. eye	Correct	,,	Correct	,,	Correct	Correct	,,	,,	right hand to left eye (correct)
R. hand to L. ear	,,	,,	,,	,,	,,	,,	,,	,,	right hand to left ear (correct)
L. hand to L. eye	,,	,,	L. hand to R. eye; corrected	,,	,,	L. hand to R. eye; corrected	,,	,,	Left hand to same eye (correct)
R. hand to R. ear	,,	,,	Correct	,,	,,	Correct	,,	,,	right hand to right ear (correct)
L. hand to R. eye	R. hand to R. eye; corrected	,,	,,	,,	,,	,,	,,	,,	Left hand to right ea
L. hand to L. ear		,,	,,	,,	,,	,,	,,	,,	Left hand to lef ear (correct)
R. hand to R. eye	Correct	,,	R. hand to L. eye; corrected	,,	,,	,,	,,	,,	right hand to right eye (correct)

first part. When you say the words, it is an immense help. If I came into the door and you said 'put your right hand on your left knee,' I should be floored; now I am strung up to right and left. Saying it aloud is a great help."

"All the time I have to say to myself 'he is going to the eye on the same side or on the opposite side.' Then I have to translate opposite into right or left. Sometimes I am so bothered I can't get any further; I have forgotten whether it was the eye or the ear by the time I have translated into right and left."

Finally, she summed up as follows: "This test would floor me or would be much slower if you made it a little harder. If you said a particular finger, I should become slow; if it is slow I can't hold it and get confused. Supposing the test was the right forefinger to the right eyelid, I think you would find I should have to refer to it three or four times before I got it right. I should have to take the right forefinger and move it; then look to see the right eyelid."

No. 26

A case of extremely severe Aphasia of vascular origin in an unusually intelligent man of sixty. Speech was reduced to meaningless sounds with "Si, si" used correctly for affirmation. He could repeat nothing. He understood what was said to him and chose familiar objects correctly, although he could not execute more complex oral commands. He read to himself with pleasure and selected common objects slowly but accurately when shown their names in print; but he failed to execute more difficult printed orders. He could write nothing spontaneously except his name and the first nine numerals; but he could copy correctly, provided he was not compelled to transcribe print into cursive script. The use of the alphabet was defective; even when given twenty-six block letters, he failed to arrange them in order. Arithmetical exercises were impossible and he could neither name coins nor express the simplest relation between any two of them. Orientation was not affected. Games, except draughts, were difficult or impossible. He enjoyed music and could sing without words.

On May 2nd, 1920, at 8 o'clock in the morning, Mr N. B., aged 60, was suddenly seized with complete inability to express himself in words. He was shaving at the time and called out "Oh! dear me. Oh! dear me." He did not lose consciousness, was not paralysed, and within ten minutes had regained his speech completely. An hour later he exclaimed, "It's going again"; but he walked downstairs unaided and in a few minutes seemed to speak as well as ever. He and his wife got into the motor-car which was waiting for them, and, after driving about four miles, he became somewhat confused and asked her where they were. She answered him, and from that moment he has neither spoken nor written normally.

On alighting from the car his right arm was found to be paralysed and the right half of the face and tongue were affected; at no time did the weakness extend to the leg. He used to complain that the right half of the body and face did not "feel" the same as the other side; but this seems to have passed away at least six months before I first saw him.

He was a Greek merchant, a man of unusual intelligence, who had lived in England all his life and could speak eight languages. At times, according to his wife, he could say a few intelligible words; but, if his attention was drawn to the fact, he ceased to be able to talk at all. He is said also to have spoken in Greek during sleep.

Condition in November 1923 (*three years and a half after the stroke*).

When I first saw him in November, 1923, he was an extremely intelligent and active elderly man, who habitually walked many miles a day.

His pulse was 80 to the minute, regular, and the systolic tension was 160 mm., the diastolic 95 mm. The arterial wall was somewhat hard, but the vessel was not tortuous. The apex beat of the heart lay a little outside the nipple line and the cardiac dulness was somewhat enlarged to the left. At the apex the first sound was loud and over the base the aortic second sound was a little exaggerated.

The urine was of a sp. gravity of 1022, and contained no albumen, sugar or other abnormal constituent.

Apart from the defects of speech, I could find no signs pointing to disease of the central nervous system. He did not suffer from headaches. There was no hemianopsia and the discs were normal. Hearing was unaffected. The pupils reacted well. Movements of the eyes and face were perfectly executed and the tongue was protruded in the middle line. All the reflexes, including the plantars and abdominals, were normal. There was no paralysis, paresis, incoordination or tremor. He could stand equally well on either foot and his gait was normal. Sensation could not be tested accurately on account of his profound inability to express himself.

Symbolic Formulation and Expression.

He was a highly educated man, anxious to perform the tasks I set him, but liable to become depressed if he failed to do so. His gestures were extremely apt and he was particularly quick in taking advantage of the slightest unwitting movement of anyone who was talking to him, such as his wife. Her vivid manner and lively gestures evidently helped him greatly. Thus, she asserted that, if the orders were given in Greek, he would be able to carry out the coin-bowl and clock tests correctly. Yet, when she was allowed to give the command, but was forbidden to move her hands or her head, he failed exactly in the same way as in the records obtained by me. The following incident shows his intelligence and quickness of apprehension. Some friends, who were discussing the Eastern question in his presence, could not remember the name of a small town in Greece; he took down the atlas, found the right page and quickly pointed to the place on the map. He still supervised his wife in her business affairs, approving or disapproving the course she was about to adopt by gestures, or by uttering "Si si" (that's so). He showed no sign in his daily conduct of mental deterioration, apart from the consequences of his loss of speech.

Articulated speech. Throughout the period of my examination, he did not utter a single intelligible word, except on rare occasions "Si si" (pronounced as in French) to express his acceptance of some suggestion. When he attempted to name an object, he employed some modification of a meaningless word "Low-la," using these sounds indifferently and with no distinctive application.

He was completely unable to repeat to order a single word or even the variants of "Low-la" he had just employed in his efforts to speak.

Understanding of spoken words. He seemed to understand most of what was said to him in conversation, provided the subject was not a complicated one and did not imply a command to action.

It was impossible to explain to him that, when we sat face to face during the hand, eye and ear tests, he had to employ what appeared to be the opposite hand. During my preliminary explanation, he held up first the right and then the left hand correctly in imitation of similar movements made by me. On his own initiative he then turned halfway round to show me that he understood that, when we were face to face, the hands would appear to be opposed, at the same time saying "Si si." But, as soon as we began the tests again in earnest, he employed the reversed hand on most occasions.

There was the same difficulty in making him understand the exact hour at which I wanted him to come to me for further examination. But, when I wrote it down on paper in simple figures, he understood perfectly.

He chose familiar objects correctly to oral commands and obviously recognised the name of each one in turn. As soon, however, as he was asked to set the clock or to carry out the complex movements of the hand, eye and ear tests, he failed lamentably. With the coin-bowl tests he frequently placed the penny into the bowl of the same number, for instance, the third into the third, oblivious of the fact that my orders never took this simple form.

Reading. He could not read a single word aloud. But there was no doubt that he understood much of what he read to himself silently. He even chose common objects correctly to printed commands, although he failed grossly to set the clock or to carry out the hand, eye and ear tests. Moreover, his answers were equally bad if the order was given in railway time, and he made many mistakes in the coin-bowl tests with commands printed in figures. The appreciation of the significance of numbers was as badly affected as that of words.

Writing. He was able to write his surname and to append the initial or even his full Christian name; this he could do both in English and Greek characters. But he was unable to add his address or to write anything else spontaneously or to dictation.

If his full name and address were written in cursive script, he reproduced it correctly, although his handwriting was extremely bad. He copied the names of common objects from print, using almost entirely printed capitals; "key" was, however, written in cursive script.

The alphabet. He could say no single letter spontaneously, simply uttering some modification of "Low-la." When he attempted to repeat the alphabet after me, he emitted a series of unintelligible sounds, which bore no relation to the letters he was trying to pronounce; but, during these efforts he somewhat modified his habitual "Low-la," although every one of these words was pure jargon.

Exactly the same results were obtained when he attempted to read the alphabet aloud, and the sounds he uttered bore no recognisable relation to the actual name of the letter, either in Greek or English; nor was it constant on two separate occasions.

He could not write the alphabet spontaneously or to dictation. But he copied printed capitals or cursive letters exactly, although he could not transcribe the former into the latter.

Given the twenty-six block letters, after many attempts he finally put together the following alphabet:

A B C D E F G I J
H L K N M O P Q
R S T V Y U X W Z.

Numbers and arithmetic. He could neither say spontaneously nor repeat after me a single number. But, asked to write them without prompting on my part, he produced the following series with great difficulty: 1 2 3 4 5 6 7 8 9 0 1 2 3 4 5 6 7 8 9 0. He then ceased and could go no further. The figures were misshapen and strokes uneven, like the writing of a child. To dictation he was less successful, and, after writing 1 2 3 4 5 6 7 8 9 0 0 8 3 7 0, he gave up all further attempts. When, however, the numbers up to 20 were placed before him in writing, he succeeded in copying them correctly and the figures were much better shaped.

He was unable to bring out the answer to even the simplest addition sum; for he could neither utter to himself nor write down any of the necessary figures with sufficient certainty to express his conclusions.

Coins and the use of money. He was unable to name a single coin, and, when I asked the relative value of any two of them, I obtained no intelligible answer. He struggled ineffectually to state it in words and seemed incapable of using his fingers or any other simple means of expressing this relation.

Games. He was said to be able to play draughts, but this I was unable to verify. He could no longer play whist or other card games.

Orientation. He walked many miles a day alone and had no difficulty in finding his way.

Singing. He could sing correctly without words and enjoyed music greatly. He had never played any instrument.

Serial Tests.

(1) *Naming and recognition of common objects.* (Table 1.)

He had no difficulty in pointing to the object shown him or placed in his hand out of sight. He also carried out oral and printed commands correctly, though somewhat slowly. But he was entirely unable to name any of the objects on the table before him and the sounds he uttered bore no relation to their usual names in any language.

Asked to write the names, he scrawled N. B., his initials, or his surname, and finally gave up after six attempts. He could, however, copy all the words correctly for the most part in printed capitals; "key" alone was written entirely in cursive script.

Table 1.

	Pointing to object shown	Naming an object indicated	Oral commands	Printed commands	Duplicate placed in hand out of sight	Writing name of object indicated	Copying from print
Knife	Perfect	"Lowla"	Correct	Correct	Perfect	Impossible	KNi
Key	,,	"Luk-ola"	,,	,,	,,	,,	Key
Penny	,,	"Lowla"	,,	,,	,,	,,	PeNNY
Matches	,,	"Low-lo"	,,	,,	,,	,,	MoTCH BOX
Scissors	,,	"S-roda"	,,	,,	,,	,,	SCISSORS
Pencil	,,	"Lowla"	,,	,,	,,	,,	PENCIL
Key	,,	"Lowla"	,,	,,	,,	,,	Key
Scissors	,,	"Lowla"	,,	Correct; slow	,,	,,	SCISSORS
Matches	,,	"Lowga"	,,	Correct	,,	,,	MATCH
Knife	,,	"Lowla"	,,	,,	,,	,,	KNIFB
Penny	,,	"Lowla"	,,	,,	,,	,,	PeNNY
Pencil	,,	"Lowla"	,,	Chose knife; then correct	,,	,,	PeNCIL

(2) *The coin-bowl tests.*

Table 2.

	Oral commands	Printed commands	
		In words only	In numbers
2nd into 3rd	1st into 2nd	3rd into 3rd	3rd into 2nd
1st into 3rd	2nd into 3rd	Correct	Correct
2nd into 1st	3rd into 4th	,,	1st into 2nd, then into 1st
3rd into 2nd	4th into 4th	2nd into 2nd	2nd into 3rd
1st into 4th	3rd into 3rd	Correct	1st into 1st, then 4th into 4th
4th into 3rd	3rd into 3rd	1st into 4th	1st into 3rd
2nd into 4th	4th into 4th	2nd into 2nd	Correct
4th into 1st	2nd into 2nd	1st into 1st	1st into 4th
3rd into 1st	1st into 3rd	3rd into 3rd	1st, then 3rd into 3rd
1st into 2nd	3rd into 3rd	2nd into 2nd	1st into 1st and then touched 2nd bowl
3rd into 4th	4th into 4th	4th into 3rd	1st into 3rd and then 4th into 4th
4th into 2nd	3rd into 3rd	2nd into 2nd	Correct

This test puzzled him greatly and yet at times he answered correctly, showing that he understood what he was expected to do. Oral commands were carried out extremely badly and he was not infrequently satisfied with placing the coin into the bowl of the same number, as for instance the 3rd into the 3rd, or the 4th into the 4th, oblivious of the fact that such an order occurred nowhere in the series.

Printed commands were given either in words (e.g. "Second penny into third bowl") or in numbers (e.g. "2nd into 3rd"). The latter form seemed to confuse him greatly; thus, he touched the 1st bowl and the 1st penny and then the 4th bowl and the 4th penny, in spite of the fact that he had previously shown he knew the sort of action he was required to perform. When the orders were printed in full, the words "penny" and "bowl" seemed to steady him and to prevent this confusion with regard to what he was intended to do.

(3) *The clock tests.*

Table 3.

	Direct imitation	Telling the time	Clock set to oral commands	Clock set to printed commands	
				Ordinary nomenclature	Railway time
5 minutes to 2	Correct	Impossible	Set 12.30	Set 12.0	Set 12.5
Half-past 1	,,	,,	Set 1.0	Set 12.30	Set 12.30
5 minutes past 8	,,	,,	Set 12.0	Set long hand at 8	Correct
20 minutes to 4	,,	,,	Set 11.50	Set nothing	Set 3.50
10 minutes past 7	,,	,,	Set 11.30	Correct	Correct
20 minutes to 6	,,	,,	Pointed to 6. Set nothing	Set nothing	Set 5.45
10 minutes to 1	,,	,,	Set 11.55	Correct	Correct
A quarter to 9	,,	,,	Set 12.50	,,	,,
20 minutes past 11	,,	,,	Set nothing	Set 20 minutes *to* 11	Set 11.25
25 minutes to 3	,,	,,	Set long hand at 3	Set 9.25	Set 6.35, then 12.35, then 10.35

He had no difficulty in setting one clock in imitation of another, but was totally unable to tell the time aloud. He uttered a series of incomprehensible sounds, such as "Lo-lo," "Trol-la," which bore no relation to the words he was seeking.

Oral and printed commands were extremely badly executed, although an occasional correct answer showed that he understood what he was expected to do. It seemed to make little or no difference whether the order was printed in the ordinary nomenclature or in railway time; both confused him gravely.

(4) *The hand, eye and ear tests.* (Table 4.)

During these tests it was impossible to explain to him that, when we sat face to face, he had to employ what appeared to be the opposite hand. During the preliminary explanation, which always preceded the actual testing, he held up first his right and then his left hand correctly in imitation of my movements. He then, on his own initiative, turned halfway round and lifted each hand in turn to show me that he understood they should be opposed when we were face to face; at the same time he said "Si si." But, as soon as we began the tests in earnest, he repeatedly employed the reversed hand to touch the wrong eye or ear.

Exactly the same form of mistake occurred with pictorial commands. But, when either my movements or the pictures were reflected in a mirror, he carried out the requisite action with rapidity and certainty.

Oral and printed commands were badly executed and he not only chose the wrong hand but frequently confused eye and ear.

Asked to write down the movements made by me he did not even attempt to make a mark upon the paper.

Table 4.

	Imitation of movements made by the observer	Imitation of movements reflected in a mirror	Pictorial commands	Pictorial commands reflected in a mirror	Oral commands	Printed commands	Writing down movements made by the observer
L. hand to L. eye	Reversed	Correct	Reversed	Correct	L. hand to R. eye	Reversed	Impossible
R. hand to R. ear	,,	,,	,,	,,	L. hand to L. *eye*	Correct	,,
R. hand to L. eye	,,	,,	,,	,,	Correct	R. hand to R. eye	,,
L. hand to R. eye	L. hand to L. eye	,,	L. hand to L. eye	,,	,,	R. hand to R. eye	,,
L. hand to L. ear	Reversed	,,	Reversed	,,	L. hand to R. *eye*	R. hand to R. *eye*; then reversed	,,
R. hand to R. eye	,,	,,	,,	,,	Reversed	Correct	,,
L. hand to R. ear	,,	,,	L. hand to L. ear	,,	L. hand to R. *eye*	R. hand to R. *eye*	,,
R. hand to L. ear	,,	,,	R. hand to R. ear	,,	R. hand to R. ear	L. hand to R. *eye*	,,
L. hand to L. eye	,,	,,	Reversed	,,	Correct	L. hand to R. eye	,,
R. hand to R. ear	,,	,,	,,	,,	L. hand to R. *eye*	L. hand to R. ear	,,
R. hand to L. eye	,,	,,	,,	,,	Reversed	Reversed	,,
L. hand to R. eye	L. hand to L. eye	,,	,,	,,	Correct	Correct	,,
L. hand to L. ear	Reversed	,,	,,	,,	L. hand to L. *eye*	L. hand to R. *eye*	,,
R. hand to R. eye	,,	,,	,,	,,	L. hand to R. eye	Correct	,,
L. hand to R. ear	L. hand to L. ear	,,	L. hand to L. ear	,,	L. hand to R. *eye*	Correct; very slow	,,
R. hand to L. ear	Reversed	,,	R. hand to R. ear	,,	Correct	Reversed	,,

REFERENCES

(1) AUBURTIN, E. "Considérations sur les localisations cérébrales, et en particulier sur le siége de la faculté du langage articulé." *Gaz. Hebdom.* 1863, X, 318–321, 348–351, 397–402, 455–458.

(2) BAGINSKY. "Aphasie in Folge schwerer Nierenerkrankungen." *Berlin. Klin. Wochenschr.* 1871, VIII, 428–431, 439–443.

(3) BASTIAN, H. CHARLTON. "On the various forms of Loss of Speech in Cerebral Disease." *Brit. and Foreign Med.-Chi. Rev.* 1869, XLIII, 209–236 and 470–492.

(4) — "The Physiology of Thinking." *Fortnightly Review*, 1869, New Series, V, 57–71.

(5) — *Brain as an Organ of Mind.* London. 1880. [Particularly pages 601–690.]

(6) — "On some problems in connexion with Aphasia and other Speech Defects." (The Lumleian Lectures.) *Lancet*, 1897, I, 933–942, 1005–1017, 1131–1137, 1187–1194.

(7) — "On a case of Amnesia and other Speech Defects of eighteen years' duration with Autopsy." *Med. Chi. Trans.* 1897, LXXX, 61–86.

(8) — *Aphasia and other Speech Defects.* London. 1898.

(9) BAZETT, H. C. and PENFIELD, W. G. "A study of the Sherrington decerebrate animal in the chronic as well as the acute condition." *Brain*, 1922, XLV, 185–265.

(10) BENARY, W. "Studien zur Untersuchung der Intelligenz bei einem Fall von Seelen-Blindheit." *Psycholog. Forschung*, 1922, II, 209–297.

(11) BOUCHARD, CH. "Aphasie sans lésion de la troisième circonvolution frontale gauche." *Comptes rend. d. Séances et Mém. d. l. Soc. d. Biologie* (année 1864), 1865, 4e Sér. I, 111–116.

(12) BOUILLAUD, J. "Recherches cliniques propres à démontrer que la perte de la parole correspond à la lésion des lobules antérieurs du cerveau," etc. *Archives Gén. de Méd.* 1825, VIII, 25–45.

(13) — *Traité clinique et physiologique de l'encéphalite ou inflammation du cerveau.* Paris, 1825.

(14) — "Exposition de nouveaux faits à l'appui de l'opinion qui localise dans les lobules antérieurs du cerveau le principe législateur de la parole," etc. *Bull. d. l'Acad. d. Méd.* 1839, IV, 282–328.

(15) — "Recherches cliniques propres à démontrer que le sens du langage articulé et le principe coordinateur des mouvements de la parole résident dans les lobules antérieurs du cerveau." *Bull. d. l'Acad. Royale d. Méd.* 1847–48, XIII, 699–719, 778–816.

(16) BROADBENT, W. H. "On the cerebral mechanism of Speech and Thought." *Med. Chi. Trans.* 1872, LV, 145–194.

(17) — "A case of peculiar affection of Speech, with Commentary." *Brain*, 1879, I, 484–503.

(18) BROCA, P. "Perte de la parole. Ramollissement chronique et destruction partielle du lobe antérieur gauche du cerveau." *Bull. d. l. Soc. d'Anthrop.* 1861, II, 235–238.

(19) — "Remarques sur le siége de la faculté du langage articulé, suivies d'une observation d'aphémie." *Bull. d. l. Soc. Anatom.* 1861, VI, 330–357.

(20) — "Nouvelle observation d'aphémie produite par une lésion de la moitié postérieure des deuxième et troisième circonvolutions frontales." *Bull. d. l. Soc. Anatom.* 1861, VI, 398–407.

(21) — Discussion on a Communication by Parrot entitled "Atrophie cérébrale," etc. *Bull. d. l. Soc. Anatom.* 1863, VIII, 379–385, 393–399.

(22) — "Deux cas d'aphémie traumatique, produite par des lésions de la troisième circonvolution frontale gauche. Diagnostic chirurgical." *Bull. d. l. Soc. d. Chirurg.* 1864, V, 51–54.

(23) — "Sur l'aphémie." *Bull. d. l. Soc. Anatom.* 1864, IX, 296–298.

(24) — Remarks on a Communication by Ange Duval entitled "Siége de la faculté du langage articulé," etc. *Bull. d. l. Soc. d'Anthrop.* 1864, V, 215–217.

(25) — "Sur les mots aphémie, aphasie, aphrasie. Lettre à M. le Professeur Trousseau." *Gaz. d. Hôp.* 1864, XXXVII, 35–36.

(26) — "Sur la faculté du langage articulé." *Bull. d. l. Soc. d'Anthrop.* 1865, VI, 493–494.

(27) — "Sur le siége de la faculté du langage articulé." *Trib. Méd.* 1869, (*a*) No. 74, 28 fév. 254–256; (*b*) No. 75, 7 mars, 265–269.

(28) BROWN, T. GRAHAM. "Studies in the physiology of the nervous system. On the phenomenon of facilitation." *Quart. Journ. of Exp. Physiol.* 1915, IX, 81–99, 101–116, 117–130, 131–145.

(29) — "Studies in the physiology of the nervous system." *Quart. Journ. of Exp. Physiol.* 1916, X, 97–102, 103–143.

(30) BROWN, T. GRAHAM, and SHERRINGTON, C. S. "On the instability of a cortical point." *Proc. Roy. Soc.* 1912, LXXXV, B. 250–277.

(31) BRUN, R. "Klinische und anatomische Studien über Apraxie." [Aus d. hirnanatomischen Institute. Prof. C. von Monakow.] Zürich, 1922. [Reprinted from *Schweiz. Archiv f. Neurolog. u. Psychiat.* 1921–22, IX, 29–64, and X, 185–210.]

(32) CHARCOT, J. M. "Sur une nouvelle observation d'aphémie." *Gaz. Hebdom.* 1863, X, 473–474.

(33) CUSHING, HARVEY. "The Field Defects produced by temporal lobe lesions." *Brain*, 1921, XLIV, 341–396.

(34) DAX, MARC. "Lésions de la moitié gauche de l'encéphale coïncidant avec l'oubli des signes de la pensée." [Lu à Montpellier en 1836.] *Gaz. Hebdom.* 1865, 2e Sér. II, 259–260.

(35) DAX, G. "Sur le même sujet." *Gaz. Hebdom.* 1865, 2e Sér. II, 260–262.

(36) DEJERINE, J. "L'aphasie sensorielle et l'aphasie motrice." *La Presse Médicale*, 1906, XIV, 437–439, 453–457.

(37) DEJERINE, J. "Aphasie et Anarthrie." *Trans. of the 17th Internat. Congress of Medicine, London*, 1913, Section XI, Neuropathology, I, 85-106.

(38) — *Sémiologie des affections du système nerveux*. Paris, 1914.

(39) DEJERINE, J. and SÉRIEUX, P. "Un cas de surdité verbale pure terminée par aphasie sensorielle suivi d'autopsie." *Comptes Rend. d. l. Soc. d. Biolog.* 1897, IV, 1074-1077.

(40) DELACROIX, H. *Le langage et la pensée*. Paris, 1924.

(41) "Discussion sur le volume et la forme du cerveau." *Bull. d. l. Soc. d'Anthrop.* 1861, II, 66-81, 139-207, 209-326, 421-449.

(42) "Discussion sur la faculté du langage articulé." *Bull. de l'Acad. Imp. de Méd.* 1864-1865, XXX, 173-175, 575-600, 604-638, 647-675, 679-703, 713-718, 724-781, 787-803, 816-832, 840-868, 888-890.

(43) "Discussion sur l'aphasie." Société de Neurologie de Paris. *Rev. Neurolog.* 1908, XVI, Séance de 11 juin, 611-636; Séance de 9 juillet, 974-1024; Séance de 23 juillet, 1025-1047.

(44) "Discussion on Aphasia." Section of Neurology of the Royal Society of Medicine. Nov. 11, 1920. *Brain*, 1920, XLIII, 412-450.

(45) FERRIER, DAVID. "Experimental Researches in Cerebral Physiology and Pathology." *West Riding Asylum Reports*, 1873, III, 30-96.

(46) — "Experiments on the Brain of Monkeys. (Second series.)" *Phil. Trans. Roy. Soc.* 1875, CLXV, 433-488.

(47) FILDES, LUCY G. "A psychological inquiry into the nature of the condition known as Congenital Word-blindness." *Brain*, 1921, XLIV, 286-307.

(48) FINKELNBURG, F. C. "Niederrheinische Gesellschaft, Sitzung vom 21. März 1870 in Bonn." *Berlin. Klin. Wochenschr.* 1870, 12 Sept. VII, 449-450, 460-462.

(49) FOSTER, MICHAEL. *Lectures on the History of Physiology*. Cambridge, 1901.

(50) GALL, F. J. "Craniologie ou découvertes nouvelles du Docteur F. J. Gall." *Ouvrage traduit de l'Allemand*. Paris, 1807.

(51) — Article "Cerveau." *Dictionnaire des Sciences Médicales*. Paris, 1813, IV, 447-479.

(52) GALL, F. J. and SPURZHEIM, G. "Recherches sur le système nerveux en général et sur celui du cerveau en particulier." *Mémoire présenté à l'Institut de France, 14 mars*, 1808. Paris, 1809.

(53) — — *Anatomie et physiologie du système nerveux en général et du cerveau en particulier, avec des observations sur la possibilité de reconnoître plusieurs dispositions intellectuelles et morales de l'homme et des animaux par la configuration de leurs têtes*. (4 vols. in quarto, atlas of 100 plates.) Paris, 1810-19.

(54) GARDINER, A. H. "The definition of the word and the sentence." *Brit. Journ. of Psychol.* 1922, XII, 352-361.

(55) GELB, A. and GOLDSTEIN, K. "Zur Psychologie des optischen Wahrnehmungs- und Erkennungsvorganges." *Zeit. f. d. gesamte Neurolog. u. Psychiat.* (Orig.) 1918, XLI, 1-142.

(56) Gelb, A. and Goldstein, K. *Psychologische Analysen hirnpathologischer Fälle.* Leipzig, 1920.

(57) —— "Ueber Farbennamenamnesie nebst Bemerkungen über das Wesen der amnestischen Aphasie überhaupt und die Beziehung zwischen Sprache und dem Verhalten zur Umwelt." *Psycholog. Forschung*, 1924, VI, 127–186.

(58) —— "Das Wesen der amnestischen Aphasie." *Verhandl. d. Gesellsch. deutsch. Nervenärz.* Sept. 1924, 132–147.

(59) Goldstein, K. "Ueber Aphasie." *Beihefte z. Mediz. Klinik.* 1910, VI, 1–32.

(60) Gordon, Hugh. "Left-handedness and mirror writing, especially among defective children." *Brain*, 1920, XLIII, 313–368.

(61) — "Hand and ear tests." *Brit. Journ. of Psychol.* 1922–23, XIII, 283–300.

(62) Head, H. *Studies in Neurology.* 2 vols. London, 1920.

(63) — "Aphasia and kindred disorders of speech." [The Linacre Lecture for 1920.] *Brain*, 1920, XLIII, 87–165.

(64) — "Aphasia; an historical review." [The Hughlings Jackson Lecture for 1920.] *Brain*, 1920, XLIII, 390–411.

(65) — "Speech and cerebral localisation." *Brain*, 1923, XLVI, 355–528.

(66) Head, H. and Holmes, Gordon. "Sensory disturbances from cerebral lesions." *Brain*, 1911–12, XXXIV, 102–254.

(67) Head, H. and Riddoch, G. "The automatic bladder, excessive sweating and some other reflex conditions in gross injuries of the Spinal Cord." *Brain*, 1917, XL, 188–263.

(68) Heilbronner, K. "Die aphasischen, apraktischen und agnostischen Störungen." Lewandowsky's *Handbuch d. Neurologie*, Berlin, 1910, I, 982–1093.

(69) Henschen, S. E. "Ueber die Hörsphäre." *Journ. f. Psycholog. u. Neurolog.* 1918, XXII, 319–474.

(70) — "On the hearing Sphere." *Acta Oto-laryngolog.* 1918, I, 423–486.

(71) — "Ueber Sinnes- und Vorstellungszentren in der Rinde des Grosshirns." *Zeit. f. d. gesamte Neurolog. u. Psychiat.* (Orig.) 1919, XLVII, 55–111.

(72) — "Ueber Sprach-, Musik- und Rechenmechanismen und ihre Lokalisationen im Grosshirn." *Zeit. f. d. gesamte Neurolog. u. Psychiat.* (Orig.) 1919, LII, 273–298.

(73) — *Klinische und anatomische Beiträge zur Pathologie des Gehirns:* [*a*] Fünfter Teil—*Ueber Aphasie, Amusie und Akalkulie.* Stockholm, 1920. [*b*] Sechster Teil—*Ueber sensorische Aphasie.* Stockholm, 1920. [*c*] Siebenter Teil—*Ueber motorische Aphasie und Agraphie.* Stockholm, 1922.

(74) — "40-jähriger Kampf um das Sehzentrum und seine Bedeutung für die Hirnforschung." *Zeit. f. d. gesamte Neurolog. u. Psychiat.* 1923, LXXXVII, 505–535.

(75) — "On the value of the discovery of the visual centre." *Scandin. Scientific Rev.* 1924, III, 10–63.

(76) Hinshelwood, J. *Congenital Word-blindness.* London, 1917.

(77) HOLMES, GORDON, and HORRAX, G. "Disturbances of Spatial orientation and Visual attention with loss of Stereoscopic vision." *Arch. of Neurolog. and Psychiat.* 1919, I, 385–407.

(78) HOLMES, GORDON, and LISTER, W. T. "Disturbances of vision from cerebral lesions with special reference to the cortical representation of the macula." *Brain*, 1916, XXXIX, 34–73.

(79) JACKSON, J. HUGHLINGS. "Case of large cerebral tumour without optic neuritis and with left hemiplegia and imperception." *Roy. Lond. Ophth. Hosp. Reports*, 1876, VIII, 434–444.

(80) — "On the Evolution and Dissolution of the Nervous System." [The Croonian Lectures for 1884.] [*a*] *Lancet*, 1884, I, 555–558, 649–652, 739–744. [*b*] *Brit. Med. Journ.* 1884, I, 591–593, 660–663, 703–707.

(81) — "Hughlings Jackson on Aphasia and kindred affections of Speech, together with a complete bibliography of his publications on Speech and a reprint of some of the more important papers." *Brain*, 1915, XXXVIII, 1–190.

(82) — *Neurological Fragments.* [With Biographical memoir by Dr James Taylor and Recollections of Sir Jonathan Hutchinson and Dr Chas. Mercier.] Oxford Univ. Press, 1925.

(83) KUSSMAUL, A. "Die Störungen der Sprache." *Ziemssen's Handbuch d. speciellen Pathologie u. Therapie*, 1877, XII. Anhang, 1–300.

(84) LEWANDOWSKY, M. "Ueber Abspaltung des Farbensinnes." *Monatschr. f. Psychiat. u. Neurolog.* 1908, XXIII, 488–510.

(85) LEYTON, A. S. F. and SHERRINGTON, C. S. "Observations on the excitable cortex of the chimpanzee, orang-utan and gorilla." *Quart. Journ. of Exp. Physiol.* 1917, XI, 135–222.

(86) LICHTHEIM, L. "On Aphasia." *Brain*, 1885, VII, 433–484.

(87) — "Ueber Aphasie." *Deut. Archiv f. Klin. Med.* 1885, XXXVI, 204–268.

(88) LIEPMANN, H. "Das Krankheitsbild der Apraxie." *Monatschr. f. Psychiat. u. Neurolog.* 1900, VIII, 15–44, 102–132, 182–197.

(89) — "Das Krankheitsbild der Apraxie." *Monatschr. f. Psychiat. u. Neurolog.* 1905, XVII, 289–311.

(90) — "Das Krankheitsbild der Apraxie." *Monatschr. f. Psychiat. u. Neurolog.* 1906, XIX, 217–243.

(91) — *Drei Aufsätze aus dem Apraxiegebiet.* Berlin, 1908.

(92) — "Motor Aphasia, Anarthria and Apraxia." *Trans. of the 17th Internat. Congress of Med. in London*, 1913, Sect. XI, Part 2, 97–106. [Also printed in *Monatschr. f. Psychiat. u. Neurolog.* 1913, XXXIV, 485–494.]

(93) — "Bemerkungen zu v. Monakows Kapitel 'Die Lokalisation der Apraxie,'" etc. *Monatschr. f. Psychiat. u. Neurolog.* 1914, XXXV, 490–516.

(94) — "Apraxie." *Ergeb. d. gesamten Medizin*, 1920, I, 516–543.

(95) LIEPMANN, H. and MAAS, O. "Fall von linksseitiger Agraphie und Apraxie bei rechtsseitiger Lähmung." *Journ. f. Psychol. u. Neurolog.* 1908, X, 214–227.

(96) LOTMAR, F. "Zur Kenntnis der erschwerten Wortfindung und ihrer Bedeutung für das Denken des Aphasischen." *Schweiz. Archiv f. Neurolog. u. Psychiatr.* 1919, V, 206–239 and 1920, VI, 3–36.

(97) MARIE, PIERRE. "La troisième circonvolution frontale gauche ne joue aucun rôle spécial dans la fonction du langage." *Semaine Médicale*, 1906, 23 mai, XXVI, 241–247.

(98) — "Que faut-il penser des aphasies sous-corticales (aphasies pures)?" *Semaine Médicale*, 1906, 17 oct. XXVI, 493–500.

(99) — "L'aphasie de 1861 à 1866." *Semaine Médicale*, 1906, 28 nov. XXVI, 565–571.

(100) — "Rectifications à propos de la question de l'aphasie." *La Presse Médicale*, 1907, 12 janv. XV, 25–26.

(101) — "Existe-t-il chez l'homme des centres préformés ou innés de langage?" *Questions Neurologiques d'Actualité*, Paris, 1922. Vingtième Conférence, 527–551.

(102) MAUDSLEY, H. "Concerning Aphasia." *Lancet*, 1868, II, 690–692, 721–723.

(103) MINGAZZINI, G. "Le nuove ricerche anatomo-cliniche di S. Henschen sulle afasie." *Il Policlinico* (Sez. Med.), 1922, XXIX, 467–488.

(104) MONAKOW, C. VON. "Neue Gesichtspunkte in der Frage nach der Lokalisation im Grosshirn." *Zeit. f. Psycholog.* 1909, LIV, 161–182. [Also published separately, Wiesbaden, 1911.]

(105) — "Aufbau und Lokalisation der Bewegungen beim Menschen." *Arbeit. a. d. hirnanatom. Institut in Zürich*, 1911, V, 1–37.

(106) — "Theoretische Betrachtungen über die Lokalisation im Zentralnervensystem insbesondere im Grosshirn." *Ergeb. d. Physiol.* 1913, XIII, 206–278.

(107) — *Die Lokalisation im Grosshirn.* Wiesbaden, 1914.

(108) — "Croonian Lectures on the Evolution and Dissolution of the Nervous System by J. Hughlings Jackson." (Translated into French, with an Introduction.) *Schweiz. Archiv f. Neurolog. u. Psychiat.* 1921, VIII, 294–302; IX, 131–152.

(109) — "Betrachtungen über Gefühl und Sprache." *Schweiz. Archiv f. Neurolog. u. Psychiat.* 1922, XI, 118–129.

(110) MOUTIER, F. *L'aphasie de Broca.* [Travail du laboratoire de M. le Professeur Pierre Marie.] Paris, 1908.

(111) NAVILLE, F. "Mémoires d'un médecin aphasique. Auto-observations et notes psychologiques du Docteur Saloz père, de Genève." *Archives de Psychologie*, 1918, XVII, 1–57.

(112) OGLE, W. "Aphasia and Agraphia." *St George's Hosp. Reports*, 1867, II, 83–122.

(113) PICK, ARNOLD. *Beiträge zur Pathologie und pathologischen Anatomie des Zentralnervensystems.* Berlin, 1898.

(114) — *Studien über motorische Apraxie.* Leipzig, 1905.

(115) — *Die agrammatischen Sprachstörungen.* [1 Teil; no second part appeared.] Berlin, 1913.

(116) PICK, ARNOLD. "Sprachpsychologische und andere Studien zur Aphasielehre." *Schweiz. Archiv f. Neurolog. u. Psychiat.* 1923, XII, 105–135, 179–200.

(117) — "Aphasie." Bethe's *Handbuch der normalen und pathologischen Physiologie.* Berlin, 1925, XV. [Seen in proof only.]

(118) RIDDOCH, G. "Dissociation of visual perceptions due to occipital injuries with especial reference to the appreciation of movement." *Brain*, 1917, XL, 15–57.

(119) — "The reflex functions of the completely divided spinal cord in man compared with those associated with less severe lesions." *Brain*, 1917, XL, 264–402.

(120) SÉRIEUX, P. "Sur un cas de surdité verbale pure." *Rev. d. Méd.* 1893, XIII, 733–750.

(121) SHERRINGTON, C. S. *The Integrative Action of the Nervous System.* London, 1906.

(122) SITTIG, O. "Störungen im Verhalten gegenüber Farben bei Aphasischen." *Monatschr. f. Psychiat. u. Neurolog.* 1921, XLIX, 63–88, 169–187.

(123) STAUFFENBERG, W. VON. "Ueber Seelenblindheit." *Arbeit. a. d. hirnanatom. Institut in Zürich*, 1913, VIII, 1–212.

(124) SUDHOFF, W. "Die Lehre von den Hirnventrikeln," etc. *Archiv f. Gesch. d. Med.* 1913, VII, 149–205.

(125) TROUSSEAU, A. "De l'Aphasie, maladie décrite récemment sous le nom impropre d'aphémie." *Gaz. des Hôp.* 1864, XXXVII, (*a*) 13–14; (*b*) 25–26; (*c*) 37–39; (*d*) 49–50.

(126) — *Clinique médicale*, 1865, 2nd ed. II, 571–626.

(127) VILLERS, C. *Lettre de Charles Villers à Georges Cuvier sur une nouvelle théorie du cerveau par le Docteur Gall: ce viscère étant considéré comme l'organe immédiat des facultés morales.* Metz, An. X, 1802.

(128) WAGNER'S *Handwörterbuch der Physiologie.* Braunschweig, 1844, II, 692–827.

(129) WERNICKE, C. *Der aphasische Symptomencomplex.* Breslau, 1874.

(130) — *Lehrbuch der Gehirnkrankheiten.* Kassel, 1881.

(131) — "Ein Fall von isolierter Agraphie." *Monatschr. f. Psychiat. u. Neurolog.* 1903, XIII, 241–265.

(132) WILSON, S. A. K. "A contribution to the study of Apraxia with a review of the Literature." *Brain*, 1908, XXXI, 164–216.

(133) WOERKOM, W. VAN. "La signification de certains éléments de l'intelligence dans la genèse des troubles aphasiques." *Journ. de Psycholog.* 1921, XVIII, 730–751.

INDEX OF AUTHORS CITED

THE REFERENCES ARE TO THE PAGES OF VOLUME I

GENERAL INDEX

THE REFERENCES ARE TO THE PAGES OF VOLUME I

INDEX OF CLINICAL REPORTS

THE REFERENCES ARE TO THE PAGES OF VOLUME II

Printed in the United States
By Bookmasters